Drugs of Choice
Drugs of Choice

2018

Selected Articles from
The Medical Letter on Drugs and Therapeutics®

Published by

The Medical Letter, Inc.
145 Huguenot St.
New Rochelle, New York 10801-7537

800-211-2769
914-235-0500
Fax 914-632-1733
www.medicalletter.org

(ISSN 1065-6596)
(ISBN 978-0-9815278 -9-5)

The Medical Letter Inc.
145 Huguenot St., Ste. 312
New Rochelle, New York 10801-7537

Contents

Tables

Introduction

The Medical Letter, Inc. is a nonprofit organization that publishes critical appraisals of new prescription drugs and comparative reviews of drugs for common diseases in its newsletter, *The Medical Letter on Drugs and Therapeutics*. It is committed to providing objective, practical, and timely information to help readers make the best decisions for their patients—without the influence of the pharmaceutical industry. The Medical Letter is supported by its readers, and does not receive any commercial support or accept advertising in any of its publications.

Many of our readers know that pharmaceutical companies and their representatives often exaggerate the therapeutic effects and understate the adverse effects of their products, but busy practitioners have neither the time nor the resources to check the accuracy of the manufacturers' claims. Our publication is intended specifically to meet the needs of busy healthcare professionals who want unbiased, reliable, and timely drug information. Our editorial process is designed to ensure that the information we provide represents an unbiased consensus of medical experts.

The editorial process used for *The Medical Letter on Drugs and Therapeutics* relies on a consensus of experts to develop prescribing recommendations. The first draft of an article is prepared by one of our in-house or contributing editors or by an outside expert. This initial draft is edited and sent to our Contributing Editors, to 10-20 other reviewers who have clinical and/or experimental experience with the drug or type of drug or disease under review, to the FDA, and to the first and last authors of all the articles cited in the text. Many critical observations, suggestions, and questions are received from the reviewers and are incorporated into the article during the revision process. Further communication as needed is followed by fact checking and editing to make sure the final appraisal is not only accurate, but also easy to read.

NOTE: The drug costs listed in the tables are based on the pricing information that was available in the month the article was originally published. When the cost of a drug has been updated or added since publication, it is designated as such.

The Medical Letter, Inc. is based in New Rochelle, NY. For more information, go to www.medicalletter.org or call 800-211-2769.

DRUGS FOR Allergic Disorders

Original publication date – May 2017 (revised March 2018)

ALLERGIC RHINITIS

Allergic rhinitis can be classified as seasonal, perennial, or episodic. It is often associated with allergic conjunctivitis, rhinosinusitis, and asthma.[1,2]

H_1-ANTIHISTAMINES — Oral – Oral second-generation H_1-antihistamines are the preferred first-line treatment for relief of the itching, sneezing, and rhinorrhea that characterize mild-to-moderate allergic rhinitis. They are less effective for nasal congestion.

Adverse Effects – Second-generation H_1-antihistamines penetrate poorly into the central nervous system (CNS) and are significantly less likely than first-generation agents to impair CNS function and cause sedation.[3,4] Fexofenadine is nonsedating and free of CNS-impairing effects, even in higher-than-recommended doses. Loratadine and desloratadine are nonimpairing and nonsedating in recommended doses, but may cause sedation at higher doses. Cetirizine and levocetirizine can cause sedation in recommended doses.

First-generation H_1-antihistamines such as diphenhydramine (*Benadryl*, and generics) can cause CNS impairment with or without sedation. They can interfere with learning and memory, impair performance on school examinations, decrease work productivity, and increase the risk of

Recommendations for Treatment of Allergic Disorders

Allergic Rhinitis and Allergic Conjunctivitis

- An oral second-generation H_1-antihistamine is the preferred first-line treatment for mild-to-moderate allergic rhinitis.
- Intranasal corticosteroids are the drugs of choice for moderate-to-severe allergic rhinitis.
- Use of an oral second-generation H_1-antihistamine or an intranasal corticosteroid for allergic rhinitis also improves symptoms of allergic conjunctivitis.
- Ophthalmic H_1-antihistamines are at least as effective as oral H_1-antihistamines for allergic conjunctivitis.
- Short-term use of an ophthalmic corticosteroid such as loteprednol can be considered for allergic conjunctivitis that fails to respond to other medications.
- Subcutaneous or sublingual allergen-specific immunotherapy can alter the natural history of allergic respiratory disease and induce long-term remission.

Atopic Dermatitis

- Topical corticosteroids are generally used to control inflammation in atopic dermatitis.
- The lowest potency topical corticosteroid that is effective should be used for maintenance treatment.
- Topical tacrolimus can be used for topical corticosteroid-resistant dermatitis, especially on the face or intertriginous areas where corticosteroid adverse effects can be troublesome. It can also be used as maintenance treatment to minimize use of topical corticosteroids.
- Subcutaneously-injected dupilumab can be used to treat moderate-to-severe atopic dermatitis that has not responded to topical therapies.
- A short course of an oral corticosteroid can be helpful in severe acute exacerbations of atopic dermatitis.

Urticaria

- An oral second-generation H_1-antihistamine is the preferred first-line treatment for acute urticaria.
- High doses (up to 4 times the usual dose) of an oral second-generation H_1-antihistamine can be used for chronic urticaria that does not respond to standard doses.
- Addition of omalizumab can reduce symptoms in patients with chronic urticaria who remain symptomatic despite H_1-antihistamine treatment.
- A short course of an oral corticosteroid can help relieve severe exacerbations of chronic urticaria.

on-the-job injuries, car accidents, and even plane crashes.[5] When these medications are taken at night, adverse effects on wakefulness and psychomotor performance can persist the next day.[6] Cumulative exposure to drugs with anticholinergic effects such as first-generation antihistamines has been associated with dementia.[7]

Intranasal – Intranasal H_1-antihistamines have a rapid onset of action. Their clinical efficacy in allergic rhinitis, including relief of nasal congestion, is equal or superior to that of oral H_1-antihistamines. An intranasal combination of the H_1-antihistamine azelastine and the corticosteroid fluticasone propionate has improved symptoms more than either drug alone in patients with seasonal allergic rhinitis.[8] Intranasal antihistamines can cause nasal discomfort, epistaxis and headache, and may cause somnolence.

INTRANASAL CORTICOSTEROIDS — Intranasal corticosteroids are the most effective drugs available for prevention and relief of allergic rhinitis symptoms, including itching, sneezing, discharge, and congestion. They are the drugs of choice for moderate-to-severe disease. Most of these agents are effective when given once daily. The onset of action typically occurs within 12 hours, but maximal effects may not be achieved for ≥7 days. In patients with seasonal allergic rhinitis, intranasal corticosteroid sprays can decrease ocular as well as nasal symptoms.[9] Several intranasal corticosteroids are now available without a prescription (see Table 2).[10]

Adverse Effects – Intranasal corticosteroids can cause mild dryness, irritation, burning and bleeding of the nasal mucosa, sore throat, epistaxis, and headache. Ulceration, mucosal atrophy, and septal perforation can occur; patients should be examined periodically to detect changes in the nasal mucosa. Increased intraocular pressure has been reported. Use of intranasal corticosteroids for ≥12 months in children has been associated with small decreases in growth velocity.

Table 1. Some Oral Drugs for Allergic Rhinitis

Drug	Some Available Formulations
Oral Second-Generation H_1-Antihistamines and Combinations	
Cetirizine[3,4] – *Zyrtec Allergy, Children's Zyrtec Allergy* (Johnson & Johnson)	5, 10 mg tabs and caps; 5, 10 mg chewable tabs; 5 mg/5 mL syrup
Cetirizine/pseudoephedrine[3,4] – *Zyrtec-D 12 hour* (Johnson & Johnson)	5 mg/120 mg ER tabs
Desloratadine – generic	5 mg tabs; 2.5, 5 mg disintegrating tabs
Clarinex (MSD)	5 mg tabs; 0.5 mg/mL syrup
Desloratadine/pseudoephedrine – *Clarinex-D 12 hour* (MSD)	2.5 mg/120 mg ER tabs
Fexofenadine[3,4] – *Allegra Allergy, Children's Allegra Allergy* (Chattem)	30, 60, 180 mg tabs; 30 mg disintegrating tabs; 30 mg/5 mL susp
Fexofenadine/pseudoephedrine[3,4] – *Allegra-D 12 hour* (Chattem)	60 mg/120 mg ER tabs
Allegra-D 24 hour	180 mg/240 mg ER tabs
Levocetirizine – generic[9] *Xyzal Allergy 24 hour, Children's Xyzal Allergy* (Chattem)[3]	5 mg tabs; 2.5 mg/5 mL oral soln
Loratadine[3,4] – *Alavert* (Pfizer)	10 mg disintegrating tabs
Claritin, Children's Claritin (Bayer)	10 mg tabs and caps; 10 mg disintegrating tabs; 5 mg chewable tabs; 1 mg/mL syrup
Loratadine/pseudoephedrine[3,4] – *Alavert-D 12 hour* (Pfizer) *Claritin-D 12 hour* (Bayer)	5 mg/120 mg ER tabs
Claritin-D 24 hour	10 mg/240 mg ER tabs

ER = extended-release

1. Dosage adjustment may be needed for renal or hepatic impairment.
2. Approximate WAC for 30 days' treatment at the lowest usual adult dosage. When multiple formulations are listed, price is for the first formulation unless otherwise indicated. WAC = wholesaler acquisition cost or manufacturer's published price to wholesalers; WAC represents a published catalogue or list price and may not represent an actual transactional price. Source: AnalySource® Monthly. April 5, 2017. Reprinted with permission by First Databank, Inc. All rights reserved. ©2017. www.fdbhealth.com/policies/drug-pricing-policy.
3. Available without a prescription. Products containing pseudoephedrine are subject to sales restrictions.

Usual Adult Dosage[1]	Usual Pediatric Dosage[1]	Cost[2]
10 mg once/d	6-11 mos: 2.5 mg once/d[5] 12-23 mos: 2.5 mg once/d-bid[5] 2-5 yrs: 2.5 or 5 mg once/d or 2.5 mg bid 6-11 yrs: 5 or 10 mg once/d	$15.90
1 tab bid	≥12 yrs: 1 tab bid	39.80
5 mg once/d	6-11 mos[6]: 1 mg once/d 1-5 yrs[6]: 1.25 mg once/d 6-11 yrs: 2.5 mg once/d	51.10 206.70
1 tab bid	≥12 yrs: 1 tab bid	284.40
60 mg bid or 180 mg once/d	6-23 mos: 15 mg bid[7] 2-11 yrs: 30 mg bid	15.60[8]
1 tab bid 1 tab once/d	≥12 yrs: 1 tab bid ≥12 yrs: 1 tab once/d	41.00 31.20
5 mg once/d	6 mos-5 yrs: 1.25 mg once/d[5] 6-11 yrs: 2.5 mg once/d	10.00 18.00[10]
10 mg once/d	2-5 yrs: 5 mg once/d ≥6 yrs: 10 mg once/d	7.80 18.60
1 tab bid 1 tab once/d	≥12 yrs: 1 tab bid ≥12 yrs: 1 tab once/d	29.40 39.90 31.50

4. Individual retailers may have their own OTC generic products.
5. The prescription product is FDA-approved for treatment of perennial allergic rhinitis and chronic urticaria in children ≥6 months old. The OTC product is recommended for children ≥2 years old.
6. Not FDA-approved for treatment of seasonal allergic rhinitis in children <2 years old.
7. The prescription product is FDA-approved for treatment of chronic idiopathic urticaria in children ≥6 months old. The OTC product is recommended for children ≥2 years old.
8. Cost of 30 days' treatment with 180 mg once/d.
9. The generic formulation is available by prescription.
10. Cost according to walgreens.com. Accessed April 27, 2017.

Continued on next page

Table 1. Some Oral Drugs for Allergic Rhinitis (continued)	
Drug	**Some Available Formulations**
Leukotriene Receptor Antagonist	
Montelukast – generic *Singulair* (Merck)	10 mg tabs; 4, 5 mg chewable tabs; 4 mg granule packets

MONTELUKAST — Release of cysteinyl leukotrienes in the nasal mucosa during allergic inflammation leads to nasal congestion. The leukotriene receptor antagonist montelukast is FDA-approved for treatment of seasonal and perennial allergic rhinitis. It provides modest relief of sneezing, itching, discharge, and congestion, but it is less effective than an intranasal corticosteroid.[11] Montelukast is generally considered safe.

DECONGESTANTS — Oral – Oral decongestants such as phenylephrine and pseudoephedrine act as vasoconstrictors in the nasal mucosa, primarily through stimulation of alpha-1 adrenergic receptors on venous sinusoids. They only relieve congestion, not sneezing, itching, or discharge. They are often used in combination with an H_1-antihistamine. Tolerance to the decongestant effect can occur.

Phenylephrine has replaced pseudoephedrine in many oral decongestant products because illicit pseudoephedrine use has resulted in sales restrictions. In an open-label, randomized, dose-ranging study, phenylephrine was no more effective than placebo for relief of nasal congestion in 539 patients with seasonal allergic rhinitis who took up to 4 times the typical dose of 10 mg.[12]

Potential adverse effects of oral decongestants include insomnia, excitability, headache, nervousness, anorexia, palpitations, tachycardia, arrhythmias, hypertension, nausea, vomiting, and urinary retention. These drugs should be used cautiously in patients with cardiovascular

Usual Adult Dosage[1]	Usual Pediatric Dosage[1]	Cost[2]
10 mg once/d	6 mos-5 yrs: 4 mg once/d 6-14 yrs: 5 mg once/d	$12.10 215.40

disease, hypertension, diabetes, hyperthyroidism, closed-angle glaucoma, or bladder neck obstruction.

Intranasal – Intranasal decongestants such as oxymetazoline (*Afrin*, and generics) are less likely than oral decongestants to cause systemic adverse effects, but they can cause stinging, burning, sneezing, and dryness of the nose and throat. In order to avoid rhinitis medicamentosa (rebound congestion), they should not be used for more than 3-5 consecutive days. Rhinitis medicamentosa associated with prolonged use is treated by discontinuing the intranasal decongestant and using an intranasal corticosteroid instead. In a cross-sectional, observational study, nasal congestion was the predominant symptom in 895 patients who self-medicated for moderate-to-severe persistent rhinitis. The prevalence of intranasal decongestant overuse was high, and was inversely related to intranasal corticosteroid use.[13]

CROMOLYN — Use of intranasal cromolyn sodium before allergen exposure inhibits mast cell degranulation and mediator release, preventing allergic rhinitis symptoms. It is relatively free from adverse effects, but must be used 3-4 times daily and is considerably less effective than an intranasal corticosteroid.[14]

IPRATROPIUM — Ipratropium bromide, a quaternary amine antimuscarinic agent, is poorly absorbed systemically and does not readily cross the blood-brain barrier. Intranasal ipratropium can be useful in patients whose primary symptom is nasal discharge. It does not relieve sneezing, itching, or congestion.

Table 2. Some Nasal Sprays for Allergic Rhinitis	
Drug	**Some Available Formulations**
H_1 -Antihistamines	
Azelastine[2] – *Astelin* 0.1% (Meda) generic	Metered-dose pump spray (137 mcg/spray)
Astepro 0.15% (Meda) generic	Metered-dose pump spray (205.5 mcg/spray)
Olopatadine 0.6%[6] – generic *Patanase* (Alcon)	Metered-dose pump spray (665 mcg/spray)
Corticosteroids	
Beclomethasone dipropionate – *Beconase AQ* (GSK)[7]	Metered-dose pump spray (42 mcg/spray)
QNASL (Teva)	HFA metered-dose aerosol (80 mcg/actuation)
QNASL Children's	HFA metered-dose aerosol (40 mcg/actuation)
Budesonide[9,10] – *Rhinocort Allergy* *Children's Rhinocort Allergy* (Johnson & Johnson)	Metered-dose pump spray (32 mcg/spray)
Ciclesonide – *Omnaris* (Sunovion)	Metered-dose pump spray (50 mcg/spray)
Zetonna (Sunovion)	HFA metered-dose aerosol (37 mcg/actuation)
Flunisolide – generic	Metered-dose pump spray (25 mcg/spray)
Fluticasone furoate[9] – *Flonase Sensimist Allergy Relief* (GSK)	Metered-dose pump spray (27.5 mcg/spray)

HFA = hydrofluoroalkane

1. Approximate WAC for 30 days' treatment at the lowest recommended adult dosage (using smallest size available). WAC = wholesaler acquisition cost or manufacturer's published price to wholesalers; WAC represents a published catalogue or list price and may not represent an actual transactional price. Source: AnalySource® Monthly. April 5, 2017. Reprinted with permission by First Databank, Inc. All rights reserved. ©2017. www.fdbhealth.com/policies/drug-pricing-policy.
2. Approved for seasonal allergic rhinitis (≥5 years old) and vasomotor rhinitis (≥12 years old).
3. Dosage for seasonal allergic rhinitis. Dosage for vasomotor rhinitis is 2 sprays per nostril bid.
4. Dosage for seasonal allergic rhinitis. Dosage for perennial allergic rhinitis is 2 sprays per nostril bid.
5. Lowest price available according to www.goodrx.com. Accessed April 27, 2017.
6. FDA-approved only for treatment of seasonal allergic rhinitis.

Usual Adult Dosage	Usual Pediatric Dosage	Cost[1]
1-2 sprays per nostril bid[3]	5-11 yrs: 1 spray per nostril bid	$142.50[5]
		43.50
1-2 sprays per nostril bid or 2 sprays per nostril once/d[4]	6-11 yrs: 1 spray per nostril bid	148.50
		111.40
2 sprays per nostril bid	6-11 yrs: 1 spray per nostril bid	216.70
	≥12 yrs: 2 sprays per nostril bid	263.30
1-2 sprays per nostril bid	6-11 yrs: 1-2 sprays per nostril bid[8]	279.40
2 sprays per nostril once/d	≥12 yrs: 2 sprays per nostril once/d	192.40
	4-11 yrs: 1 spray per nostril once/d	192.40
2 sprays per nostril once/d[8,11]	6-11 yrs: 1-2 sprays per nostril once/d[8,12]	11.10
2 sprays per nostril once/d	≥6 yrs[13]: 2 sprays per nostril once/d	234.10
1 spray per nostril once/d	≥12 yrs: 1 spray per nostril once/d	234.10
2 sprays per nostril bid-tid	6-14 yrs: 1 spray per nostril tid or 2 sprays per nostril bid	55.00
2 sprays per nostril once/d x 7 days, then 1-2 sprays per nostril once/d[11]	2-11 yrs: 1 spray per nostril once/d[12]	13.60

7. Also FDA-approved for treatment of vasomotor rhinitis.
8. A dose of 2 sprays/nostril should only be used until symptoms improve; then the dose should be reduced to 1 spray/nostril.
9. Available without a prescription.
10. Individual retailers may have their own OTC generic products.
11. OTC intranasal corticosteroids should not be used daily for >6 months without consulting a physician.
12. OTC intranasal corticosteroids should not be used daily for >2 months/year in children <12 years old without consulting a physician.
13. Not FDA-approved for treatment of perennial allergic rhinitis in children <12 years old.

Continued on next page

Table 2. Some Nasal Sprays for Allergic Rhinitis (continued)	
Drug	**Some Available Formulations**
Corticosteroids (continued)	
Fluticasone propionate[9,10] – *Flonase Allergy Relief*, *Children's Flonase Allergy Relief* (GSK) *Clarispray Nasal Allergy Spray* (Bayer)	Metered-dose pump spray (50 mcg/spray)
Mometasone furoate – generic *Nasonex* (Merck)[14]	Metered-dose pump spray (50 mcg/spray)
Triamcinolone acetonide[9,10] – *Nasacort Allergy 24 hour*, *Children's Nasacort Allergy 24 hour* (Chattem)	Metered-dose pump spray (55 mcg/spray)
H_1-Antihistamine/Corticosteroid	
Azelastine/fluticasone propionate – *Dymista* (Meda)[6]	Metered-dose pump spray (137 mcg/50 mcg per spray)
Mast Cell Stabilizer	
Cromolyn sodium – generic *Nasalcrom*[9] (Prestige)	Metered-dose pump spray (5.2 mg/spray)
Anticholinergic	
Ipratropium bromide – generic	Metered-dose pump spray (21 or 42 mcg/spray)

14. Also FDA-approved for prophylaxis of seasonal allergic rhinitis in patients ≥12 years old.
15. Dosage of 0.03% formulation is 2 sprays (42 mcg) per nostril bid-tid in patients ≥6 years old with allergic or nonallergic perennial rhinitis; dosage of 0.06% formulation is 2 sprays (84 mcg) per nostril qid in patients ≥5 years old with seasonal allergic rhinitis.

Adverse Effects – Ipratropium can cause dry nose and mouth, epistaxis, and pharyngeal irritation. After inadvertent instillation in the eye, it can increase intraocular pressure and should be used with caution in patients with glaucoma.

OMALIZUMAB — Omalizumab *(Xolair)*, a monoclonal antibody approved by the FDA for treatment of allergic asthma and chronic urticaria, has a dose-dependent beneficial effect in seasonal allergic rhinitis.

Usual Adult Dosage	Usual Pediatric Dosage	Cost[1]
2 sprays per nostril once/d x 7 days, then 1-2 sprays per nostril once/d[11]	4-11 yrs: 1 spray per nostril once/d[12]	$11.80
		10.20
2 sprays per nostril once/d	2-11 yrs: 1 spray per nostril once/d	162.40 237.30
2 sprays per nostril once/d[8,11]	2-5 yrs: 1 spray per nostril once/d[12] 6-11 yrs: 1-2 sprays per nostril once/d[8,12]	11.20
1 spray per nostril bid	≥6 yrs: 1 spray per nostril bid	170.20
1 spray per nostril tid-qid	≥2 yrs: 1 spray per nostril tid-qid	7.00 11.60
2 sprays per nostril bid-qid[15]	≥5 yrs: 2 sprays per nostril bid-qid[15]	30.00

Injected subcutaneously every 2-4 weeks, it decreases free IgE levels in serum and the number of IgE receptors on mast cells and basophils. In a systematic review and meta-analysis of 11 studies that included 2870 patients with inadequately controlled allergic rhinitis, injection of omalizumab significantly reduced daily nasal symptom severity scores and rescue medication use and improved quality of life. Adverse effects did not differ from placebo.[15] Omalizumab is generally well tolerated, but it has caused anaphylaxis in about 0.1% of patients with asthma.

ORAL CORTICOSTEROIDS — A short course of an oral corticosteroid can be effective in patients with severe allergic rhinitis or rhinitis medicamentosa who cannot tolerate or do not respond to other drugs.

ALLERGEN-SPECIFIC IMMUNOTHERAPY — Immunotherapy can alter the natural history of allergic respiratory disease (see page 24).

PREGNANCY — In a systematic review and meta-analysis of 37 studies that included >50,000 women exposed to H_1-antihistamines during the first trimester of pregnancy, use of these drugs was not associated with an increased risk of major malformations, spontaneous abortions, prematurity, or low birth weight.[16] Nasal saline irrigations, cromolyn sodium, and intranasal corticosteroids are also considered safe for pregnant women with allergic rhinitis.[17]

ALLERGIC CONJUNCTIVITIS

Allergic conjunctivitis, although underreported, probably occurs in the majority of patients with allergic rhinitis. Symptoms such as itching, redness, tearing, and photophobia are frequently seasonal. Nonpharmacologic management includes allergen identification and avoidance, use of cool compresses, and avoidance of eye rubbing and contact lens wearing during symptomatic periods. Optimal management of allergic rhinitis with an oral second-generation H_1-antihistamine and an intranasal corticosteroid can benefit concomitant allergic conjunctivitis as well.[18]

OPHTHALMIC DRUGS — Ophthalmic **antihistamines** are at least as effective as oral H_1-antihistamines for treatment of allergic conjunctivitis. Onset of action occurs within a few minutes. Starting treatment before the pollen season may be more beneficial in controlling symptoms than waiting for them to occur. Alcaftadine,[19] azelastine, bepotastine, epinastine, and olopatadine are marketed as having both H_1-antihistamine and mast-cell-stabilizing activity, as is ketotifen, which is available over the counter. A meta-analysis of four studies in a total of 204 patients has suggested that olopatadine may be more effective than ketotifen in improving some ocular symptoms.[20]

The ophthalmic **mast cell stabilizers** cromolyn, lodoxamide, and nedocromil have a slower onset of action than ophthalmic H_1-antihistamines and are mostly used for treatment of mild-to-moderate symptoms.

The topical **nonsteroidal anti-inflammatory** drug ketorolac is less effective than ophthalmic H_1-antihistamines.

Ophthalmic **decongestants** such as naphazoline reduce erythema, congestion, itching, and eyelid edema, but they have a short duration of action and can cause burning, stinging, rebound hyperemia, and conjunctivitis medicamentosa. Ophthalmic **antihistamine/decongestant combinations** available over the counter such as pheniramine/naphazoline (*Visine A*, and generics) and antazoline/naphazoline *(Vasocon-A)* have similar adverse effects.

Ophthalmic **corticosteroids** can be considered for use in allergic conjunctivitis that fails to respond to other medications. Loteprednol is inactivated rapidly in the anterior chamber of the eye and has been associated with significantly lower rates of intraocular pressure elevation than ophthalmic administration of prednisolone or dexamethasone.[21] Treatment with ophthalmic corticosteroids should be limited to two weeks, and even during this brief exposure, patients should be monitored for exacerbations of conjunctival or corneal viral infections and for increased intraocular pressure. With longer treatment, cataract formation is a concern.

STINGING AND BURNING — Patients who find that application of any topical ophthalmic preparation leads to stinging or burning should try refrigerating the drug before use. Compounding pharmacies can prepare preservative-free formulations for patients with ocular hypersensitivity to preservatives in ophthalmic drugs. A novel filter device

Table 3. Some Ophthalmic Drugs for Allergic Conjunctivitis

Drug	Some Formulations
H_1-Antihistamines	
Alcaftadine – *Lastacaft* (Allergan)	0.25% soln*
Azelastine – generic	0.05% soln*
Bepotastine – *Bepreve* (Valeant)	1.5% soln*
Cetirizine – *Zerviate* (Nicox)	0.24% soln*
Emedastine difumarate – *Emadine* (Alcon)	0.05% soln*
Epinastine – generic *Elestat* (Allergan)	0.05% soln*
Ketotifen fumarate[3] – generic *Zaditor* (Novartis) *Alaway* (Valeant)	0.025% soln*
Olopatadine – generic *Patanol* (Alcon) *Pataday* (Alcon) *Pazeo* (Alcon)	 0.1% soln* 0.2% soln* 0.7% soln*
Mast Cell Stabilizers	
Cromolyn sodium[4] – generic	4% soln*
Lodoxamide tromethamine – *Alomide*[4] (Alcon)	0.1% soln*
Nedocromil – *Alocril* (Allergan)	2% soln*
Nonsteroidal Anti-Inflammatory Drug (NSAID)	
Ketorolac tromethamine – generic *Acular* (Allergan)	0.5% soln*
Corticosteroids	
Loteprednol etabonate – *Lotemax* (Valeant) *Alrex* (Valeant)	0.5% susp* 0.2% susp*
Prednisone acetate – *Pred Mild* (Allergan)	0.12% susp*

soln = solution; susp = suspension; N.A. = Cost not yet available (March 2018)
*Contains benzalkonium chloride (preservative).
1. Approximate WAC for one bottle. WAC = wholesaler acquisition cost or manufacturer's published price to wholesalers; WAC represents a published catalogue or list price and may not represent an actual transactional price. Source: AnalySource® Monthly. April 5, 2017. Reprinted with permission by First Databank, Inc. All rights reserved. ©2017. www.fdbhealth.com/policies/drug-pricing-policy.

Available Sizes	Usual Dosage	Minimum Age	Cost[1]
3 mL	1 drop once/d	2 yrs	$196.20
6 mL	1 drop bid	3 yrs	50.00
5, 10 mL	1 drop bid	2 yrs	187.90[2]
5, 7.5 mL	1 drop bid (q8h)	2 yrs	N.A.
5 mL	1 drop qid	3 yrs	125.20
5 mL	1 drop bid	3 yrs	85.50
			227.40
5 mL	1 drop bid (q8-12h)	3 yrs	6.10
5 mL			8.10
10 mL			8.60
			40.50
5 mL	1 drop bid (q6-8h)	3 yrs	249.40
2.5 mL	1 drop once/d	3 yrs	166.10
2.5 mL	1 drop once/d	2 yrs	164.10
10 mL	1 drop q4-6h	4 yrs	22.50
10 mL	1 drop qid	2 yrs	161.40
5 mL	1 drop bid	3 yrs	195.30
3, 5, 10 mL	1 drop qid	3 yrs	32.10[2]
5 mL			249.80
5, 10, 15 mL	1-2 drops qid[5]	See footnote 6	205.40[2]
5, 10 mL	1 drop qid[5]	See footnote 6	195.30[2]
5, 10 mL	1-2 drops bid-qid[5]	See footnote 6	126.70[2]

2. Cost of a 5-mL bottle.
3. Available without a prescription.
4. FDA-approved for treatment of vernal keratoconjunctivitis, vernal conjunctivitis, and vernal keratitis.
5. Ophthalmic corticosteroids should not be used for >2 weeks.
6. Safety and effectiveness in pediatric patients have not been established.

has been developed for removal of benzalkonium chloride, the most common offender.[22]

ATOPIC DERMATITIS

Atopic dermatitis (also known as atopic eczema) commonly presents in infancy and early childhood and is frequently associated with allergic rhinitis and asthma. Skin hydration followed by application of moisturizers and emollients is highly recommended and can reduce disease severity when combined with topical drugs.[23] Avoidance of irritating soaps, detergents or clothing, extremes of temperature and humidity, and keeping fingernails trimmed are all helpful in the management of atopic dermatitis symptoms. In some patients with atopic dermatitis exacerbated by food or other allergens, confirmation of the trigger and elimination of the relevant allergen may be helpful.

TOPICAL DRUGS — Corticosteroids – A medium- or high-potency topical corticosteroid may be needed to achieve control of skin inflammation in atopic dermatitis. For maintenance treatment, the lowest potency topical corticosteroid that is effective in a given patient should be used. High-potency corticosteroids such as betamethasone dipropionate 0.05% ointment or cream should only be applied to the trunk and extremities for short periods of time and should never be applied to the face or intertriginous areas such as the axillae and groin. Low-potency corticosteroids such as hydrocortisone cream are safe for use on the face and intertriginous areas.

Use of topical corticosteroids can lead to development of striae and skin atrophy. When applied to the eyelids for prolonged periods, they can potentially cause glaucoma and cataracts. The risks of systemic adverse effects, including adrenal suppression and possibly lymphoma, increase with corticosteroid potency, percentage of body surface covered, and duration of treatment. The risks are greatest when high-potency corticosteroids are applied under occlusive dressings in infants and young children with widespread skin involvement who require long-term treatment.

Calcineurin Inhibitors – Topically applied tacrolimus and pimecrolimus can reduce inflammation and itching associated with atopic dermatitis within a few days. Topical tacrolimus 0.1% is similar in efficacy to a medium-potency topical corticosteroid and may be considered for use in patients with topical corticosteroid-resistant atopic dermatitis, especially on the face or intertriginous areas where corticosteroid adverse effects can be troublesome. It can also be used as maintenance treatment to minimize use of topical corticosteroids. After control of inflammation is achieved, applying tacrolimus ointment 2-3 times weekly increases the number of flare-free days and the time to relapse. Pimecrolimus is not as effective as a medium-potency topical corticosteroid, but it can be useful as steroid-sparing therapy for mild-to-moderate atopic dermatitis.

Tacrolimus and, less often, pimecrolimus can cause mild, transient itching, burning, stinging, and erythema, and both have been associated with an increased risk of viral skin infections such as herpes simplex and varicella zoster, but they do not cause cutaneous atrophy. Rare postmarketing reports of malignancies in patients treated with topical calcineurin inhibitors led the FDA to include a boxed warning in the labels of these drugs about possible risks of lymphoma and other cancers with prolonged treatment. A causal relationship has not been established.[24]

Crisaborole – Crisaborole *(Eucrisa)*, a topical phosphodiesterase type-4 (PDE4) inhibitor, has been approved by the FDA for treatment of atopic dermatitis in patients ≥2 years old. It acts in part by increasing levels of cyclic adenosine monophosphate (cAMP) to suppress production of proinflammatory cytokines in the skin. Systemic absorption is minimal.[25] In two randomized controlled trials in patients with mild-to-moderate atopic dermatitis, crisaborole 2% ointment applied twice daily to affected areas of skin was compared to its vehicle alone. A significantly higher percentage of patients using crisaborole achieved clear or almost-clear skin in both trials (33% vs 25% and 31% vs 18%).[26] Adverse effects have been mainly stinging and burning at the application site. The drug's long-term adverse effects are unknown. How crisaborole compares to topical corticosteroids or calcineurin inhibitors remains to be established.

Table 4. Some Topical Drugs for Atopic Dermatitis

Drug	Vehicle	Cost[1]
CALCINEURIN INHIBITORS		
Pimecrolimus 1%		
Elidel (Novartis)	cream	$517.20[2]
Tacrolimus 0.03%, 0.1%		
generic	oint	416.70[2]
Protopic (Astellas)		486.20[2]
PDE4 INHIBITOR		
Crisaborole 2%		
Eucrisa (Pfizer)	oint	580.00[2]
CORTICOSTEROIDS		
Super-High Potency		
Betamethasone dipropionate augmented 0.05%		
generic	oint	105.70
Diprolene		170.70
Clobetasol propionate 0.05%		
generic	cream, oint, gel	124.50
	lotion, soln	149.00
	foam	292.30
Clobex (Galderma)	lotion	500.10
	spray	442.50
Olux, Olux-E (Prestium/Mylan)	foam	493.00
Fluocinonide 0.1%		
generic	cream	323.80
Vanos (Valeant)		952.30
Halobetasol propionate 0.05%		
generic	cream, oint	153.10[3]
Ultravate (Ranbaxy)	cream, oint, lotion	916.00[3]

oint = ointment; soln = solution

1. Approximate WAC. WAC = wholesaler acquisition cost or manufacturer's published price to wholesalers; WAC represents a published catalogue or list price and may not represent an actual transactional price. Source: AnalySource® Monthly. April 5, 2017. Reprinted with permission by First Databank, Inc. All rights reserved. ©2017. www.fdbhealth.com/policies/drug-pricing-policy. When multiple formulations are listed, the price of the first formulation is provided (30 g of cream, ointment, or gel, 50 or 60 mL of lotion, solution, or spray, 118 mL of shampoo, and 50 g of foam).
2. Cost of 60 g.
3. Cost of 50 g.

Continued on next page

Table 4. Some Topical Drugs for Atopic Dermatitis (continued)

Drug	Vehicle	Cost[1]
High Potency		
Amcinonide 0.1%	oint	$324.00[2]
Betamethasone dipropionate 0.05% augmented		
generic	cream	42.40
Diprolene AF (Merck)		170.70
Betamethasone dipropionate 0.05%	oint	87.00[4]
Desoximetasone 0.25%		
generic	cream, oint	87.40
Topicort (Taro)	cream, oint, spray	343.80[2]
Desoximetasone 0.05%	gel	147.00
Diflorasone diacetate 0.05%	oint	335.50
Fluocinonide 0.05%	oint, gel	111.20
	cream, soln	72.90
Halcinonide 0.1%		
Halog (Ranbaxy)	cream, oint	452.80
Mometasone furoate 0.1%	oint	32.00
Medium-High Potency		
Amcinonide 0.1%	cream	189.00
	lotion	271.40
Betamethasone dipropionate 0.05%	cream	84.50
Betamethasone valerate 0.1%, 0.12%	oint, cream	32.50
	foam	261.50
Desoximetasone 0.05%	cream	87.40
Diflorasone diacetate 0.05%	cream	335.50
Fluocinonide emollient 0.05%	cream	77.10
Fluticasone propionate 0.005%	oint	57.20
Triamcinolone acetonide 0.5%	oint, cream	16.40
Medium Potency		
Betamethasone dipropionate 0.05%		
Sernivo (Promius)	spray	780.00[5]
Betamethasone valerate 0.12%		
generic	foam	261.50
Luxiq (Prestium/Mylan)		411.60

4. Cost of 120 g.
5. Cost of 120 mL.

Continued on next page

Table 4. Some Topical Drugs for Atopic Dermatitis (continued)		
Drug	**Vehicle**	**Cost[1]**
Medium Potency (continued)		
Fluocinolone acetonide 0.025%	oint	$56.30
Flurandrenolide 0.05%		
generic	oint	523.00[2]
Cordran (Aqua)		581.00[2]
Hydrocortisone valerate 0.2%	oint	157.40
Mometasone furoate 0.1%	cream, soln	35.00
Triamcinolone acetonide 0.1%	oint, cream	9.00
Triamcinolone acetonide 0.05%		
Trianex (Promius)	oint	860.00[6]
Medium-Low Potency		
Betamethasone dipropionate 0.05%	lotion	38.00
Betamethasone valerate 0.1%	cream	44.80
Desonide 0.05%	oint	96.20
Fluocinolone acetonide 0.025%	cream	58.50
Flurandrenolide 0.05%		
generic	cream, lotion	412.70[2]
Cordran (Aqua)		962.00[4]
Fluticasone propionate 0.05%		
generic	cream	25.80
Cutivate (PharmaDerm)		113.10
Hydrocortisone butyrate 0.1%		
generic	cream, oint	100.20
	soln	191.20
Locoid (Onset)	cream, oint	328.40[7]
	lotion, soln	483.30
Locoid Lipocream	cream	689.60[7]
Hydrocortisone probutate 0.1%		
Pandel (Sandoz)	cream	984.10[8]
Hydrocortisone valerate 0.2%	cream	143.20
Prednicarbate 0.1%	cream, oint	114.30
Triamcinolone acetonide 0.025%	oint	10.00
Triamcinolone acetonide 0.1%	lotion	29.00

6. Cost of a 430-g jar.
7. Cost of 45 g.
8. Cost of 80 g.

Continued on next page

Table 4. Some Topical Drugs for Atopic Dermatitis (continued)		
Drug	**Vehicle**	**Cost**[1]
Low Potency		
Alclometasone dipropionate 0.05%	cream, oint	$76.90
Betamethasone valerate 0.1%	lotion	60.00
Clocortolone pivalate 0.1%		
generic	cream	268.70[7]
Cloderm (Promius)		325.50[7]
Desonide 0.05%		
generic	cream	128.50
	lotion	236.90
Desonate (Bayer)	gel	513.40[2]
Verdeso (Stiefel)	foam	780.00
Fluocinolone acetonide 0.01%	cream	74.20
	soln	125.30
Triamcinolone acetonide 0.025%	cream	7.20
	lotion	29.00
Lowest Potency (may be ineffective for some indications)		
Hydrocortisone 2.5%	cream, oint	2.70
	lotion	16.40
Hydrocortisone 1.0%[9]	cream, oint	6.80[10]
	lotion	8.00[10]
Hydrocortisone 0.5%[9]	cream	5.00[10]

9. Available without a prescription.
10. Price according to walgreens.com (0.5% cream, 1% cream and lotion). Accessed April 27, 2017.

Coal Tar – Coal tar preparations have antipruritic and anti-inflammatory effects, but they are messy and odoriferous and are now seldom used except in shampoo formulations. Adverse effects include skin irritation, folliculitis, and photosensitivity.

Antipruritic Therapy – Pruritus is optimally controlled by regular applications of topical anti-inflammatory medications to the skin. Although the efficacy of oral H_1-antihistamines in atopic dermatitis has not been confirmed in randomized controlled trials, some physicians recommend a first-generation sedating H_1-antihistamine such as diphenhydramine or hydroxyzine (*Vistaril*, and generics) at bedtime. Topical H_1-antihistamines are potentially sensitizing and are therefore contraindicated for use in atopic dermatitis.[27]

SYSTEMIC DRUGS — Dupilumab *(Dupixent)*, a subcutaneously-injected, fully human monoclonal antibody that inhibits the signaling of the inflammatory cytokines interleukin (IL)-4 and IL-13, has been approved by the FDA for treatment of adults with moderate-to-severe atopic dermatitis that has not responded to topical therapies.[28] In two randomized, double-blind, 16-week trials in 1379 adults, dupilumab monotherapy significantly improved measures of skin clearing, overall extent and severity of disease, and pruritus compared to placebo. A score of clear or almost clear on the Investigator's Global Assessment scale and a reduction of ≥2 points on that score from baseline, the primary endpoint, occurred in 38% and 36% of patients treated with dupilumab every other week in the two trials versus 10% and 8% of those who received placebo.[29] Administration of dupilumab in combination with topical corticosteroids for 52 weeks significantly improved skin clearing and overall disease severity compared to use of topical corticosteroids alone.[30] Adverse effects have included injection-site reactions, conjunctivitis, blepharitis, keratitis, and oral herpes and other herpes simplex virus infections.

Cyclosporine (*Neoral*, and generics) is not FDA-approved for use in atopic dermatitis, but it has been recommended for short-term treatment of moderate-to-severe atopic dermatitis that is refractory to topical therapy.[31] In multiple randomized controlled trials, it significantly decreased disease activity within 2 to 6 weeks.[32] The usual dosage is 3-6 mg/kg/day (150-300 mg/day in adults). Cyclosporine can cause hypertension, nephrotoxicity, GI disturbances, hirsutism, headache, paresthesias, hypertriglyceridemia, and musculoskeletal or joint pain. It also increases the risks of infection and cutaneous and lymphoproliferative malignancies, and it interacts with many other drugs.

Short courses of an **oral corticosteroid** such as prednisone can be helpful in severe acute exacerbations of atopic dermatitis, but the drug should be tapered quickly and intensified treatment with topical corticosteroids and calcineurin inhibitors should be started.

PHOTOTHERAPY — Phototherapy in moderation has been effective in some patients after failure of topical drugs. It can be used alone or in combination with emollients and topical corticosteroids.[31]

URTICARIA

Acute urticaria is a self-limited condition that responds well to treatment with an oral H_1-antihistamine. **Chronic urticaria** (≥6 weeks) can last for months, years, or decades.

H_1-ANTIHISTAMINES — Randomized controlled trials have shown that oral second-generation H_1-antihistamines consistently decrease itching and reduce the number, size, and duration of wheals in acute and chronic urticaria.[33] Taken regularly, they can prevent new wheals from appearing. Cetirizine and levocetirizine are more potent in suppressing histamine-induced wheals than fexofenadine, and fexofenadine is more potent than loratadine and desloratadine. High doses (up to 4 times the usual dose) of a second-generation H_1-antihistamine are recommended (off-label) for treatment of chronic urticaria that does not respond to standard doses.[34] Despite decades of use in urticaria, first-generation H_1-antihistamines have never been optimally studied in randomized controlled trials, and they can cause CNS impairment with or without sedation. Nevertheless, when even higher-than-usual doses of an oral second-generation H_1-antihistamine fail to adequately control symptoms, some clinicians have found that hydroxyzine or diphenhydramine can be helpful.

OMALIZUMAB — Omalizumab is FDA-approved for treatment of chronic idiopathic urticaria refractory to H_1-antihistamines.[35] In randomized placebo-controlled trials, subcutaneous injections of omalizumab every 4 weeks significantly reduced itch and wheal scores and significantly increased rates of complete response; the highest response rates occurred with a 300-mg dose.[36] Omalizumab also significantly reduced the angioedema that was associated with urticaria in some patients.[37,38] Adverse events were similar to those with placebo. No patients developed anaphylaxis, which has occurred with use of omalizumab in patients with asthma.

OTHER DRUGS — A short course (3-7 days) of an **oral corticosteroid** such as prednisone 1 mg/kg (maximum dose 50 mg) can be helpful in relieving severe exacerbations of itching and whealing in chronic urticaria. Topical corticosteroids are not effective.

Cyclosporine is recommended in guidelines as a low-cost alternative to omalizumab in H_1-antihistamine-refractory chronic urticaria. Although not FDA-approved for this indication, it has been effective in randomized controlled trials.[39] Patients taking cyclosporine require monitoring of blood pressure and renal function. In one small randomized controlled trial, use of **dapsone** 100 mg/day to treat antihistamine-refractory chronic urticaria led to a significant improvement in symptoms[40]; monitoring of complete blood counts and hepatic function is required, and dapsone should not be used in G6PD-deficient patients.

In some randomized controlled trials, the leukotriene receptor antagonist **montelukast** had a beneficial effect in H_1-antihistamine-refractory chronic urticaria, but results have been inconsistent. Montelukast is not FDA-approved for treatment of urticaria, but it has been recommended in some guidelines as an alternative when other treatments have failed.[41]

Other immunomodulators such as systemic tacrolimus, mycophenolate mofetil, and hydroxychloroquine have been recommended for treatment of urticaria based on anecdotal experience.[41,42]

ALLERGEN-SPECIFIC IMMUNOTHERAPY

Sublingual immunotherapy (SLIT) has been approved by the FDA for treatment of allergic rhinitis induced by grass pollen, ragweed pollen, and dust mites.[43,57] Both subcutaneous immunotherapy (SCIT) and SLIT are effective in altering the natural history of allergic respiratory disease and inducing long-term remission, but SCIT has been used much longer, and has been highly effective in preventing future anaphylactic reactions to insect stings. Both SCIT and SLIT may be beneficial in decreasing symptoms and rescue medication use in patients with allergic rhinitis. Definitive randomized controlled trials comparing SCIT with SLIT are needed.[44]

Local adverse effects of SCIT include pain and swelling at injection sites. Anaphylaxis and, very rarely, death can occur. SCIT should only be administered under medical supervision. After dose buildup, maintenance injections are typically continued at monthly intervals for 4-5 years.

SLIT can cause local adverse effects such as mouth and ear pruritus, mouth edema, and throat irritation. Systemic adverse effects include nausea and mild abdominal pain. Anaphylaxis is rare and fatalities have not been reported.[45] Maintenance treatment is self-administered at home.

Advances have been made in immunotherapy for prevention of allergic reactions to peanuts and other foods. Oral, sublingual, and epicutaneous routes of administration are being investigated.[46] No immunotherapy is currently approved by the FDA for treatment of food allergy.

ANAPHYLAXIS

Anaphylaxis, a multi-system allergic reaction that is rapid in onset and may cause death, often occurs in community settings where it is typically triggered by a food, insect sting, or medication. The incidence of anaphylaxis is increasing in the US population. The greatest increase has been reported in food-related anaphylaxis, which occurs most commonly in the pediatric population.[47] Vaccine-triggered anaphylaxis remains rare.[48] Patients at risk for anaphylaxis in community settings should receive printed information about how to avoid their relevant triggers.[49] Those who have had an anaphylactic reaction triggered by stinging insects should be instructed in insect avoidance measures and referred to an

Table 5. Epinephrine Auto-Injectors		
Drug	**Formulations**[1]	**Cost**[2]
Epinephrine injection, USP –		
generic (Mylan)[3]	0.15 mg/0.3 mL, 0.3 mg/0.3 mL	$300.00
		300.00
EpiPen Jr (Mylan)	0.15 mg/0.3 mL	608.60
EpiPen	0.3 mg/0.3 mL	608.60
Epinephrine injection, USP[4] –		
generic (Impax)	0.15 mg/0.15 mL, 0.3 mg/0.3 mL	395.20[5,6]
Adrenaclick (Impax)[7]		460.90[5]
Epinephrine injection, USP – *Auvi-Q* (Kaléo)[8]	0.1 mg/0.1 mL, 0.15 mg/0.15 mL, 0.3 mg/0.3 mL	See footnote 9
Epinephrine injection, USP –		
Symjepi (Adamis)	0.3 mg/0.3 mL	N.A.

N.A. = Cost not yet available (March 2018)

1. The dose of epinephrine is 0.15 mg for patients who weigh 15-30 kg and 0.3 mg for those who weigh ≥30 kg.
2. Approximate WAC for one package containing two auto-injectors. WAC = wholesaler acquisition cost or manufacturer's published price to wholesalers; WAC represents a published catalogue or list price and may not represent an actual transactional price. Source: AnalySource® Monthly. April 5, 2017. Reprinted with permission by First Databank, Inc. All rights reserved. ©2017. www.fdbhealth.com/policies/drug-pricing-policy.
3. Interchangeable with *EpiPen* and *EpiPen Jr*.
4. *Adrenaclick* and its generic equivalent are similar to *EpiPen* and *EpiPen Jr* in size and functionality, but they are not considered interchangeable due to differences in device design and instructions for use.
5. Both strengths cost the same.
6. Both strengths are available at CVS for a cash price of $110.00 for two auto-injectors.
7. *Adrenaclick* is no longer being manufactured; its generic equivalent will continue to be marketed after supplies of *Adrenaclick* are depleted.
8. *Auvi-Q* is not interchangeable with other currently available epinephrine auto-injectors.
9. Manufacturer's list price (WAC) is $4500.00. However, according to the manufacturer, the out-of-pocket cost is $0 for all commercially insured patients, whether or not their insurer covers the device. The cash price for patients without government or commercial insurance is $360 for those with a household income ≥$100,000/year and $0 for those with a household income <$100,000/year.

allergy/immunology specialist for immunotherapy with standardized extracts of insect venom or whole-body extract from fire ants.[50]

EPINEPHRINE — All patients at risk for anaphylaxis recurrence in community settings and caregivers of children at risk should be equipped with one or more epinephrine auto-injectors such as *EpiPen* or *Auvi-Q* (or generic epinephrine for injection) and trained to recognize anaphylaxis and use the auto-injector correctly and safely. There are no absolute contraindications to epinephrine injection in anaphylaxis.

Concerns about potential adverse effects in the elderly and in patients with cardiovascular disease need to be weighed against the possibility of death from anaphylaxis.[51]

Injection of epinephrine 0.3 mg from either *Auvi-Q* or *EpiPen* results in similar peak epinephrine levels and total epinephrine exposure.[52] *Auvi-Q*, reintroduced in the US in 2017, has a compact rectangular shape and provides visual signals and step-by-step audio instructions for use. Compared with pen-type auto-injectors, it is more convenient to carry and easier to use, has additional safety features including an automatic fully retractable needle, and is less likely to cause unintentional injuries.[53,54]

The recommended dose of epinephrine is 0.01 mg/kg (0.5 mg maximum) intramuscularly. Until recently, epinephrine auto-injectors provided epinephrine only in fixed doses of 0.15 or 0.3 mg. The FDA has now approved *Auvi-Q* 0.1 mg for use in infants and small children weighing 7.5-15 kg. Auto-injectors containing 0.15 mg are labeled for children weighing 15-30 kg, and those containing 0.3 mg are labeled for adults and children weighing ≥30 kg. No auto-injector provides an optimal dose for children weighing between 15 and 30 kg; some clinicians prescribe an auto-injector containing 0.3 mg for children who weigh ≥25 kg.[55]

After injection of epinephrine, patients should be taken to the nearest emergency department for observation because anaphylaxis symptoms recur within hours in up to 20% of patients. Intravenous fluids and oxygen may be required in cases of severe anaphylaxis. H_1-antihistamines and corticosteroids are not recommended for treatment of anaphylaxis in community settings; they do not prevent or relieve airway obstruction, hypotension or shock, or prevent death.

INSECT STINGS AND BITES

Small local allergic reactions to insect stings and bites (itchy red swellings) are self-limited. Large local reactions that occur at the sites of stings from honeybees, yellowjackets, wasps, and fire ants, or bites from mosquitoes, deer flies, and other insects, can involve a large portion of the face or an entire extremity and cause extreme discomfort. For prevention and treatment of large local reactions, an oral second-generation H_1-antihistamine such as cetirizine should be used as soon as possible after the sting or bite. For mild or moderate large local reactions, a topical corticosteroid cream can be applied to the affected area for 5-7 days. Oral prednisone 1 mg/kg once daily (maximum daily dose 50 mg) for 5-7 days may be needed for severe large local reactions. Although the risk of anaphylaxis in patients with large local reactions to stinging insects is <5%, epinephrine auto-injectors are often prescribed for these patients. Venom immunotherapy is effective in preventing large local reactions and can be considered for those with occupational or other unavoidable exposure to stinging insects who frequently require treatment for reactions to stings.[56]

1. MD Seidman et al. Clinical practice guideline: allergic rhinitis executive summary. Otolaryngol Head Neck Surg 2015; 152:197.
2. GK Scadding. Optimal management of allergic rhinitis. Arch Dis Child 2015; 100:576.
3. FE Simons and KJ Simons. Histamine and H_1-antihistamines: celebrating a century of progress. J Allergy Clin Immunol 2011; 128:1139.
4. MK Church et al. Risk of first-generation H(1)-antihistamines: a GA(2)LEN position paper. Allergy 2010; 65:459.
5. MP McKay and L Groff. 23 years of toxicology testing fatally injured pilots: implications for aviation and other modes of transportation. Accid Anal Prev 2016; 90:108.
6. Y Katayose et al. Carryover effect on next-day sleepiness and psychomotor performance of nighttime administered antihistaminic drugs: a randomized controlled trial. Hum Psychopharmacol 2012; 27:428.
7. SL Gray et al. Cumulative use of strong anticholinergics and incident dementia: a prospective cohort study. JAMA Intern Med 2015; 175:401.
8. BM Prenner. A review of the clinical efficacy and safety of MP-AzeFlu, a novel intranasal formulation of azelastine hydrochloride and fluticasone propionate, in clinical studies conducted during different allergy seasons in the US. J Asthma Allergy 2016; 9:135.
9. P Ratner et al. Efficacy of daily intranasal fluticasone propionate on ocular symptoms associated with seasonal allergic rhinitis. Ann Allergy Asthma Immunol 2015; 114:141.
10. OTC fluticasone furoate nasal spray (Flonase Sensimist) for allergic rhinitis. Med Lett Drugs Ther 2017; 59:e70.
11. A Nayak and RB Langdon. Montelukast in the treatment of allergic rhinitis: an evidence-based review. Drugs 2007; 67:887.
12. In brief: Oral phenylephrine for nasal congestion. Med Lett Drugs Ther 2015; 57:174.
13. E Mehuys et al. Self-medication in persistent rhinitis: overuse of decongestants in half of the patients. J Allergy Clin Immunol Pract 2014; 2:313.

14. B Lange et al. Efficacy, cost-effectiveness, and tolerability of mometasone furoate, levocabastine, and disodium cromoglycate nasal sprays in the treatment of seasonal allergic rhinitis. Ann Allergy Asthma Immunol 2005; 95:272.
15. S Tsabouri et al. Omalizumab for the treatment of inadequately controlled allergic rhinitis: a systematic review and meta-analysis of randomized clinical trials. J Allergy Clin Immunol Pract 2014; 2:332.
16. F Etwel et al. The risk of adverse pregnancy outcome after first trimester exposure to H_1-antihistamines: a systematic review and meta-analysis. Drug Saf 2017; 40:121.
17. I Pali-Schöll et al. Allergic diseases and asthma in pregnancy, a secondary publication. World Allergy Organ J 2017; 10:10.
18. M Shaker and E Salcone. An update on ocular allergy. Curr Opin Allergy Clin Immunol 2016; 16:505.
19. Alcaftadine (Lastacaft) for allergic conjunctivitis. Med Lett Drugs Ther 2011; 53:19.
20. M Castillo et al. Topical antihistamines and mast cell stabilisers for treating seasonal and perennial allergic conjunctivitis. Cochrane Database Syst Rev 2015; 6:CD009566.
21. JD Sheppard et al. Impact of the topical ophthalmic corticosteroid loteprednol etabonate on intraocular pressure. Adv Ther 2016; 33:532.
22. KH Hsu and A Chauhan. Rapid and selective removal of preservative from ophthalmic formulations during eyedrops instillation. Eur J Pharm Biopharm 2015; 97:30.
23. EJ van Zuuren et al. Emollients and moisturisers for eczema. Cochrane Database Syst Rev 2017; 2:CD012119.
24. DJ Margolis et al. Association between malignancy and topical use of pimecrolimus. JAMA Dermatol 2015; 151:594.
25. Crisaborole (Eucrisa) for atopic dermatitis. Med Lett Drugs Ther 2017; 59:34.
26. AS Paller et al. Efficacy and safety of crisaborole ointment, a novel, nonsteroidal phosphodiesterase 4 (PDE4) inhibitor for the topical treatment of atopic dermatitis (AD) in children and adults. J Am Acad Dermatol 2016; 75:494.
27. L Schneider et al. Atopic dermatitis: a practice parameter update 2012. J Allergy Clin Immunol 2013; 131:295.
28. Dupilumab (Dupixent) for moderate to severe atopic dermatitis. Med Lett Drugs Ther 2017; 59:64.
29. EL Simpson et al. Two phase 3 trials of dupilumab versus placebo in atopic dermatitis. N Engl J Med 2016; 375:2335.
30. A Blauvelt et al. Long-term management of moderate-to-severe atopic dermatitis (AD) with dupilumab and concomitant topical corticosteroids (TCS): a 1-year, randomized, placebo-controlled phase 3 trial (CHRONOS). Presented at the 75th American Academy of Dermatology (AAD) Annual Meeting, Orlando, FL, March 3-7, 2017. Abstract 5267.
31. R Sidbury et al. Guidelines of care for the management of atopic dermatitis: section 3. Management and treatment with phototherapy and systemic agents. J Am Acad Dermatol 2014; 71:327.
32. E Roekevisch et al. Efficacy and safety of systemic treatments for moderate-to-severe atopic dermatitis: a systematic review. J Allergy Clin Immunol 2014; 133:429.
33. G Deza and AM Giménez-Arnau. Itch in urticaria management. Curr Probl Dermatol 2016; 50:77.

34. T Zuberbier et al. The EAACI/GA(2) LEN/EDF/WAO Guideline for the definition, classification, diagnosis, and management of urticaria: the 2013 revision and update. Allergy 2014; 69:868.
35. Omalizumab (Xolair) for chronic urticaria. Med Lett Drugs Ther 2013; 55:43.
36. ZT Zhao et al. Omalizumab for the treatment of chronic spontaneous urticaria: a meta-analysis of randomized clinical trials. J Allergy Clin Immunol 2016; 137:1742.
37. JL Zazzali et al. Angioedema in the omalizumab chronic idiopathic/spontaneous urticaria pivotal studies. Ann Allergy Asthma Immunol 2016; 117:370.
38. P Staubach et al. Effect of omalizumab on angioedema in H1-antihistamine-resistant chronic spontaneous urticaria patients: results from X-ACT, a randomized controlled trial. Allergy 2016; 71:1135.
39. DR Doshi and MM Weinberger. Experience with cyclosporine in children with chronic idiopathic urticaria. Pediatr Dermatol 2009; 26:409.
40. M Morgan et al. Double-blind placebo-controlled trial of dapsone in antihistamine refractory chronic idiopathic urticaria. J Allergy Clin Immunol Pract 2014; 2:601.
41. LA Beck et al. A review of international recommendations for the diagnosis and management of chronic urticaria. Acta Derm Venereol 2017; 97:149.
42. M Maurer et al. Current and future therapies for treating chronic spontaneous urticaria. Expert Opin Pharmacother 2016; 17:1131.
43. Sublingual immunotherapy for allergic rhinitis. Med Lett Drugs Ther 2014; 56:47.
44. SR Durham and M Penagos. Sublingual or subcutaneous immunotherapy for allergic rhinitis? J Allergy Clin Immunol 2016; 137:339.
45. TG Epstein et al. Current evidence on safety and practical considerations for administration of sublingual allergen immunotherapy (SLIT) in the United States. J Allergy Clin Immunol Pract 2017; 5:34.
46. RA Wood. Food allergen immunotherapy: current status and prospects for the future. J Allergy Clin Immunol 2016; 137:973.
47. S Lee et al. Trends, characteristics, and incidence of anaphylaxis in 2001-2010: a population-based study. J Allergy Clin Immunol 2017; 139:182.
48. MM McNeil et al. Risk of anaphylaxis after vaccination in children and adults. J Allergy Clin Immunol 2016; 137:868.
49. P Lieberman et al. Anaphylaxis – a practice parameter update 2015. Ann Allergy Asthma Immunol 2015; 115:341.
50. TB Casale and AW Burks. Hymenoptera-sting hypersensitivity. N Engl J Med 2014; 370:1432.
51. P Lieberman and FE Simons. Anaphylaxis and cardiovascular disease: therapeutic dilemmas. Clin Exp Allergy 2015; 45:1288.
52. ES Edwards et al. Epinephrine 0.3 mg bioavailability following a single injection with a novel epinephrine auto-injector, e-cue, in healthy adults, with reference to a single injection using EpiPen 0.3 mg. J Allergy Clin Immunol 2012; 129:AB179.
53. M Anshien et al. Unintentional epinephrine auto-injector injuries: a national poison center observational study. Am J Ther 2016 Nov 24 (epub).
54. Auvi-Q epinephrine auto-injector returns. Med Lett Drugs Ther 2017; 59:33.
55. SH Sicherer et al. Epinephrine for first-aid management of anaphylaxis. Pediatrics 2017; 139:e20164006.

56. DB Golden. Large local reactions to insect stings. J Allergy Clin Immunol Pract 2015; 3:331.
57. Odactra--sublingual immunotherapy for house dust mite-induced allergic rhinitis. Med Lett Drugs Ther 2018; 60:37.

DRUGS FOR Asthma

Original publication date – August 2017 (revised March 2018)

The goal of asthma treatment is to control symptoms and prevent exacerbations.[1] Management of acute exacerbations of asthma is not discussed here.

INHALED SABAs — The inhaled short-acting beta$_2$-agonists (SABAs) albuterol and levalbuterol are used for rapid relief of asthma symptoms. Their effect begins within 5 minutes, peaks within 30-60 minutes and lasts for 4-6 hours. They do not decrease airway inflammation and should only be used as needed for relief of symptoms or for prevention of exercise-induced bronchoconstriction (EIB). SABAs should be needed infrequently (≤2 days/week) for symptom relief in patients whose asthma is well controlled. The safety and efficacy of racemic albuterol and levalbuterol are comparable.[2]

Adverse Effects – Inhaled SABAs can cause paradoxical bronchospasm, tremor, tachycardia, QT interval prolongation, hyperglycemia, hypokalemia, and hypomagnesemia, especially if used in high doses. Tolerance can develop with regular use.[3]

INHALED SAMA — Ipratropium bromide is an inhaled short-acting muscarinic antagonist (SAMA) approved only for treatment of chronic obstructive pulmonary disease (COPD). It has been used off-label in asthma as an alternative reliever medication for patients who cannot use a

Recommendations for Treatment of Asthma
▸ Inhaled short-acting beta$_2$-agonists (SABAs) are used as needed for acute relief.
▸ Patients with persistent symptoms should be treated with an inhaled corticosteroid (ICS). Low daily doses of an ICS suppress airway inflammation and reduce the risk of exacerbations.
▸ For patients who remain symptomatic despite adherence to ICS treatment and good inhalational technique, addition of an inhaled long-acting beta$_2$-agonist (LABA) is recommended.
▸ Patients who continue to have uncontrolled asthma may need to take higher doses of ICSs.
▸ For patients with severe asthma that is unreponsive to high ICS doses, addition of the inhaled long-acting muscarinic antagonist (LAMA) tiotropium or a phenotype-targeted biologic agent can improve asthma control.
▸ Failure of pharmacologic treatment often results from poor inhaler technique, lack of adherence to prescribed medications, uncontrolled comorbid conditions such as allergic rhinitis, misdiagnosis, or continued exposure to allergens, tobacco smoke, or other airborne pollutants or irritants.

SABA and in combination with a SABA for treatment of acute bronchoconstriction. SABAs have a more rapid onset of action than ipratropium.

Adverse Effects – Ipratropium can cause dry mouth, pharyngeal irritation, increased intraocular pressure, and urinary retention.

INHALED CORTICOSTEROIDS — An inhaled corticosteroid (ICS) is the most effective long-term treatment for control of persistent asthma of any severity. In randomized controlled trials, ICSs have been significantly more effective than long-acting beta$_2$-agonists, leukotriene modifiers, or theophylline in improving pulmonary function, preventing symptoms and exacerbations, reducing the need for emergency department treatment, and decreasing deaths due to asthma. Patients with well-controlled asthma who stop using ICSs have an increased risk of exacerbations compared to those who continue using them.[4]

Most of the beneficial effects of ICSs are achieved at relatively low doses. Patients should receive the lowest dose that maintains asthma control; this dose may change seasonally and over time. Current evidence suggests that, at usual doses, all ICSs are similar in efficacy; they are not interchangeable, however, on a per-microgram or per-inhalation basis because the dose varies with the drug, formulation, and delivery device.

Adverse Effects – Local adverse effects of ICSs include oral candidiasis (thrush), dysphonia, and reflex cough and bronchospasm. Their incidence may be reduced by use of a spacer (with a metered-dose inhaler) and by mouth-rinsing after inhalation. Ciclesonide, a prodrug that is activated in the lungs, is less likely to cause oropharyngeal and systemic side effects than other ICSs.[5]

Regular administration of low or medium doses of ICSs may reduce growth slightly during the first year of treatment, especially in prepubescent children. In the Childhood Asthma Management Study (CAMP) in children 5 to 13 years old, which used a medium dose of budesonide (400 mcg/day for 4-6 years), the effect on growth was not progressive or cumulative; mean adult height was 1.2 cm less with the ICS compared to placebo.[6] Newer ICSs such as fluticasone, mometasone, and ciclesonide have lower oral bioavailability and improved lipophilicity compared to budesonide and beclomethasone and are less likely to affect growth velocity when used in low doses.[7]

Clinically relevant adverse effects on hypothalamic-pituitary-adrenal (HPA) axis function generally do not occur with low or medium doses of ICSs.

Patients who require high-dose ICS treatment should be monitored for HPA axis suppression, changes in bone density, and development of cataracts or glaucoma. ICSs do not increase the risk of pneumonia in patients with asthma.[8]

INHALED LABAs — Addition of an inhaled long-acting beta$_2$-agonist (LABA) such as salmeterol or formoterol to an ICS improves lung function, decreases symptoms and exacerbations, and reduces rescue use of SABAs. Several ICS/LABA combination inhalers (see Table 3)

Table 1. Treatment of Persistent Asthma

Asthma Severity		Recommended Regimen[1]
Mild		
Preferred		Low-dose ICS[2]
Alternative		Montelukast
Moderate		
Preferred		Low-dose ICS[2] + a LABA[3,4]
Alternatives		Medium-dose ICS[2]
	or	Low-dose ICS[2] + a leukotriene modifier[4]
Severe		
Preferred		Medium- or high-dose ICS[2] + a LABA[3-5]
Alternatives		Medium- or high-dose ICS[2] + a LABA and/or a LAMA[4-6]
	or	High-dose ICS[2] + a leukotriene modifier or theophylline[4,6]

ICS = inhaled corticosteroid; LABA = inhaled long-acting beta$_2$-agonist; LAMA = long-acting muscarinic antagonist

1. For patients ≥12 years old. Treatment should be adjusted based on response. All regimens include use of a an inhaled short-acting beta$_2$-agonist (SABA) as needed.
2. The ideal dose of an ICS is the lowest dose that maintains asthma control. Recommended low, medium, and high ICS doses can be found at http://medicalletter.org/TML-article-1528b.
3. The FDA recommends stopping a LABA once symptoms are controlled, but the recommendation is controversial (S Ahmad et al. Cochrane Database Syst Rev 2015; 19(6):CD011306).
4. Consider sublingual immunotherapy for adult patients with allergic rhinitis or allergy to house dust mites.
5. Tiotropium *(Spiriva Respimat)* is the only LAMA that is FDA-approved for maintenance treatment of asthma.
6. For patients with severe asthma that remains uncontrolled, omalizumab can be added in those with allergic asthma and an anti-interleukin-5 antibody can be added in those with eosinophilic asthma. Addition of a low-dose oral corticosteroid is an alternative. When other therapies fail, bronchial thermoplasty could be considered.

are FDA-approved for use in patients with persistent asthma that is not well-controlled on an ICS alone or is severe enough to require starting treatment with both an ICS and a LABA. Monotherapy with an inhaled LABA is contraindicated. LABAs are not indicated for relief of acute asthma symptoms.

Adverse Effects – LABAs, especially if used in higher-than-recommended doses, can cause tremor, hypokalemia, tachycardia, and other cardiac effects.

An FDA meta-analysis that found use of a LABA to be associated with an increased risk of asthma-related hospitalization, intubation, and death prompted the FDA to recommend that LABAs be discontinued once asthma is controlled. However, four FDA-mandated safety trials comparing the use of a LABA in combination with an ICS to an ICS alone in >41,000 adults and children with persistent asthma found that use of the combination was not associated with an increased risk of asthma-related adverse events. Therefore, the FDA has decided to remove the boxed warning about an increase in asthma-related death from the labels of inhaled corticosteroid/LABA combination products.[9-11,46]

INHALED LAMAs — Tiotropium bromide, an inhaled long-acting muscarinic antagonist (LAMA) previously approved for use in COPD, is now approved for maintenance treatment of asthma. In patients with moderate-to-severe asthma, addition of tiotropium to ICS therapy improves lung function and decreases symptoms.[12] Addition of tiotropium to combination treatment with an ICS and a LABA can improve lung function in patients with poorly-controlled severe asthma and reduce the need for rescue oral corticosteroids.[13]

Other inhaled LAMAs such as umeclidinium *(Incruse Ellipta)* may also be effective for treatment of asthma, but more data are needed.[14,15]

Adverse Effects – LAMAs have limited systemic bioavailability and are generally well tolerated.[16] They can cause dry mouth and pharyngeal irritation.

LEUKOTRIENE MODIFIERS — The leukotriene receptor antagonists montelukast and zafirlukast are alternatives to low-dose ICS treatment for patients who are unable or unwilling to use an ICS, but they are generally less effective than ICSs for asthma control. Leuko-

Table 2. Inhalation Devices

Metered-Dose Inhalers (MDIs)

Many products – see Table 3
- Use a hydrofluoroalkane (HFA) propellent
- Generally require hand/breath coordination
- Spacers help some patients, especially young children and the elderly, use MDIs effectively by minimizing the need to coordinate actuation and inhalation; valved spacers have one-way valves that prevent the patient from exhaling into the device
- Priming generally required
- Indicator shows how many doses are left

Dry Powder Inhalers (DPIs)

Advair Diskus **(fluticasone propionate/salmeterol),** ***Flovent Diskus*** **(fluticasone propionate),** ***Serevent Diskus*** **(salmeterol)**
- Drug delivery to lungs is dependent upon ability to perform a rapid, deep inhalation
- Indicator shows how many doses are left
- Twice-daily dosing

Arnuity Ellipta **(fluticasone furoate),** ***Breo Ellipta*** **(fluticasone furoate/vilanterol)**
- Drug delivery to lungs is dependent upon ability to perform a rapid, deep inhalation
- No assembly or priming required
- Indicator shows how many doses are left
- Doses may be wasted if inhaler is opened/closed accidentally
- Once-daily dosing

ProAir Respiclick **(albuterol),** ***AirDuo Respiclick*** **(fluticasone propionate/salmeterol),** ***ArmonAir Respiclick*** **(fluticasone propionate)**
- Drug delivery to lungs is dependent upon ability to perform a rapid, deep inhalation
- No priming required
- Indicator shows how many doses are left
- Doses may be wasted if inhaler is opened/closed accidentally

Asmanex Twisthaler **(mometasone)**
- Drug delivery to lungs is dependent upon ability to perform a rapid, deep inhalation
- No priming required
- Indicator shows how many doses are left

Continued on next page

Table 2. Inhalation Devices (continued)
Inhalation Spray (Soft Mist) Inhaler (ISI)
Spiriva Respimat **(tiotropium)** ▸ Drug delivery to lungs is not dependent on strength of breath intake ▸ Uses a spring to generate mechanical power to aerosolize the drug solution into a soft mist ▸ Assembly may be difficult for some patients ▸ Indicator shows approximately how much medicine is left ▸ Once-daily dosing
Nebulizers
▸ Delivers aerosolized medication with a face mask or mouthpiece ▸ Less dependent on the patient's coordination and cooperation, but more time-consuming, less efficient, and more costly than delivery through an MDI or DPI

triene modifiers are also generally less effective than inhaled LABAs as add-on therapy for patients whose asthma is not well controlled on an ICS alone. Leukotriene modifiers are not recommended for treatment of acute asthma symptoms.

Adverse Effects – Montelukast is considered safe for long-term use. Both zafirlukast and (especially) zileuton have been reported to cause life-threatening, hepatic injury; liver function tests should be monitored and patients should be advised to discontinue the drug immediately if abdominal pain, nausea, jaundice, itching, or lethargy occur. Churg-Strauss vasculitis has been reported rarely with montelukast and zafirlukast; in some cases, this was probably a consequence of corticosteroid withdrawal rather than a direct effect of the leukotriene modifier.[17]

THEOPHYLLINE — The availability of safer alternatives has significantly reduced the use of theophylline for persistent asthma. It is occasionally used in patients whose asthma is not controlled with an ICS and a LABA.[18] Monitoring serum theophylline concentrations is recommended to maintain peak levels between 8 and 15 mcg/mL.

Adverse Effects – Theophylline can cause nausea, vomiting, nervousness, headache, and insomnia, and it interacts with many other drugs. At high serum concentrations, hypokalemia, hyperglycemia, tachycardia, cardiac arrhythmias, tremor, neuromuscular irritability, seizures, and death can occur.

ORAL CORTICOSTEROIDS — Oral glucocorticoids should only be used as long-term controller medications in the small minority of patients with poorly-controlled severe persistent asthma despite proper inhalation technique and compliance with an optimal treatment regimen, comorbidity management, and environmental control. In this situation, an oral glucocorticoid should be given at the lowest effective dose, preferably on alternate mornings.

FAILURE OF STANDARD TREATMENT — Failure of pharmacologic treatment often results from lack of adherence to prescribed medications, improper inhalation technique, uncontrolled comorbid conditions, misdiagnosis, or continued exposure to allergens, tobacco smoke, and other airborne pollutants or irritants.[19] Smoking and exposure to second-hand smoke can cause airway hyperresponsiveness and decrease the effectiveness of ICSs. Some patients with asthma who take aspirin or other NSAIDs may experience acute asthma symptoms. Oral or ophthalmic nonselective beta-adrenergic blockers, such as propranolol (*Inderal*, and others) or timolol, can decrease the bronchodilating effect of both endogenous and exogenous $beta_2$-agonists in patients with asthma.

PHENOTYPE-TARGETED THERAPIES — Severe asthma, a heterogeneous condition consisting of phenotypes with certain biological and clinical features, may be unresponsive to high doses of ICSs plus a second asthma controller. A phenotype-targeted approach to treatment includes allergen immunotherapy and the anti-IgE antibody omalizumab for allergic asthma and use of other biologic agents such as the anti-interleukin-5 antibodies mepolizumab and reslizumab for eosinophilic asthma. For patients who fail or cannot tolerate these therapies, bronchial thermoplasty could be considered.[20]

IMMUNOTHERAPY — In selected patients with allergic asthma, specific immunotherapy (subcutaneous injections and sublingual tablets) may provide long-lasting benefits in reducing asthma symptoms and the need for medications.[21]

OMALIZUMAB — Omalizumab *(Xolair)*, a recombinant anti-IgE monoclonal antibody, is FDA-approved for use in patients ≥6 years old with moderate-to-severe persistent asthma not well controlled on an ICS who have well-documented specific sensitizations to airborne allergens, such as mold, pollen, or animal dander.

Subcutaneous injection of omalizumab every 2 or 4 weeks reduces asthma exacerbations and has a modest ICS-sparing effect. In adults and adolescents, omalizumab added to standard treatment improves symptoms and reduces exacerbations.[22,23] When added to standard treatment in children with allergic asthma, omalizumab can improve asthma control and decrease exacerbations and maintenance ICS doses.[24] Use of omalizumab does not preclude simultaneous use of allergen immunotherapy.

Adverse Effects – Injection-site pain and bruising can occur. The labeling of omalizumab includes a boxed warning regarding a risk of anaphylaxis. The drug should be administered in a healthcare setting by providers prepared to manage potentially life-threatening anaphylaxis. Symptoms of anaphylaxis can occur more than 2 hours post-injection. Patients receiving omalizumab should be instructed on how to recognize anaphylaxis and advised to self-inject epinephrine promptly if it occurs.[25]

ANTI-INTERLEUKIN-5 (IL-5) ANTIBODIES — Three anti-IL-5 antibodies, mepolizumab *(Nucala)*, reslizumab *(Cinqair)*, and benralizumab *(Fasenra)*, are approved by the FDA for treatment of severe asthma in patients who have elevated eosinophil levels.[26,27]

In a randomized, placebo-controlled trial in 576 patients ≥12 years old with severe eosinophilic asthma, **mepolizumab** 100 mg SC every 4 weeks for 32 weeks reduced the annualized frequency of clinically

Table 3. Some Drugs for Asthma	
Drug	**Some Available Formulations**
Inhaled Short-Acting Beta$_2$-Agonists (SABAs)	
Albuterol –	
ProAir HFA (Teva) *Proventil HFA* (Merck) *Ventolin HFA* (GSK)	HFA MDI (60[2] or 200 inh/unit) 90 mcg/inh
ProAir Respiclick (Teva)	DPI (200 inh/unit) 90 mcg/inh
generic – single-dose vials	Solution for nebulization[4] 0.63, 1.25, 2.5 mg/3 mL
Levalbuterol –	
Xopenex HFA (Sunovion)	HFA MDI (80, 200 inh/unit) 45 mcg/inh
Xopenex (Sunovion) generic – single-dose vials	Solution for nebulization[4] 0.31, 0.63, 1.25 mg/3 mL
Inhaled Short-Acting Muscarinic Antagonist (SAMA)	
Ipratropium[7] – *Atrovent HFA* (Boehringer Ingelheim)	HFA MDI (200 inh/unit) 17 mcg/inh
generic – single-dose vials	Solution for nebulization 200 mcg/mL
Inhaled Short-Acting Beta$_2$-Agonist/Short-Acting Muscarinic Antagonist Combination	
Albuterol/ipratropium[7] – *Combivent Respimat* (Boehringer Ingelheim)	ISI 120 inh/unit 100 mcg/20 mcg/inh
generic	Solution for nebulization 2.5 mg/0.5 mg/3 mL

DPI = dry powder inhaler; ER = extended-release; HFA = hydrofluoroalkane; inh = inhalation; ISI = inhalation spray inhaler; MDI = metered-dose inhaler

1. Approximate WAC for 30 days' treatment at the lowest recommended adult dosage. WAC = wholesaler acquisition cost or manufacturer's published price to wholesalers; WAC represents a published catalogue or list price and may not represent an actual transactional price. Source: AnalySource® Monthly. August 5, 2017. Reprinted with permission by First Databank, Inc. All rights reserved. ©2017. www.fdbhealth.com/policies/drug-pricing-policy.
2. Only *Ventolin HFA* is available in a 60 inhalations/unit formulation.

Usual Adult Dosage	Usual Pediatric Dosage	Cost[1]
90-180 mcg q4-6h PRN	≥4 yrs: 90-180 mcg q4-6h PRN	$56.20[3]
		75.40[3]
		52.20[3]
90-180 mcg q4-6h PRN	≥4 yrs: 90-180 mcg q4-6h PRN	53.00[3]
1.25-5 mg q4-8h PRN	2-4 yrs: 0.63-2.5 mg q4-6h PRN	21.30[5]
90 mcg q4-6h PRN	≥4 yrs: 90 mcg q4-6h PRN	68.20[3]
0.63-1.25 mg tid q6-8h PRN	6-11 yrs: 0.31-0.63 mg tid q6-8h PRN ≥12 yrs: 0.63-1.25 mg tid q6-8h PRN	950.00[6] 537.00[6]
2 inh (34 mcg) qid PRN	--	332.70[3]
500 mcg qid PRN	--	18.10[6]
1 inh qid PRN	--	344.90[8]
2.5 mg/0.5 mg qid PRN	--	73.10[8]

3. Cost of 200 inhalations.
4. Nebulized solutions may be used for very young, very old, and other patients unable to use pressurized aerosols. More time is required to administer the drug and the device may not be portable.
5. Cost of 100 2.5-mg doses.
6. Cost of 100 doses.
7. Not FDA-approved for use in asthma.
8. Cost of 120 doses.

Continued on next page

Table 3. Some Drugs for Asthma (continued)	
Drug	**Some Available Formulations**
Inhaled Corticosteroids (ICSs)[9]	
Beclomethasone dipropionate –	
QVAR (Teva)	HFA MDI (100 or 120 inh/unit) 40, 80 mcg/inh
QVAR Redihaler (Teva)	HFA MDI (120 inh/unit)[10a] 40, 80 mcg/inh
Budesonide – *Pulmicort Flexhaler* (AstraZeneca)	DPI (60, 120 inh/unit) 90, 180 mcg/inh
Pulmicort Respules (AstraZeneca) single-dose ampules generic	Suspension for nebulization 0.25, 0.5 mg, 1 mg/2 mL
Ciclesonide – *Alvesco* (Sunovion)	HFA MDI (60 inh/unit) 80, 160 mcg/inh
Flunisolide – *Aerospan HFA* (Acton)	HFA MDI (60, 120 inh/unit) 80 mcg/inh
Fluticasone furoate – *Arnuity Ellipta* (GSK)	DPI (30 inh/unit) 100, 200 mcg/inh
Fluticasone propionate –	
Flovent Diskus (GSK)	DPI (60 inh/unit) 50, 100, 250 mcg/blister
Flovent HFA (GSK)	HFA MDI (120 inh/unit) 44, 110, 220 mcg/inh
ArmonAir Respiclick (Teva)	DPI (60 inh/unit) 55, 113, 232 mcg/inh
Mometasone furoate –	
Asmanex HFA (Merck)	HFA MDI (120 inh/unit) 100, 200 mcg/inh
Asmanex Twisthaler (Merck)	DPI (30, 60, 120 inh/unit) 110, 220 mcg/inh
Inhaled Long-Acting Beta$_2$-Agonists (LABAs)[13]	
Formoterol – *Perforomist* (Mylan)[8]	Solution for nebulization[4] 20 mcg/2 mL
Salmeterol – *Serevent Diskus* (GSK)	DPI (60 inh/unit) 50 mcg/blister

9. Recommended low, medium, and high ICS doses can be found at http://medicalletter.org/TML-article-1528b.
10. Dose is based on disease severity and/or prior asthma therapy. See package insert for specific dosing instructions.
10a. The *Redihaler* is a breath-actuated MDI that does not require hand/breath coordination or priming and should not be used with a spacer.

Usual Adult Dosage	Usual Pediatric Dosage	Cost[1]
40-320 mcg bid[10]	5-11 yrs: 40-80 mcg bid[9]	$169.30[11]
40-320 mcg bid[10]	4-11 yrs: 40-80 mcg bid	169.30[11]
180-720 mcg bid	6-17 yrs: 180-360 mcg bid	216.50
--	1-8 yrs: 0.25 mg bid or 0.5 mg once/d or bid or 1 mg once/d[10]	872.00[12] 753.00[12]
80-320 mcg bid[10]	≥12 yrs: 80-320 mcg bid[10]	228.90
160-320 mcg bid[10]	6-11 yrs: 80-160 mcg bid[10]	196.10
100-200 mcg once/d[10]	≥12 yrs: 100-200 mcg once/d[10]	159.00
100-1000 mcg bid[10]	4-11 yrs: 50-100 mcg bid[10]	171.40
88-880 mcg bid[10]	4-11 yrs: 88 mcg bid	171.40
55-232 mcg bid[10]	≥12 yrs: 55-232 mcg bid[10]	169.30[11]
200-400 mcg bid[10]	≥12 yrs: 200-400 mcg bid[10]	191.40
220-880 mcg once/d in evening or 220 mcg bid[10]	4-11 yrs: 110 mcg once/d in evening[10]	191.60
20 mcg bid	--	893.40
50 mcg bid	≥4 yrs: 50 mcg bid	351.60

11. Approximate WAC for 30 days' treatment at the lowest recommended adult dosage. Source: AnalySource® Monthly. March 5, 2018.
12. Cost of 100 0.25-mg doses.
13. Only FDA-approved for concomitant use with a long-term controller medication in the treatment of asthma.

Continued on next page

Table 3. Some Drugs for Asthma (continued)	
Drug	**Some Available Formulations**
Inhaled Corticosteroid/Long-Acting Beta$_2$-Agonist Combinations	
Budesonide/formoterol –	
Symbicort (AstraZeneca)	HFA MDI (60, 120 inh/unit) 80, 160 mcg/4.5 mcg/inh
Fluticasone furoate/vilanterol – *Breo Ellipta* (GSK)	DPI (30 inh/unit) 100, 200 mcg/25 mcg/inh
Fluticasone propionate/salmeterol –	
Advair Diskus (GSK)	DPI (60 inh/unit) 100, 250, 500 mcg/50 mcg/blister[14]
Advair HFA (GSK)	HFA MDI (60, 120 inh/unit) 45, 115, 230 mcg/21 mcg/inh
AirDuo Respiclick (Teva) generic	DPI (60 inh/unit) 55, 113, 232 mcg/14 mcg/inh
Mometasone/formoterol –	
Dulera (Merck)	HFA MDI (60, 120 inh/unit) 100, 200 mcg/5 mcg/inh
Inhaled Long-Acting Muscarinic Antagonist (LAMA)	
Tiotropium – *Spiriva Respimat* (Boehringer Ingelheim)	ISI (60 inh/unit) 1.25 mcg/inh
Leukotriene Modifiers[15]	
Montelukast – generic *Singulair* (Merck)	10 mg tabs; 4, 5 mg chew tabs; 4 mg oral granules
Zafirlukast – generic *Accolate* (AstraZeneca)	10, 20 mg tabs
Zileuton – *Zyflo* (Chiesi)	600 mg tabs
extended-release –	
generic *Zyflo CR* (Chiesi)	600 mg ER tabs
Anti-IgE Antibody	
Omalizumab – *Xolair* (Genentech)	Powder for injection 150 mg/5 mL vial

14. Only the 100 mcg/50 mcg formulation is approved for use in children.
15. Montelukast is taken once daily in the evening, with or without food. Montelukast granules must be taken within 15 minutes of opening the packet. Zafirlukast is taken 1 hour before or 2 hours after a meal. Zileuton is taken within one hour after morning and evening meals.
16. For exercise-induced broncoconstriction (EIB), dose is one 10-mg tab for patients ≥15 years old and one 5-mg chewable tab for children 6-14 years old, taken at least 2 hours before exercise.

Usual Adult Dosage	Usual Pediatric Dosage	Cost[1]
2 inh bid	6-11 yrs: 2 inh (80/4.5 mcg) bid	$270.00
1 inh once/d	--	321.70
1 inh bid	4-11 yrs: 1 inh (100/50 mcg)[14] bid	290.90
2 inh bid	≥12 yrs: 2 inh bid	290.90
1 inh bid	≥12 yrs: 1 inh bid	285.00 90.00
2 inh bid	≥12 yrs: 2 inh bid	290.60
2 inh once/d	≥6 yrs: 2 inh once/d	368.20
10 mg PO once/d[16]	≥1 yr: 4 or 5 mg PO once/d[16,17]	11.20 228.30
20 mg PO bid	5-11 yrs: 10 mg PO bid ≥12 yrs: 20 mg PO bid	99.60 227.60
600 mg PO qid	≥12 yrs: 600 mg PO qid	3580.00
1200 mg PO bid	≥12 yrs: 1200 mg PO bid	3220.30 3580.00
150-300 mg SC q4 wks or 225-375 mg SC q2 wks[18]	6-11 yrs: 75-300 mg SC q4 wks or 225-375 mg q2 wks[18]	1022.50

17. Dosage for 12-23 months: one packet of 4-mg oral granules; for 2-5 yrs: 4-mg chewable tab or one packet of 4-mg oral granules once/d; for 6-14 yrs: 5-mg chewable tab once/d.
18. Dose depends on the patient's body weight and total serum IgE level. See package insert for specific dosing instructions.

Continued on next page

Table 3. Some Drugs for Asthma (continued)	
Drug	**Some Available Formulations**
Anti-Interleukin-5 Antibodies	
Benralizumab – *Fasenra* (AstraZeneca)	30 mg/mL single-dose prefilled syringe
Mepolizumab – *Nucala* (GSK)	100 mg single-dose vials
Reslizumab – *Cinqair* (Teva)	100 mg/10 mL single-use vials
Theophylline[20]	
generic	100, 200, 300 mg ER tabs; 80 mg/15 mL oral elixir
Theo-24 (Auxilium)	100, 200, 300, 400 mg ER caps
Theochron (Caraco)	100, 200 mg ER tabs

19. Cost of a single treatment. With reslizumab, cost is for a patient weighing 70 kg (3 vials). Benralizumab cost based on published price as of March 5, 2018.
20. Extended-release formulations may not be interchangeable.

significant exacerbations by 53% compared to placebo.[28] A post-hoc analysis found that the largest reductions in exacerbations occurred in patients with high baseline eosinophil levels.[29] In a study in patients with severe oral glucocorticoid-dependent eosinophilic asthma, those treated with mepolizumab 100 mg SC every 4 weeks for 20 weeks were 2.39 times more likely than those randomized to placebo to have their oral glucocorticoid dose reduced. Treatment was also associated with a reduction in the annual asthma exacerbation rate (1.44 vs 2.12).[30]

In two randomized, placebo-controlled trials in a total of 953 patients 12-75 years old with moderate-to-severe eosinophilic asthma, **reslizumab** 3 mg/kg IV every 4 weeks significantly reduced the frequency of clinically significant asthma exacerbations by 54% compared to placebo. The mean increase from baseline in forced expiratory volume in 1 second (FEV_1) was also significantly greater among patients treated with reslizumab (110 mL vs placebo).[31] Because a post-hoc analysis of patients 12-17 years old (n=25) found that the annual asthma exacerbation rate in those treated with reslizumab was twice as high as the rate in the pla-

Usual Adult Dosage	Usual Pediatric Dosage	Cost[1]
30 mg SC q4 wks x 3, then q8 wks	≥12 yrs: 30 mg SC q4 wks x 3, then q8 wks	$4752.00[19]
100 mg SC q4 wks	≥12 yrs: 100 mg SC q4 wks	2785.10[19]
3 mg/kg IV q4 wks	--	2580.00[19]
300-600 mg once/d or divided bid	10 mg/kg/d divided bid[21] (max 300 mg/d)	16.50
300-600 mg once/d[22]		99.60
300-600 mg once/d		17.30

21. Starting dose. Usual maximum dose is 16 mg/kg/day (max 600 mg/day) in children >1 year old; in infants 0.2 x (age in weeks) + 5 = dose in mg/kg/day.
22. If *Theo-24* is taken <1 hr before a meal, the entire 24-hour dose can be released in a 4-hour period.

cebo group (2.86 vs 1.37), reslizumab is FDA-approved for use only in patients ≥18 years old.

Benralizumab, an anti-IL-5 receptor alpha monoclonal antibody,[47] is administered subcutaneously once every 4 weeks for the first 3 doses, then every 8 weeks. It significantly reduced annual asthma exacerbation rates by 28-51% in two randomized, double-blind, placebo-controlled trials in >1000 patients 12-75 years old with severe asthma and blood eosinophil counts ≥300 cells/mL.[32,33] In another randomized trial in 220 adults with severe eosinophilic asthma, use of benralizumab reduced oral glucocorticoid doses by 75% compared to a reduction of 25% with placebo, a statistically significant difference.[34]

Adverse Effects – The most common adverse effects of mepolizumab have been injection-site reactions, headache, back pain, and fatigue. Reslizumab has been associated with oropharyngeal pain, creatine phosphokinase elevations, myalgia, and, rarely, malignancies. Adverse effects that occurred more often with benralizumab than with placebo in clinical trials included headache, pyrexia, and pharyngitis. Hypersensitivity reactions have occurred with all three drugs; the reslizumab package insert includes a boxed warning about a risk of anaphylaxis.

BRONCHIAL THERMOPLASTY — Approved by the FDA for use in adults with severe persistent asthma not well controlled on an ICS and a LABA, bronchial thermoplasty leads to modest improvements in respiratory symptoms and exacerbation rates,[35] which can last for up to 5 years.[36] The long-term efficacy and safety of the procedure are unknown.

Patients undergo fiberoptic bronchoscopy on 3 separate occasions 3 weeks apart. During the procedure, the airway walls are treated with radiofrequency energy that is converted to heat (target tissue temperature 65°C), resulting in ablation of airway smooth muscle. Adverse effects, mainly transient worsening of asthma, are common in the weeks immediately following bronchial thermoplasty.

AZITHROMYCIN — In a 48-week, randomized, placebo-controlled, parallel group trial in 420 patients with symptomatic asthma despite treatment with an ICS and a LABA, treatment with azithromycin 500 mg three times per week resulted in fewer asthma exacerbations compared to placebo. Diarrhea was common in azithromycin-treated patients and antimicrobial resistance is a concern.[37] More data on the effects of long-term treatment with azithromycin are needed.

EXERCISE-INDUCED BRONCHOCONSTRICTION — Exercise-induced bronchoconstriction (EIB) may be the only manifestation of asthma in patients with mild disease. EIB may also be a transient phenomenon in non-asthmatic athletes.[38] SABAs used just before exercise will prevent EIB for 2-4 hours after inhalation in most patients. Daily use of these drugs may lead to a reduction in the duration of protection. Montelukast can decrease EIB within 2 hours after administration; the protection may last for up to 24 hours and does not wane with repeated use. In patients who continue to have symptoms despite use of a SABA before exercise or who require daily use of a SABA, possibly because of poorly-controlled persistent asthma, daily anti-inflammatory medications should be started or increased in dosage. ICSs are the most effective anti-inflammatory agents for EIB.[3]

PREGNANCY — Poorly controlled asthma increases the risk of pregnancy-related complications including pre-eclampsia, perinatal mortality, preterm birth, and low birth weight.[39]

Albuterol is the preferred SABA for use in pregnancy. ICSs (budesonide and fluticasone are the best studied) are the preferred long-term controller medications during pregnancy; they do not appear to have any effects on fetal adrenal function.[40-42] In a cohort study of 13,280 pregnancies, the incidence of major congenital malformations was increased with use of higher ICS doses (>1000 mcg/day beclomethasone equivalent) during the first trimester in women with more severe or uncontrolled asthma, but not with low-to-moderate doses of ICSs.[43] LABAs (used with ICSs) and montelukast appear to be safe for use during pregnancy.[44,45] Teratogenicity in animals has been reported with zileuton.

Allergen immunotherapy (without dose escalation) can be continued in pregnancy. Omalizumab appears to be safe for use during pregnancy. There are no adequate studies of mepolizumab or reslizumab in pregnant women; there was no evidence of fetal harm in animal studies. The passage of monoclonal antibodies across the placenta increases linearly as pregnancy progresses.

1. JL McCracken et al. Diagnosis and management of asthma in adults: a review. JAMA 2017; 318:279.
2. KR Jat and A Khairwa. Levalbuterol versus albuterol for acute asthma: a systematic review and meta-analysis. Pulm Pharmacol Ther 2013; 26:239.
3. JP Parsons et al. An official American Thoracic Society clinical practice guideline: exercise-induced bronchoconstriction. Am J Respir Crit Care Med 2013; 187:1016.
4. MA Rank et al. The risk of asthma exacerbation after stopping low-dose inhaled corticosteroids: a systematic review and meta-analysis of randomized controlled trials. J Allergy Clin Immunol 2013; 131:724.
5. JK Mukker et al. Ciclesonide: a pro-soft drug approach for mitigation of side effects of inhaled corticosteroids. J Pharm Sci 2016; 105:2509.

6. HW Kelly et al. Effect of inhaled glucocorticoids in childhood on adult height. N Engl J Med 2012; 367:904.
7. AL Fuhlbrigge and HW Kelly. Inhaled corticosteroids in children: effects on bone mineral density and growth. Lancet Respir Med 2014; 2:487.
8. PM O'Byrne et al. Risks of pneumonia in patients with asthma taking inhaled corticosteroids. Am J Respir Crit Care Med 2011; 183:589.
9. DA Stempel et al. Serious asthma events with fluticasone plus salmeterol versus fluticasone alone. N Engl J Med 2016; 374:1822.
10. SP Peters et al. Serious asthma events with budesonide plus formoterol vs. budesonide alone. N Engl J Med 2016; 375:850.
11. DA Stempel et al. Safety of adding salmeterol to fluticasone propionate in children with asthma. N Engl J Med 2016; 375:840.
12. D Radovanovic et al. The evidence on tiotropium bromide in asthma: from the rationale to the bedside. Multidiscip Respir Med 2017; 12:12.
13. KM Kew and K Dahri. Long-acting muscarinic antagonists (LAMA) added to combination long-acting beta2-agonists and inhaled corticosteroids (LABA/ICS) versus LABA/ICS for adults with asthma. Cochrane Database Syst Rev 2016; 1:CD011721.
14. LA Lee et al. The effect of fluticasone furoate/umeclidinium in adult patients with asthma: a randomized, dose-ranging study. Respir Med 2015; 109:54.
15. TE Albertson et al. Muscarinic antagonists in early stage clinical development for the treatment of asthma. Expert Opin Investig Drugs 2017; 26:35.
16. HA Kerstjens et al. Tiotropium for the treatment of asthma: a drug safety evaluation. Expert Opin Drug Saf 2016; 15:1115.
17. G Calapai et al. Montelukast-induced adverse drug reactions: a review of case reports in the literature. Pharmacology 2014; 94:60.
18. Global Initiative for Asthma. Global strategy for asthma management and prevention, 2017. Available at: http://ginasthma.org/2017-gina-report-global-strategy-for-asthma-management-and-prevention. Accessed August 17, 2017.
19. SK Medrek et al. Fungal sensitization is associated with increased risk of life-threatening asthma. J Allergy Clin Immunol Pract 2017; 5:1025.
20. KF Chung et al. International ERS/ATS guidelines on definition, evaluation, and treatment of severe asthma. Eur Respir J 2014; 43:343.
21. MA Calderón et al. Allergen-specific immunotherapy for respiratory allergies: from meta-analysis to registration and beyond. J Allergy Clin Immunol 2011; 127:30.
22. GJ Rodrigo et al. Efficacy and safety of subcutaneous omalizumab vs placebo as add-on therapy to corticosteroids for children and adults with asthma: a systematic review. Chest 2011; 139:28.
23. NA Hanania et al. Omalizumab in severe allergic asthma inadequately controlled with standard therapy: a randomized trial. Ann Intern Med 2011; 154:573.
24. BE Chipps et al. Omalizumab in children with uncontrolled allergic asthma: review of clinical trial and real-world experience. J Allergy Clin Immunol 2017; 139:1431.
25. L Cox et al. American Academy of Allergy, Asthma & Immunology/American College of Allergy, Asthma & Immunology Omalizumab-Associated Anaphylaxis Joint Task Force follow-up report. J Allergy Clin Immunol 2011; 128:210.
26. Mepolizumab (Nucala) for severe eosinophilic asthma. Med Lett Drugs Ther 2016; 58:11.

27. Reslizumab (Cinqair) for severe eosinophilic asthma. Med Lett Drugs Ther 2016; 58:81.
28. HG Ortega et al. Mepolizumab treatment in patients with severe eosinophilic asthma. N Engl J Med 2014; 371:1198.
29. HG Ortega et al. Severe eosinophilic asthma treated with mepolizumab stratified by baseline eosinophilic thresholds: a secondary analysis of the DREAM and MENSA studies. Lancet Respir Med 2016; 4:549.
30. EH Bel et al. Oral glucocorticoid-sparing effect of mepolizumab in eosinophilic asthma. N Engl J Med 2014; 371:1189.
31. M Castro et al. Reslizumab for inadequately controlled asthma with elevated blood eosinophil counts: results from two multicentre, parallel, double-blind, randomised, placebo-controlled, phase 3 trials. Lancet Respir Med 2015; 3:355.
32. ER Bleecker et al. Efficacy and safety of benralizumab for patients with severe asthma uncontrolled with high-dosage inhaled corticosteroids and long-acting β2-agonists (SIROCCO): a randomised, multicentre, placebo-controlled phase 3 trial. Lancet 2016; 388:2115.
33. JM FitzGerald et al. Benralizumab, an anti-interleukin-5 receptor α monoclonal antibody, as add-on treatment for patients with severe, uncontrolled, eosinophilic asthma (CALIMA): a randomised, double-blind, placebo-controlled phase 3 trial. Lancet 2016; 388:2128.
34. P Nair et al. Oral glucocorticoid-sparing effect of benralizumab in severe asthma. N Engl J Med 2017; 376:2448.
35. M Pretolani et al. Effectiveness of bronchial thermoplasty in patients with severe refractory asthma: clinical and histopathologic correlations. J Allergy Clin Immunol 2017; 139:1176.
36. A Trivedi et al. Bronchial thermoplasty and biological therapy as targeted treatments for severe uncontrolled asthma. Lancet Respir Med 2016; 4:585.
37. PG Gibson et al. Effect of azithromycin on asthma exacerbations and quality of life in adults with persistent uncontrolled asthma (AMAZES): a randomised, double-blind, placebo-controlled trial. Lancet 2017 July 4 (epub).
38. V Bougault et al. Airway hyperresponsiveness in elite swimmers: is it a transient phenomenon? J Allergy Clin Immunol 2011; 127:892.
39. JA Namazy and M Schatz. Pharmacological difficulties in the treatment of asthma in pregnant women. Expert Rev Clin Pharmacol 2017; 10:285.
40. NA Hodyl et al. Fetal glucocorticoid-regulated pathways are not affected by inhaled corticosteroid use for asthma during pregnancy. Am J Respir Crit Care Med 2011; 183:716.
41. B Cossette et al. Relative perinatal safety of salmeterol vs formoterol and fluticasone vs budesonide use during pregnancy. Ann Allergy Asthma Immunol 2014; 112:459.
42. RA Charlton et al. Safety of fluticasone propionate prescribed for asthma during pregnancy: a UK population-based cohort study. J Allergy Clin Immunol Pract 2015; 3:772.
43. L Blais et al. High doses of inhaled corticosteroids during the first trimester of pregnancy and congenital malformations. J Allergy Clin Immunol 2009; 124:1229.
44. LN Bakhireva et al. Safety of leukotriene receptor antagonists in pregnancy. J Allergy Clin Immunol 2007; 119:618.
45. B Cossette et al. Impact of maternal use of asthma-controller therapy on perinatal outcomes. Thorax 2013; 68:724.

46. FDA Drug Safety Communication: FDA review finds no significant increase in risk of serious asthma outcomes with long-acting beta agonists (LABAs) used in combination with inhaled corticosteroids (ICS). December 20, 2017. Available at: www.fda.gov/Drugs/DrugSafety/ucm589587.htm. Accessed March 20, 2018.
47. Benralizumab (Fasenra) for severe eosinophilic asthma. Med Lett Drugs Ther 2018; 60:33.

DRUGS FOR Common Bacterial Infections in Adults

Original publication date – October 2017 (revised March 2018)

Bacterial infections in adults are generally treated empirically, with the antibiotic covering most, but not all, of the potential causative pathogens. For some infections, culture and sensitivity testing can guide treatment, allowing for use of narrower-spectrum antibiotics. The recommended dosages and durations of antibiotic treatment for common respiratory, skin, and urinary tract infections are listed in Tables 1-3. Infectious disease experts now recommend shorter treatment durations for many infections to reduce the development of antimicrobial resistance and minimize adverse effects.

RESPIRATORY TRACT INFECTIONS

ACUTE PHARYNGITIS — Most cases of acute pharyngitis in adults are caused by viruses, such as influenza, Epstein-Barr, or rhinovirus, and should not be treated with antibiotics. Group A *Streptococcus* is the causative pathogen in 5-15% of adult cases. Other possible pathogens include group C and group G *Streptococcus*, *Fusobacterium necrophorum*, and *Neisseria gonorrhoeae*.

Diagnosis of group A *Streptococcus* pharyngitis in adults should be made using a rapid antigen detection test; throat culture can be performed if the rapid test is negative and the clinical presentation strongly suggests bacterial infection. Patients with a positive rapid test should be treated with

Table 1. Empiric Treatment of Respiratory Tract Infections in Adults

Type of Infection (Suspected Pathogens)	Regimen(s) of Choice[1]
Pharyngitis[2,3] (Group A *Streptococcus*)	Penicillin VK 250 mg PO qid or 500 mg PO bid x 10 days Amoxicillin 500 mg PO bid x 10 days Penicillin G benzathine 1.2 million units IM x 1 dose
Sinusitis[2] (*Streptococcus pneumoniae, Haemophilus influenzae, Moraxella catarrhalis*)	Amoxicillin/clavulanate 875/125 mg PO bid x 5-7 days[7,8]
Bronchitis (AECB)[2] (*Streptococcus pneumoniae, Haemophilus influenzae, Moraxella catarrhalis*)	Amoxicillin/clavulanate 875/125 mg PO bid x 5-7 days[7,8]
Community-Acquired Pneumonia (*Streptococcus pneumoniae, Mycoplasma pneumoniae*[12])	
Outpatient[13]	Doxycycline 100 mg PO bid[14] x ≥5 days[15] Amoxicillin 1 g tid or amoxicillin/clavulanate 2 g bid x ≥5 days[15,16] **plus** azithromycin 500 mg PO x 1, then 250 mg once/d x 4 d (or 500 mg once/d x 3 days)[17] Levofloxacin 750 mg PO once/d x ≥5 days[15] Moxifloxacin 400 mg PO once/d x ≥5 days[15]

AECB = Acute exacerbation of chronic bronchitis

1. Usual adult dosage. Dosage adjustments may be needed for renal or hepatic impairment.
2. Most cases of pharyngitis, sinusitis, and bronchitis are viral and should not be treated with antibiotics.
3. Fluoroquinolones, tetracyclines, and trimethoprim/sulfamethoxazole should not be used.
4. For patients with non-anaphylactic penicillin allergy.
5. Other oral cephalosporins such as cefdinir or cefpodoxime are also effective, but their broader spectrum of activity is unnecessary for treatment of group A *Streptococcus* pharyngitis and they are generally more expensive.
6. For patients with severe beta-lactam allergy. Group A *Streptococcus* may be resistant to macrolides and clindamycin.
7. 500 mg/125 mg tid is an alternative.
8. High-dose amoxicillin/clavulanate (two 1000/62.5 mg extended-release tablets bid) should be considered for patients with severe disease and for those at risk of infection with *Streptococcus pneumoniae* with reduced susceptibility to penicillin.
9. For patients who are allergic to penicillin.
10. 200 mg once/d is an alternative.
11. Only for patients who lack other treatment options. The FDA has warned that the risk of serious adverse effects with fluoroquinolones outweighs their benefits for treatment of uncomplicated infections such as sinusitis, bronchitis, and acute cystitis.

Some Alternative Regimens[1]
Cefadroxil 1 g PO once/d x 10 days[4,5] Cephalexin 500 mg PO bid x 10 days[4,5] Clindamycin 300 mg PO tid x 10 days[6] Azithromycin 500 mg PO x 1, then 250 mg once/d x 4 days[6] Clarithromycin 250 mg PO bid x 10 days[6,17a]
Cefpodoxime 200 mg PO bid x 5-7 days[4] Doxycycline 100 mg PO bid x 5-7 days[9,10] Levofloxacin 500 mg PO once/d x 5-7 days[11] Moxifloxacin 400 mg PO once/d x 5-7 days[11]
Cefpodoxime 200 mg PO bid x 5-7 days[4] Doxycycline 100 mg PO bid x 5-7 days[9,10] Levofloxacin 500 mg PO once/d x 5-7 days[11] Moxifloxacin 400 mg PO once/d x 5-7 days[11]

12. Other possible pathogens include *Staphylococcus aureus, Haemophilus influenzae, Chlamydia pneumoniae, Moraxella catarrhalis, Legionella spp.*, and anaerobic mouth organisms.
13. Monotherapy with a macrolide such as azithromycin has been a regimen of choice for treatment of community-acquired pneumonia (CAP) in otherwise healthy adults without recent antibiotic exposure. While a macrolide would be effective for treatment of CAP caused by atypical pathogens or *Haemophilus influenzae*, the rate of macrolide-resistant *Streptococcus pneumoniae* in the US is >40% and use of macrolide monotherapy for empiric treatment of CAP could result in treatment failure in patients with pneumococcal infection.
14. For patients without comorbidities or recent antibiotic exposure. Should not be used for empiric treatment in areas where the rate of doxycycline-resistant *Streptococcus pneumoniae* is ≥25% or in pregnant women.
15. Patient should be clinically stable and afebrile for 48-72 hours before stopping therapy.
16. Alternatives include ceftriaxone, cefpodoxime, and cefuroxime (500 mg bid).
17. Clarithromycin 500 mg PO bid (or clarithromycin ER 1000 mg PO once/day) is an alternative. Clarithromycin may increase the risk of cardiac adverse effects and death in patients with coronary artery disease (FDA Drug Safety Communication, February 2018). Doxycycline 100 mg PO bid can be used instead of a macrolide.

17a. Clarithromycin may increase the risk of cardiac adverse effects and death in patients with coronary artery disease (FDA Drug Safety Communication, February 2018).

Continued on next page

Table 1. Empiric Treatment of Respiratory Tract Infections in Adults (continued)

Type of Infection (Suspected Pathogens)	Regimen(s) of Choice[1]
Community-Acquired Pneumonia (continued)	
Hospitalized (not ICU)[18]	Ceftriaxone 1-2 g IV once/d or cefotaxime 1-2 g IV q8h or ceftaroline 600 mg IV q12h or ampicillin/sulbactam 3 g IV q8h **plus** azithromycin[17] 500 mg IV or PO once/d x ≥5 days[15]
	Levofloxacin 750 mg IV or PO once/d x ≥5 days[15]
	Moxifloxacin 400 mg IV or PO once/d x ≥5 days[15]

18. In severe cases, empiric treatment of MRSA is recommended. Vancomycin or linezolid can be added to a recommended regimen.

a 10-day course of penicillin.[1] Clindamycin or a macrolide can be used in patients with severe penicillin allergy, but pharyngeal isolates of group A *Streptococcus* may be resistant to these drugs.[2] Fluoroquinolones, tetracyclines, and trimethoprim/sulfamethoxazole should not be used for treatment of streptococcal pharyngitis.

SINUSITIS — Acute sinusitis in adults is often viral and generally should not be treated with antibiotics; symptoms can be managed with analgesics, a nasal corticosteroid, and/or nasal saline irrigation. Acute bacterial sinusitis is usually caused by *Streptococcus pneumoniae* (pneumococcus), *Haemophilus influenzae*, or *Moraxella catarrhalis*. Otherwise healthy patients with acute bacterial sinusitis often improve within 10 days without antibiotic therapy.[3,4] Antibiotic treatment can be considered for patients who present with severe symptoms or high fever. Amoxicillin/clavulanate is the drug of choice[5]; addition of clavulanate to amoxicillin improves its coverage of beta-lactamase-producing organisms. Doxycycline is an option for adults who are allergic to penicillin, but resistance to doxycycline has increased, par-

Some Alternative Regimens[1]
Ertapenem 1 g IV once/d **plus** azithromycin[17] 500 mg IV or PO once/d x ≥5 days[15]

ticularly among isolates of *S. pneumoniae* with reduced susceptibility to penicillin.[3-5]

A respiratory fluoroquinolone (levofloxacin or moxifloxacin) has been used in penicillin-allergic patients, but the FDA recently required changes in the labeling of systemic fluoroquinolones to warn that their risk of rare but serious adverse effects, including tendinitis and tendon rupture, peripheral neuropathy, and CNS effects, generally outweighs their benefits for treatment of uncomplicated infections such as acute sinusitis. They should be considered only for patients who lack other treatment options.[6]

Macrolides and trimethoprim/sulfamethoxazole are not recommended for treatment of acute sinusitis because of increasing resistance among pneumococci.

BRONCHITIS — Acute bronchitis in otherwise healthy adults is usually viral. Symptoms are self-limited and routine use of antibiotics is not recommended. Acute exacerbations of chronic bronchitis (AECB) are also often viral in origin, but moderate to severe exacerbations in patients with COPD are usually treated with antibacterial drugs. Like sinusitis, bacterial AECB are often caused by *S. pneumoniae*, *H. influenzae*, or *M. catarrhalis* and treated with amoxicillin/clavulanate. Doxycycline can be considered for adults who are allergic to penicillin. Because of the risk of serious adverse effects, fluoroquinolones should be reserved for patients who lack other treatment options.[6]

COMMUNITY-ACQUIRED PNEUMONIA — The organisms responsible for community-acquired bacterial pneumonia (CAP) are usually not confirmed, but *S. pneumoniae* and *Mycoplasma pneumoniae* are common pathogens. Among hospitalized patients with CAP, *S. pneumoniae* is probably the most common. Other causative pathogens include *Staphylococcus aureus*, *H. influenzae, M. catarrhalis*, *Legionella* spp., and anaerobic mouth organisms.

Monotherapy with a macrolide such as azithromycin has been a regimen of choice for treatment of CAP in otherwise healthy adults without recent antibiotic exposure. While a macrolide would be effective for treatment of CAP caused by atypical pathogens or *H. influenzae*, the rate of macrolide-resistant *S. pneumoniae* in the US is >40% and use of macrolide monotherapy for empiric treatment of CAP could result in treatment failure in patients with pneumococcal infection. Doxycycline is a reasonable alternative in areas where the pneumococcal rate of resistance to the drug is <25%.[7] A respiratory fluoroquinolone (levofloxacin or moxifloxacin) is often used for adults with comorbidities or exposure to other antibiotics during the previous 90 days. It can also be considered for use in otherwise healthy adults in areas where the rates of pneumococcal resistance to macrolides and doxycycline are ≥25%. Combining a beta-lactam (such as high-dose amoxicillin or cefpodoxime) with a macrolide or doxycycline is another alternative.[8]

Macrolides and respiratory fluoroquinolones can prolong the QT interval and rarely cause life-threatening ventricular arrhythmias; these drugs should be used with caution in patients with cardiovascular disease or risk factors for QT interval prolongation and arrhythmia.[9] Although clinical data are limited, some expert clinicians would combine doxycycline with a beta-lactam in such patients.

Update 3/7/2018: The FDA updated the labeling of clarithromycin (*Biaxin*, and others) to warn about an increased risk of adverse cardiac events and death in patients with coronary artery disease who were treated with the drug.[26]

In CAP requiring hospitalization (not ICU), empiric treatment with an IV beta-lactam (such as ceftriaxone, cefotaxime, ceftaroline, or ampicillin/sulbactam) plus a macrolide (or doxycycline) or monotherapy with a respiratory fluoroquinolone (levofloxacin or moxifloxacin) is recommended pending culture results. In severe cases, methicillin-resistant *S. aureus* (MRSA) should be considered as a possible causative pathogen and addition of vancomycin or linezolid is recommended (daptomycin should not be used for treatment of pneumonia).[8] If aspiration pneumonia is suspected, metronidazole or clindamycin should be added; ampicillin/sulbactam is a reasonable alternative.

SKIN AND SOFT TISSUE INFECTIONS

Uncomplicated skin and soft tissue infections in immunocompetent patients are most frequently caused by *S. aureus*, *Streptococcus pyogenes,* or other beta-hemolytic streptococci.

Purulent Infection – MRSA, a healthcare-associated pathogen that is now also prevalent in the community, is the predominant cause of suppurative skin and soft tissue infections in many parts of the US.[10,11] Community-associated MRSA (CA-MRSA) usually causes furunculosis, purulent cellulitis, and abscesses, but necrotizing fasciitis can also occur.

Table 2. Empiric Treatment of Skin and Soft Tissue Infections in Adults	
Type of Infection (Suspected Pathogens)	**Regimen(s) of Choice[1]**
Purulent[2]	
(MRSA, MSSA)	
Outpatient	Trimethoprim/sulfamethoxazole 1-2 DS[3] tablets PO q12h x 5 days Doxycycline 100 mg PO q12h x 5 days[4] Clindamycin 300-450 mg PO tid-qid x 5 days[5]
Hospitalized	Vancomycin 15-20 mg/kg (max 2 g) IV q8-12h x 5-14 days
Nonpurulent (cellulitis)	
(Beta-hemolytic streptococci, MSSA)[8]	
Outpatient, mild, nonsystemic symptoms	Dicloxacillin 250 mg PO q6h x 5 days[9] Cephalexin 500 mg PO q6h x 5 days[9] Cefadroxil 500 mg PO bid or 1 g PO once/d x 5 days[9]
Hospitalized, nonsevere	Penicillin 2-4 million units IV q4-6h[11] x 5-14 days Nafcillin 1-2 g IV q4-6h x 5-14 days Cefazolin 1-2 g IV q8h x 5-14 days Ceftriaxone 1-2 g IV q24h x 5-14 days

MRSA = methicillin-resistant *Staphylococcus aureus*; MSSA = methicillin-susceptible *Staphylococcus aureus*

1. Usual adult dosage. Dosage adjustments may be needed for renal or hepatic impairment.
2. Incision, drainage, and culture should be performed if possible. For small, simple abscesses, incision and drainage alone may be effective. Addition of an antibiotic can improve cure rates. Fluoroquinolones (except possibly delafloxacin) should not be used for empiric treatment of MRSA infections.
3. DS tablets contain 160 mg trimethoprim and 800 mg sulfamethoxazole.
4. Or minocycline 200 mg PO x 1, then 100 mg bid is an alternative.
5. Local rates of MRSA resistance to clindamycin can vary. Clindamycin is more likely than other empiric choices to cause *Clostridium difficile* infection.

Some Alternative Regimens[1]
Linezolid 600 mg PO q12h x 5 days Dalbavancin 1500 mg IV x 1 dose
Linezolid 600 mg IV q12h x 5-14 days[6] Daptomycin 4 mg/kg IV q24h x 5-14 days Dalbavancin 1500 mg IV x 1 dose[7] Ceftaroline fosamil 600 mg IV q12h x 5-14 days
Clindamycin 300-450 mg PO q6-8h[10] x 5 days[9] Linezolid 600 mg PO q12h[10] x 5 days[9]
Clindamycin 600-900 mg IV q8h[10] x 5-14 days Vancomycin 15-20 mg/kg (max 2 g) IV q8-12h[10] x 5-14 days

6. Tedizolid 200 mg IV is an alternative.
7. Oritavancin 1200 mg IV once and telavancin 10 mg/kg IV q24h are alternatives.
8. If erysipelas (clear demarcation, raised area of infection) is strongly suspected, treatment for streptococcal infection with penicillin VK or amoxicillin is an alternative. MRSA is also a potential pathogen, but adding MRSA coverage does not appear to increase cure rates (GJ Moran et al. JAMA 2017; 317:2088).
9. A longer duration may be needed for severe or slow-responding infections.
10. For patients with severe beta-lactam allergy.
11. If infection with group A *Streptococcus* is known or erysipelas (clear demarcation, raised area of infection) is strongly suspected. Not for treatment of *Staphylococcus aureus* infection.

Unlike healthcare-associated strains, which are often resistant, CA-MRSA strains have generally been susceptible to trimethoprim/sulfamethoxazole, tetracyclines, and clindamycin (local clindamycin resistance rates vary). Both types of MRSA strains are susceptible *in vitro* to vancomycin, daptomycin, and linezolid. Resistance to fluoroquinolones is common and is increasing in both healthcare and community settings.

For small abscesses typically caused by *S. aureus*, incision and drainage alone may be sufficient. Addition of oral trimethoprim/sulfamethoxazole, clindamycin, or doxycycline can improve abscess cure rates.[12,13] Linezolid is an alternative for oral treatment. Fluoroquinolones (except possibly delafloxacin) should not be used empirically to treat skin and soft tissue infections.[14,15]

Purulent skin and soft tissue infections requiring hospitalization are usually treated empirically with IV vancomycin. Some alternatives include linezolid, daptomycin, ceftaroline fosamil, and dalbavancin.[16-19]

Nonpurulent Infection – Nonpurulent skin and soft tissue infections (cellulitis, erysipelas) are usually caused by *S. pyogenes* and *S. aureus*. Empiric coverage of MRSA does not appear to improve cure rates.[20] Mild infection can be treated with an oral penicillin or first-generation cephalosporin. Clindamycin is an alternative for patients with severe beta-lactam allergy. Doxycycline should not be used for treatment of streptococcal skin infections. Patients hospitalized for nonpurulent skin and soft tissue infections can usually be treated empirically with IV penicillin, cefazolin, or ceftriaxone.[21] Vancomycin or clindamycin can be used in patients with severe beta-lactam allergy.

Group A *Streptococcus, S. aureus,* or *Clostridium* spp., with or without other anaerobes, can cause fulminant soft tissue infections and necrosis, particularly in patients with diabetes. If such infections are suspected, rapid treatment with clindamycin plus a penicillin is recommended. In severely ill patients, vancomycin, linezolid, or daptomycin should be added until MRSA is ruled out. Surgical debridement is essential to the management of necrotizing skin and soft tissue infections.

URINARY TRACT INFECTIONS

ACUTE UNCOMPLICATED CYSTITIS — Most episodes of acute uncomplicated cystitis are caused by *Escherichia coli*. The remaining cases are generally caused by *Staphylococcus saprophyticus*, *Klebsiella pneumoniae*, *Proteus* spp., other gram-negative rods, or enterococci. Asymptomatic bacteriuria and pyuria in nonpregnant women should generally not be treated with antibiotics.[22]

Trimethoprim/sulfamethoxazole is a drug of choice for empiric treatment of acute uncomplicated cystitis in nonpregnant women, as long as the local rate of resistance to it among urinary pathogens is <20%. Nitrofurantoin is an equally effective alternative with a low rate of resistance among *E. coli*. A single dose of fosfomycin, which has a broad spectrum of activity against the usual uropathogens, is another first-line alternative. Beta-lactams such as amoxicillin/clavulanate, cefdinir, cefpodoxime, or ceftibuten are second-line options.[23]

Fluoroquinolones (especially ciprofloxacin) have been the most common class of antibiotics prescribed for urinary tract infections, but they should no longer be used for empiric treatment, unless no other treatment options exist.[24] In 2016, the FDA required changes in the labeling of systemic fluoroquinolones to warn that their risk of serious adverse effects, including tendinitis and tendon rupture, peripheral neuropathy and CNS effects, generally outweighs their benefits for treatment of uncomplicated infections such as acute cystitis.[6]

Based on the results of sensitivity testing, nitrofurantoin, amoxicillin, or a cephalosporin could be used to treat uncomplicated cystitis in pregnant women, but nitrofurantoin should not be given in the third trimester or during labor because it can cause hemolytic anemia in the newborn.

Table 3. Empiric Treatment of Urinary Tract Infections in Adults

Type of Infection (Suspected Pathogens)	Regimen(s) of Choice[1]
Acute Uncomplicated Cystitis[2]	
(Escherichia coli, Staphylococcus saprophyticus, Klebsiella pneumoniae, Proteus spp.)	Trimethoprim/sulfamethoxazole 1 DS tablet PO bid x 3 days[3,4] Nitrofurantoin monohydrate/macrocrystals 100 mg PO bid x 5 days[5] Fosfomycin tromethamine 3 g PO once
Acute Pyelonephritis	
(same as acute cystitis)	
Outpatient	Ciprofloxacin 500 mg PO bid or 1000 mg extended-release once/d x 7 days[6] Levofloxacin 750 mg once/d x 5-7 days[6]

1. Usual adult dosage. Dosage adjustments may be needed for renal or hepatic impairment.
2. In women. Fluoroquinolones should not be used as first-line (or primary alternative) agents for empiric treatment of acute uncomplicated cystitis. Other drugs are preferred due to concerns over emerging resistance, adverse effects, and cost effectiveness.
3. As long as the local rate of resistance among urinary pathogens is <20%.
4. DS tablets contain 160 mg trimethoprim and 800 mg sulfamethoxazole.
5. Contraindicated in patients with a CrCl ≤60 mL/min according to the manufacturer. Short-term use for cystitis in patients with a CrCl ≥30 mL/min is probably safe.
6. If the local rate of resistance among uropathogens is <10%. Starting treatment with a single IV dose of ciprofloxacin 400 mg or ceftriaxone 1 g should be considered. If fluoroquinolone resistance is thought to be >10%, IV ceftriaxone or an aminoglycoside (5-7 mg/kg of gentamicin or tobramycin) can be used pending culture results.

ACUTE PYELONEPHRITIS — Increasing rates of resistance of *E. coli* to fluoroquinolones has made acute pyelonephritis more difficult to treat with oral therapy. In areas where the prevalence of resistance to fluoroquinolones among uropathogens is <10%, ciprofloxacin or levofloxacin can be used for empiric outpatient treatment of nonpregnant women or men with acute uncomplicated pyelonephritis. Trimethoprim/sulfamethoxazole is an alternative for treatment of susceptible uropatho-

Alternative Regimens[1]
Amoxicillin/clavulanate 500/125 mg PO q12h x 3-7 days Cefdinir 300 mg PO bid x 3-7 days Cefpodoxime 100 mg PO q12h x 3-7 days
Trimethoprim/sulfamethoxazole 1 DS tablet PO bid x 7-10 days[4,7] Amoxicillin/clavulanate 500/125 mg PO q12h x 7-10 days[8] Cefdinir 300 mg PO bid x 7-10 days[8] Cefpodoxime 100 mg PO q12h x 7-10 days[8]

7. If the pathogen is known to be susceptible. If used empirically, starting treatment with a single IV dose of ceftriaxone 1 g or an aminoglycoside (5-7 mg/kg of gentamicin or tobramycin) should be considered. IV aztreonam is another alternative.
8. Beta-lactams are generally considered to be less effective than fluoroquinolones or trimethoprim/sulfamethoxazole for empiric treatment. Nitrofurantoin and fosfomycin should not be used to treat pyelonephritis.

gens. Another alternative is a single IV dose of the third-generation cephalosporin ceftriaxone, followed by 7-14 days of an oral antimicrobial to which the pathogen is susceptible. Oral beta-lactams are generally considered less effective for treatment of pyelonephritis than fluoroquinolones or trimethoprim/sulfamethoxazole.[25] Nitrofurantoin and fosfomycin do not achieve therapeutic concentrations in the kidney and should not be used for treatment of pyelonephritis.[23]

Table 4. Adverse Effects and Toxicity in Pregnancy of Some Antibacterial Drugs[1]

AZITHROMYCIN *(Zithromax)*

Occasional: GI disturbance; headache; dizziness; vaginitis
Rare: QT interval prolongation; torsades de pointes; angioedema; cholestatic jaundice; photosensitivity; reversible dose-related hearing loss; CDI
Toxicity in Pregnancy: none known[2]

CARBAPENEMS[3]

Occasional: phlebitis; pain at injection site; fever; urticaria; rash; pruritus; GI disturbance and transient hypotension during intravenous infusion
Rare: seizures (primarily with imipenem); CDI
Toxicity in Pregnancy: Meropenem and doripenem: unknown, no studies in pregnant women; ertapenem: decreased weight in animals; imipenem/cilastatin: toxic in some pregnant animals, use only for strong clinical indication in absence of a suitable alternative

CEPHALOSPORINS[4]

Frequent: thrombophlebitis with IV use; serum-sickness-like reaction with prolonged parenteral administration; moderate to severe diarrhea, especially with cefixime
Occasional: hypersensitivity reactions, rarely anaphylactic; pain at injection site; GI disturbance; rash; hypoprothrombinemia, hemorrhage with cefotetan; rash and arthritis ("serum-sickness") with cefaclor or cefprozil, especially in children; cholelithiasis with ceftriaxone; vaginal candidiasis (especially with cefdinir); CDI
Rare: hemolytic anemia; hematologic abnormalities; hepatic dysfunction; renal damage; acute interstitial nephritis; seizures; encephalopathy; toxic epidermal necrolysis
Toxicity in Pregnancy: none known

CDI = *Clostridium difficile* infection

1. Adverse effects of antimicrobial drugs vary with dosage, duration of administration, concomitant therapy, renal and hepatic function, immune competence, and the age of the patient. The adverse effects of some antibacterial drugs are listed in the table. The designation of adverse effects as "frequent," "occasional," or "rare" is based on published reports and on the experience of Medical Letter reviewers.
2. In a nested, case-control study, after adjustment for potential confounders, use during early pregnancy was associated with an increased risk of spontaneous abortion (PT Muanda et al. CMAJ 2017; 189:E625).
3. Doripenem *(Doribax)*, ertapenem *(Invanz)*, imipenem/cilastatin *(Primaxin)*, and meropenem *(Merrem)*.
4. Cefaclor *(Raniclor)*, cefadroxil *(Duricef)*, cefazolin *(Ancef*, others), cefdinir *(Omnicef)*, cefditoren *(Spectracef)*, cefepime *(Maxipime)*, cefixime *(Suprax)*, cefoperazone *(Cefobid)*, cefotaxime *(Claforan)*, cefotetan *(Cefotan)*, cefoxitin *(Mefoxin)*, cefpodoxime *(Vantin)*, cefprozil *(Cefzil)*, ceftaroline fosamil, *(Teflaro)*, ceftazidime *(Fortaz)*, ceftazidime/avibactam *(Avycaz)*, ceftibuten *(Cedax)*, ceftizoxime *(Cefizox)*, ceftolozane/tazobactam *(Zerbaxa)*, ceftriaxone *(Rocephin)*, cefuroxime *(Zinacef)*, cefuroxime axetil *(Ceftin)*, cephalexin *(Keflex)*. Experience with newer agents is limited.

Continued on next page

Table 4. Adverse Effects and Toxicity in Pregnancy of Some Antibacterial Drugs[1] (continued)

CLARITHROMYCIN *(Biaxin)*

Occasional: GI disturbance; abnormal taste; headache; dizziness; QT interval prolongation

Rare: reversible dose-related hearing loss; pancreatitis; torsades de pointes; psychotic disturbance (mania); CDI

Toxicity in Pregnancy: teratogenic in animals[2]; contraindicated

CLINDAMYCIN *(Cleocin)*

Frequent: diarrhea; hypersensitivity reactions

Occasional: CDI

Rare: hematologic abnormalities; esophageal ulceration; hepatotoxicity; polyarthritis

Toxicity in Pregnancy: none known; no studies on use during first trimester; use only for strong clinical indication in absence of a suitable alternative

DALBAVANCIN *(Dalvance)*

Frequent: nausea; diarrhea; headache; constipation

Occasional: rash; pruritus

Rare: infusion-related reactions ("red man" syndrome); hypersensitivity reactions; increased aminotransferases; hypokalemia; hypotension; CDI

Toxicity in Pregnancy: delayed fetal maturation; embryolethality, and increased death of offspring 1 week postpartum; use only for strong clinical indication in absence of a suitable alternative

DAPTOMYCIN *(Cubicin)*

Occasional: GI disturbance; rash; injection site reaction; fever; headache; insomnia; dizziness

Rare: increased creatine phosphokinase and rhabdomyolysis; eosinophilic pneumonia; peripheral neuropathy; hypersensitivity reactions; CDI

Toxicity in Pregnancy: none known; limited data in pregnant women

FLUOROQUINOLONES[5]

Occasional: GI disturbance; dizziness; headache; tremors; restlessness; confusion; rash; oral/vaginal *Candida* infections; eosinophilia; neutropenia; leukopenia; increased aminotransferases; hyper- and hypoglycemia; increased serum creatinine; insomnia; photosensitivity reactions, QT interval prolongation; peripheral neuropathy; tendinitis or tendon rupture; CDI

CDI = *Clostridium difficile* infection

5. Ciprofloxacin *(Cipro)*, delafloxacin *(Baxdela)*, levofloxacin *(Levaquin)*, and moxifloxacin *(Avelox)*.

Continued on next page

Table 4. Adverse Effects and Toxicity in Pregnancy of Some Antibacterial Drugs[1] (continued)

FLUOROQUINOLONES[5] (continued)

Rare: hallucinations; delirium; psychosis; vertigo; seizures; paresthesias; blurred vision and photophobia; retinal detachment; severe hepatitis; hyper- and hypoglycemia; interstitial nephritis; vasculitis; possible exacerbation of myasthenia gravis; serum-sickness-like reaction; anaphylaxis; Stevens-Johnson syndrome and toxic epidermal necrolysis; anemia; ventricular tachycardia and torsades de pointes

Toxicity in Pregnancy: Ciprofloxacin: arthropathy in immature animals, available data suggest teratogenic risk unlikely[2]; levofloxacin and moxifloxacin: decreased fetal weight and increased mortality,[2] use only for strong clinical indication in absence of a suitable alternative

---

FOSFOMYCIN *(Monurol)*

Frequent: diarrhea

Occasional: vaginitis

Toxicity in Pregnancy: fetal toxicity in rabbits with maternally toxic doses

---

LINEZOLID *(Zyvox)*

Frequent: GI disturbance; bone marrow suppression particularly thrombocytopenia, risk greater with treatment for >10 days; increased aminotransferases

Rare: peripheral and optic neuropathy; bradycardia; seizures

Toxicity in Pregnancy: decreased fetal survival in rats; use only for strong clinical indication in absence of a suitable alternative

---

NITROFURANTOIN *(Macrobid)*

Frequent: GI disturbance; allergic reactions, including pulmonary infiltrates

Occasional: lupus-like syndrome; hematologic abnormalities; hemolytic anemia; peripheral neuropathy, sometimes severe; interstitial pneumonitis and pulmonary fibrosis

Rare: cholestatic jaundice; chronic active hepatitis, sometimes fatal; focal nodular hyperplasia of liver; pancreatitis; lactic acidosis; parotitis; trigeminal neuralgia; crystalluria; increased intracranial pressure; severe hemolytic anemia in G6PD deficiency

Toxicity in Pregnancy: hemolytic anemia in newborn; use only for strong clinical indication in absence of a suitable alternative

---

ORITAVANCIN *(Orbactiv)*

Frequent: nausea; vomiting; headache

Occasional: limb and subcutaneous abscess; diarrhea

Rare: hypersensitivity reactions; infusion-related reactions; CDI

Toxicity in Pregnancy: none known; no studies in pregnant women

---

CDI = *Clostridium difficile* infection

Continued on next page

Table 4. Adverse Effects and Toxicity in Pregnancy of Some Antibacterial Drugs[1] (continued)

PENICILLINS[6]

Frequent: allergic reactions, rarely anaphylaxis, erythema multiforme, or Stevens Johnson syndrome; rash; diarrhea; nausea and vomiting with amoxicillin/clavulanate

Occasional: hemolytic anemia; neutropenia; platelet dysfunction with high doses of piperacillin or nafcillin; cholestatic hepatitis with amoxicillin/clavulanate; CDI

Rare: hepatic damage with semisynthetic penicillins; granulocytopenia or agranulocytosis with semisynthetic penicillins; renal damage with semi-synthetic penicillins and penicillin G; muscle irritability and seizures, usually after high doses in patients with impaired renal function; hyperkalemia and arrhythmias with IV potassium penicillin G given rapidly; bleeding diathesis; hypokalemic alkalosis and/or sodium overload with high doses of nafcillin; hemorrhagic cystitis with methicillin; GI bleeding with dicloxacillin; tissue damage with extravasation of nafcillin

Toxicity in Pregnancy: none known

TEDIZOLID PHOSPHATE *(Sivextro)*

Frequent: nausea; headache

Occasional: diarrhea; vomiting; dizziness; hematologic abnormalities

Rare: peripheral and optic neuropathy; CDI

Toxicity in Pregnancy: fetal developmental effects in animals, including reduced fetal weight; costal cartilage anomalies and skeletal variations; use only for strong clinical indication in absence of a suitable alternative

TELAVANCIN *(Vibativ)*

Frequent: taste disturbance; nausea; vomiting; foamy urine

Occasional: renal failure

Rare: QT interval prolongation; infusion-related reactions ("red man" syndrome)

Toxicity in Pregnancy: decreased fetal weight and limb and digit malformations in animals; use only for strong clinical indication in absence of a suitable alternative

TETRACYCLINES[7]

Frequent: GI disturbance; bone lesions and staining and deformity of teeth in children up to 8 years old, and in the newborn when given to pregnant women after the fourth month of pregnancy

Occasional: malabsorption; enterocolitis; photosensitivity reactions; vestibular toxicity with minocycline; increased azotemia with renal insufficiency

CDI = *Clostridium difficile* infection

6. Amoxicillin, amoxicillin/clavulanate *(Augmentin)*, ampicillin/sulbactam *(Unasyn)*, dicloxacillin *(Dycill)*, nafcillin *(Nafcil)*, oxacillin, penicillin, piperacillin/tazobactam *(Zosyn)*.
7. Doxycycline *(Doryx, Vibramycin)* and minocycline *(Minocin)*.

Continued on next page

Table 4. Adverse Effects and Toxicity in Pregnancy of Some Antibacterial Drugs[1] (continued)

TETRACYCLINES[7] (continued)

(except doxycycline, but exacerbation of renal failure with doxycycline has been reported); hepatitis; parenteral doses may cause serious liver damage, especially in pregnant women and patients with renal disease receiving ≥1 gram/day; esophageal ulcerations; cutaneous and mucosal hyperpigmentation; tooth discoloration in adults with minocycline

Rare: hypersensitivity reactions, including serum sickness and anaphylaxis; CDI; hemolytic anemia and other hematologic abnormalities; drug-induced lupus with minocycline; autoimmune hepatitis; increased intracranial pressure; fixed drug eruptions; transient acute myopia; blurred vision, diplopia, papilledema; photoonycholysis and onycholysis; acute interstitial nephritis with minocycline; aggravation of myasthenic symptoms with IV injection, reversed with calcium; possibly transient neuropathy

Toxicity in Pregnancy: Doxycycline and tetracycline hydrochloride: tooth discoloration and dysplasia; inhibition of bone growth in fetus; hepatic toxicity and azotemia with IV use in pregnant patients with decreased renal function or with overdosage[2]; contraindicated

---

TRIMETHOPRIM/SULFAMETHOXAZOLE *(Bactrim, Septra)*

Frequent: hypersensitivity reactions (rash, photosensitivity, fever); nausea; vomiting; anorexia

Occasional: hemolysis in G6PD deficiency; hematologic abnormalities; CDI; kernicterus in newborn; hyperkalemia

Rare: hepatotoxicity; pancreatitis; Stevens-Johnson syndrome; aseptic meningitis; fever; confusion; depression; hallucinations; intrahepatic cholestasis; methemoglobinemia; ataxia; CNS toxicity in patients with AIDS; deterioration in renal disease; renal tubular acidosis; sudden death in patients also taking ACE inhibitors or ARBs

Toxicity in Pregnancy: Trimethoprim: folate antagonism; teratogenic in rats; sulfamethoxazole: teratogenic in some animal studies; hemolysis in newborn with G6PD deficiency; increased risk of kernicterus in newborn[2]; use only for strong clinical indication in absence of a suitable alternative, contraindicated at term

CDI = *Clostridium difficile* infection

Continued on next page

Table 4. Adverse Effects and Toxicity in Pregnancy of Some Antibacterial Drugs[1] (continued)
VANCOMYCIN *(Vancocin)*
Frequent: thrombophlebitis; fever; chills
Occasional: eighth-nerve damage (mainly hearing) especially with large or continued doses (>10 days), in presence of renal damage, and in the elderly; neutropenia; renal damage; hypersensitivity reactions; rash; "red man" syndrome
Rare: peripheral neuropathy; hypotension with rapid IV administration; exfoliative dermatitis; thrombocytopenia
Toxicity in Pregnancy: unknown; limited data in pregnant women; use only for strong clinical indication in absence of a suitable alternative[8]

8. Oral vancomycin capsules are poorly absorbed and may be safer for use in pregnancy.

1. ST Shulman et al. Clinical practice guideline for the diagnosis and management of Group A streptococcal pharyngitis: 2012 update by the Infectious Diseases Society of America. Clin Infect Dis 2012; 55:1279.
2. GP DeMuri et al. Macrolide and clindamycin resistance in group A streptococci isolated from children with pharyngitis. Pediatr Infect Dis J 2017; 36:342.
3. AW Chow et al. IDSA clinical practice guideline for acute bacterial rhinosinusitis in children and adults. Clin Infect Dis 2012; 54:e72.
4. RM Rosenfeld et al. Clinical practice guideline (update): adult sinusitis executive summary. Otolaryngol Head Neck Surg 2015; 152:598.
5. AM Harris et al. Appropriate antibiotic use for acute respiratory tract infection in adults: advice for high-value care from the American College of Physicians and the Centers for Disease Control and Prevention. Ann Intern Med 2016; 164:425.
6. FDA Drug Safety Communication: FDA advises restricting fluoroquinolone antibiotic use for certain uncomplicated infections; warns about disabling side effects that can occur together. Available at: www.fda.gov/Drugs/DrugSafety/ucm500143.htm. Accessed October 12, 2017.
7. J Aspa et al. Pneumococcal antimicrobial resistance: therapeutic strategy and management in community-acquired pneumonia. Expert Opin Pharmacother 2008; 9:229.
8. LA Mandell et al. Infectious Diseases Society of America/American Thoracic Society consensus guidelines on the management of community-acquired pneumonia in adults. Clin Infect Dis 2007; 44 Suppl 2:S27.
9. AD Mosholder et al. Cardiovascular risks with azithromycin and other antibacterial drugs. N Engl J Med 2013; 368:1665.
10. DA Talan et al. Comparison of *Staphylococcus aureus* from skin and soft-tissue infections in US emergency department patients, 2004 and 2008. Clin Infect Dis 2011; 53:144.
11. R Dantes et al. National burden of invasive methicillin-resistant *Staphylococcus aureus* infections, United States, 2011. JAMA Intern Med 2013; 173:1970.
12. DA Talan et al. Trimethoprim-sulfamethoxazole versus placebo for uncomplicated skin abscess. N Engl J Med 2016; 374:823.

13. RS Daum et al. A placebo-controlled trial of antibiotics for smaller skin abcesses. N Engl J Med 2017; 376:2545.
14. AJ Singer and DA Talan. Management of skin abscesses in the era of methicillin-resistant *Staphylococcus aureus*. N Engl J Med 2014; 370:1039.
15. C Liu et al. Clinical practice guidelines by the Infectious Diseases Society of America for the treatment of methicillin-resistant *Staphylococcus aureus* infections in adults and children: executive summary. Clin Infect Dis 2011; 52:285.
16. Telavancin (Vibativ) for gram-positive skin infections. Med Lett Drugs Ther 2010; 52:1.
17. Ceftaroline fosamil (Teflaro) - a new IV cephalosporin. Med Lett Drugs Ther 2011; 53:5.
18. Two new drugs for skin and skin structure infections. Med Lett Drugs Ther 2014; 56:73.
19. Oritavancin (Orbactiv) for skin and skin structure infections. Med Lett Drugs Ther 2015; 57:3.
20. GS Moran et al. Effect of cephalexin plus trimethoprim/sulfamethoxazole vs. cephalexin alone in clinical cure of uncomplicated cellulitis: a randomized clinical trial. JAMA 2017; 317:2088.
21. DL Stevens et al. Practice guidelines for the diagnosis and management of skin and soft tissue infections: 2014 update by the Infectious Diseases Society of America. Clin Infect Dis 2014; 59:147.
22. LE Nicolle et al. Infectious Diseases Society of America guidelines for the diagnosis and treatment of asymptomatic bacteriuria in adults. Clin Infect Dis 2005; 40:643.
23. K Gupta et al. International clinical practice guidelines for the treatment of acute uncomplicated cystitis and pyelonephritis in women: a 2010 update by the Infectious Diseases Society of America and the European Society for Microbiology and Infectious Diseases. Clin Infect Dis 2011; 52:e103.
24. Alternatives to fluoroquinolones. Med Lett Drugs Ther 2016; 58:75.
25. TM Hooton. Clinical practice. Uncomplicated urinary tract infection. N Engl J Med 2012; 366:1028.
26. FDA Drug Safety Communication: FDA review finds additional data supports the potential for increased long-term risks with antibiotic clarithromycin (Biaxin) in patients with heart disease. Available at: www.fda.gov/drugs/drugsafety/ucm597289.htm. Accessed March 7, 2018.

DRUGS FOR COPD

Original publication date – April 2017 (revised March 2018)

The main goals of treatment for chronic obstructive pulmonary disease (COPD) are to relieve symptoms, reduce the frequency and severity of exacerbations, and prevent disease progression. Updated guidelines for treatment of COPD have been published in recent years.[1,2]

SMOKING CESSATION — Cigarette smoking is the primary cause of COPD in the US. Smoking cessation offers health benefits at all stages of the disease and can slow the decline of lung function. Counseling and pharmacotherapy can help patients stop smoking. Varenicline *(Chantix)* appears to be the most effective drug for treatment of tobacco dependence. Nicotine replacement therapy and bupropion (*Zyban*, and others) are also effective.[3] Use of $\geq$2 medications has been more effective than monotherapy.[4,5]

SHORT-ACTING BRONCHODILATORS — For patients with occasional dyspnea, an inhaled short-acting bronchodilator can provide acute relief. Short-acting drugs, which include inhaled **beta$_2$-agonists** such as albuterol and the **antimuscarinic** (anticholinergic) ipratropium, can relieve symptoms and improve FEV_1 (forced expiratory volume in one second). Short-acting beta$_2$-agonists have a more rapid onset of action than ipratropium, but ipratropium has a longer duration of action (6-8 hrs vs ~4 hrs).

Some Recommendations for Treatment of COPD
▸ Patients with COPD should stop smoking; pharmacotherapy can be helpful, especially with varenicline *(Chantix)*.
▸ Patients with occasional dyspnea can use inhaled short-acting bronchodilators as needed for acute symptom relief.
▸ For patients who have moderate to severe dyspnea or symptoms, or who are at increased risk of exacerbations, regular treatment with an inhaled long-acting bronchodilator (an antimuscarinic or a beta$_2$-agonist) can relieve symptoms, improve lung function, and reduce the frequency of exacerbations.
▸ An inhaled long-acting beta$_2$-agonist plus an inhaled long-acting antimuscarinic can be used in patients with moderate to severe dyspnea or symptoms who are at increased risk for exacerbations and in those inadequately controlled on monotherapy.
▸ Addition of an inhaled corticosteroid is recommended for patients with moderate to severe COPD who experience frequent exacerbations despite treatment with bronchodilators.
▸ All patients should be assessed for proper inhalation technique.
▸ Oxygen therapy can improve survival in patients with severe hypoxemia.
▸ Pulmonary rehabilitation should be considered for all patients.

Combining a short-acting beta$_2$-agonist with ipratropium is more effective than either drug alone.[6] The combination of ipratropium and albuterol is available in a single inhaler (see Table 1).

Regular use of an inhaled short-acting bronchodilator is not recommended for treatment of COPD. Patients on maintenance treatment for COPD should have a short-acting bronchodilator available for use as needed for acute relief.

INHALED LONG-ACTING BRONCHODILATORS — Regular treatment with an inhaled long-acting bronchodilator (either a beta$_2$-agonist or an antimuscarinic agent) is recommended for patients who have moderate to severe dyspnea or other symptoms or who are at increased risk of exacerbations. Long-acting antimuscarinic agents (LAMAs; also called long-acting anticholinergics) may be more effective than long-acting beta$_2$-agonists (LABAs) in preventing exacerbations in patients with moderate to very severe COPD.[7,8] In patients with less severe COPD, there is no strong evidence supporting the use of one over the other.[9,10]

LABAs can provide sustained bronchodilation for at least 12 hours. They have been shown to improve lung function and quality of life, and to reduce the frequency of exacerbations in patients with COPD.[11] Several inhaled LABAs are available alone or in fixed-dose combinations with other agents for treatment of COPD in the US (see Tables 1 and 3).

Inhaled beta$_2$-agonists can cause tachycardia, palpitations, prolongation of the QT interval, hypokalemia, skeletal muscle tremors and cramping, headache, insomnia, and increases in serum glucose concentrations. Unstable angina and myocardial infarction have been reported. Tolerance can develop with continued use. All LABAs in the US include a boxed warning about an increased risk of asthma-related death; there is no evidence to date that patients with COPD are at risk.

Four inhaled **LAMAs** are available alone or in combination with other agents for the treatment of COPD (see Table 1). Tiotropium, the longest available and best studied LAMA, has been shown to improve lung function and reduce exacerbation and hospitalization rates, but it may not reduce the rate of lung function decline.[12,13] The other three LAMAs are generally considered similar in safety and efficacy to tiotropium.[14-16]

Inhaled antimuscarinics have limited systemic absorption. They commonly cause dry mouth. Pharyngeal irritation, urinary retention, and increases in intraocular pressure may occur; antimuscarinic inhalers should be used with caution in patients with narrow-angle glaucoma and in those with symptomatic prostatic hypertrophy or bladder neck obstruction.

Long-Acting Bronchodilator Combinations – Combining a LAMA with a LABA can improve lung function and reduce symptoms, and may decrease exacerbation rates in patients with COPD. Dual bronchodila-

Table 1. Some Inhaled Bronchodilators for COPD	
Drug	**Some Available Formulations**
Inhaled Short-Acting Antimuscarinic	
Ipratropium – *Atrovent HFA* (Boehringer Ingelheim)	17 mcg/inh
generic – single-dose vials	200 mcg/mL soln
Inhaled Short-Acting Beta$_2$-Agonists	
Albuterol – *ProAir HFA* (Teva)	90 mcg/inh
Proventil HFA (Merck)	
Ventolin HFA (GSK)	
ProAir Respiclick (Teva)	90 mcg/inh
generic	0.63, 1.25, 2.5 mg/3 mL soln
Levalbuterol –	
Xopenex HFA (Sunovion)	45 mcg/inh
Xopenex (Akorn)	0.31, 0.63, 1.25 mg/3 mL soln
generic	
Inhaled Short-Acting Beta$_2$-Agonist/Short-Acting Antimuscarinic Combination	
Albuterol/ipratropium –	
Combivent Respimat (Boehringer Ingelheim)	100 mcg/20 mcg/inh
generic	2.5 mg/0.5 mg/3 mL soln
Inhaled Long-Acting Beta$_2$-Agonists (LABAs)	
Arformoterol – *Brovana* (Sunovion)	15 mcg/2 mL soln
Indacaterol – *Arcapta Neohaler* (Sunovion)	75 mcg/cap
Olodaterol – *Striverdi Respimat* (Boehringer Ingelheim)	2.5 mcg/inh
Salmeterol – *Serevent Diskus* (GSK)	50 mcg/blister
Formoterol – *Perforomist* (Mylan)	20 mcg/2 mL soln

DPI = dry powder inhaler; ER = extended-release; HFA = hydrofluoroalkane; inh = inhalation; ISI = inhalation spray inhaler; MDI = metered-dose inhaler

1. All patients should be assessed for proper inhalation technique.
2. Approximate WAC for 30 days' treatment at the lowest recommended adult dosage. For short-acting beta$_2$-agonists and *Atrovent HFA*, cost is for 200 inhalations. WAC = wholesaler acquisition cost or manufacturer's published price to wholesalers; WAC represents a published catalogue or list price and may not represent an actual transactional price. Source: AnalySource® Monthly. March 5, 2017. Reprinted with permission by First Databank, Inc. All rights reserved. ©2017. www.fdbhealth.com/policies/drug-pricing-policy.

Delivery Device[1]	Usual Adult Dosage	Cost[2]
HFA MDI (200 inh/unit)	2 inh qid PRN	$332.70
Nebulizer[3]	500 mcg qid PRN	18.10[4]
HFA MDI (60[5] or 200 inh/unit)	90-180 mcg q4-6h PRN	56.20
		75.40
		52.20
DPI (200 inh/unit)	90-180 mcg q4-6h PRN	53.00
Nebulizer[3]	1.25-5 mg q4-8h PRN	21.30[6]
HFA MDI (80, 200 inh/unit)	90 mcg q4-6h PRN	68.20
Nebulizer[3]	0.63-1.25 mg tid PRN	855.00
		439.90
ISI (120 inh/unit)	1 inh qid PRN	344.90[7]
Nebulizer[3]	2.5 mg/0.5 mg qid PRN	73.10[7]
Nebulizer[3]	15 mcg bid	871.20
DPI (30 inh/unit)	1 inh once/d	213.60
ISI (60 inh/unit)	2 inh once/d	181.60
DPI (28, 60 inh/unit)	1 inh bid	351.60
Nebulizer[3]	20 mcg bid	838.80

3. Nebulized solutions may be used for very young, very old, and other patients unable to use handheld inhalers. More time is required to administer the drug and the device may not be portable. Nebulizers and nebulized drugs may be covered as durable medical equipment (DME) under Medicare part B.
4. Cost for 100 doses.
5. Only *Ventolin HFA* is available in an inhaler containing 60 inh/unit.
6. Cost for 100 2.5-mg doses.
7. Cost for 120 doses.

Continued on next page

Table 1. Some Inhaled Bronchodilators for COPD (continued)

Drug	Some Available Formulations
Inhaled Long-Acting Antimuscarinic Agents (LAMAs)[8]	
Aclidinium – *Tudorza Pressair* (AstraZeneca)	400 mcg/inh
Glycopyrrolate – *Seebri Neohaler* (Sunovion)	15.6 mcg/cap
Lonhala Magnair (Sunovion)	25 mcg/mL soln
Tiotropium –	
Spiriva Handihaler (Boehringer Ingelheim)	18 mcg/cap
Spiriva Respimat	2.5 mcg/inh
Umeclidinium – *Incruse Ellipta* (GSK)	62.5 mcg/inh
Inhaled Long-Acting Antimuscarinic Agents/Long-Acting Beta$_2$-Agonist Combinations (LAMA/LABA Combinations)	
Glycopyrrolate/formoterol – *Bevespi Aerosphere* (AstraZeneca)	9 mcg/4.8 mcg/inh
Glycopyrrolate/indacaterol – *Utibron Neohaler* (Sunovion)	15.6 mcg/27.5 mcg/cap
Tiotropium/olodaterol – *Stiolto Respimat* (Boehringer Ingelheim)	2.5 mcg/2.5 mcg/inh
Umeclidinium/vilanterol – *Anoro Ellipta* (GSK)	62.5 mcg/25 mcg/inh

DPI = dry powder inhaler; ER = extended-release; HFA = hydrofluoroalkane; inh = inhalation; ISI = inhalation spray inhaler; MDI = metered-dose inhaler

8. Also called inhaled long-acting anticholinergics.

tor therapy is recommended for patients who have moderate to severe dyspnea or symptoms and are at increased risk for exacerbations and for those with persistent symptoms or exacerbations despite use of a single long-acting bronchodilator.[17,18] Four fixed-dose combinations of a LAMA and a LABA have been approved by the FDA (see Table 1).

INHALED CORTICOSTEROIDS (ICSs) — ICSs do not slow the progression of COPD or reduce mortality.[19] They are less effective than inhaled long-acting bronchodilators for treatment of COPD and should not be used as monotherapy. Use of an ICS in addition to a long-acting bronchodilator can improve lung function and reduce exacerbations.[20] Addition of an ICS is recommended for patients with moderate to very

Delivery Device[1]	Usual Adult Dosage	Cost[2]
DPI (30, 60 inh/unit)	1 inh bid	$322.20
DPI (6, 60 inh/unit)	1 inh bid	394.20
Nebulizer[3,10]	25 mcg bid	566.40
DPI (5, 30, 90 inh/unit)	18 mcg[9] once/d	368.20
ISI (60 inh/unit)	2 inh once/d	368.20
DPI (7, 30 inh/unit)	1 inh once/d	324.10
HFA MDI (120 inh/unit)	2 inh bid	334.60
DPI (60 inh/unit)	1 inh bid	340.20
ISI (60 inh/unit)	2 inh once/d	340.90
DPI (7, 30 inh/unit)	1 inh once/d	340.90

9. Contents of one capsule; two inhalations of the powder are required to deliver the full dose.
10. Glycopyrrolate inhalation solution should only be used with the *Magnair* handheld nebulizer. Each dose should be administered over a period of 2-3 minutes.

severe COPD who continue to have exacerbations while receiving long-acting bronchodilators. Various combinations of ICSs and LABAs are available (see Table 3).

Adverse Effects – Local effects of ICSs on the mouth and pharynx include candidiasis and dysphonia. Systemic absorption of ICSs has been associated with skin bruising, cataracts, reduced bone mineral density, and an increased risk of fractures. Use of ICSs in patients with COPD is associated with an increased risk of pneumonia.[21]

ICS Withdrawal – In one study, 2485 patients with COPD on triple therapy with tiotropium, salmeterol, and fluticasone propionate were ran-

Table 2. Some Long-Acting Bronchodilator Inhalers: Ease of Use

***Aerosphere* Inhaler**

Bevespi Aerosphere **(glycopyrrolate/formoterol)**
- ► Metered-dose inhaler; requires coordination of inhalation with hand-actuation; drug delivery is not dependent on strength of breath intake
- ► Easy to assemble; requires priming
- ► Indicator shows approximately how many doses are left
- ► Twice-daily dosing

***Ellipta* Inhalers**

Anoro Ellipta **(umeclidinium/vilanterol),** ***Breo Ellipta*** **(fluticasone furoate/vilanterol),** ***Incruse Ellipta*** **(umeclidinium),** ***Trelegy Ellipta*** **(fluticasone furoate/umeclidinium/vilanterol)**
- ► Dry powder inhaler; drug delivery to lungs is dependent upon ability to perform a rapid, deep inhalation
- ► No assembly or priming required
- ► Indicator shows how many doses are left
- ► Doses may be wasted if inhaler is opened/closed accidentally
- ► Once-daily dosing

***Respimat* Inhalers**

Spiriva Respimat **(tiotropium),** ***Striverdi Respimat*** **(olodaterol),** ***Stiolto Respimat*** **(tiotropium/olodaterol)**
- ► Inhalation spray inhaler; drug delivery to lungs is not dependent on strength of breath intake
- ► Assembly may be difficult for some patients
- ► Indicator shows approximately how many doses are left
- ► Once-daily dosing

***Neohaler* Inhalers**

Arcapta Neohaler **(indacaterol),** ***Seebri Neohaler*** **(glycopyrrolate),** ***Utibron Neohaler*** **(glycopyrrolate/indacaterol)**
- ► Dry powder inhaler; drug delivery to lungs is dependent upon ability to perform a rapid, deep inhalation
- ► Removal of the capsule from the foil pack and insertion of the capsule into the inhaler may be difficult for some patients
- ► Transparent capsules may be helpful in determining if the full dose was inhaled
- ► Once-daily dosing *(Arcapta)*; twice-daily dosing *(Utibron, Seebri)*

Continued on next page

Table 2. Some Long-Acting Bronchodilator Inhalers: Ease of Use (continued)
***Pressair* Inhaler**
***Tudorza Pressair* (aclidinium)** ► Dry powder inhaler; drug delivery to lungs is dependent upon ability to perform a rapid, deep inhalation ► No assembly required ► Twice-daily dosing
***Handihaler* Inhaler**
***Spiriva Handihaler* (tiotropium)** ► Dry powder inhaler; drug delivery to lungs is dependent upon ability to perform a rapid, deep inhalation ► Inserting the capsules into the device may be difficult for some patients ► Once-daily dosing
***Diskus* Inhalers**
***Advair Diskus* (fluticasone propionate/salmeterol), *Serevent Diskus* (salmeterol)** ► Dry powder inhaler; drug delivery to lungs is dependent upon ability to perform a rapid, deep inhalation ► Indicator shows how many doses are left ► Twice-daily dosing

domized to either continue triple therapy or taper the ICS over 12 weeks. The time to the first moderate or severe exacerbation within 12 months was similar in both groups, but a statistically significant decrease in trough FEV_1 occurred in the corticosteroid taper group; the clinical significance is unclear.[22] A post-hoc analysis found that the risk of exacerbation was higher in the corticosteroid taper group compared to the continuation group in patients who had blood eosinophil levels ≥300 cells/mcL at baseline.[23]

LABA/LAMA vs ICS/LABA — In patients who are at increased risk of exacerbations, the combination of a LABA and a LAMA appears to be more effective than an ICS/LABA combination in reducing exacerbations.[24] In a 52-week study comparing the combination of glycopyrronium and indacaterol with fluticasone and salmeterol, patients who received the LAMA/LABA combination had 11% fewer exacerba-

Table 3. Some Inhaled Corticosteroids and Other Drugs for COPD

Drug	Some Available Formulations
Inhaled Corticosteroids (ICSs)[3]	
Beclomethasone dipropionate –	
QVAR (Teva)	40, 80 mcg/inh
QVAR Redihaler	40, 80 mcg/inh
Budesonide[4] – *Pulmicort Flexhaler* (AstraZeneca)	90, 180 mcg/inh
Ciclesonide – *Alvesco* (Sunovion)	80, 160 mcg/inh
Flunisolide – *Aerospan HFA* (Meda)	80 mcg/inh
Fluticasone furoate – *Arnuity Ellipta* (GSK)	100, 200 mcg/inh
Fluticasone propionate –	
Flovent Diskus (GSK)	50, 100, 250 mcg/blister
Flovent HFA	44, 110, 220 mcg/inh
ArmonAir Respiclick (Teva)	55, 113, 232 mcg/inh
Mometasone furoate –	
Asmanex HFA (Merck)	100, 200 mcg/inh
Asmanex Twisthaler (Merck)	110, 220 mcg/inh
Inhaled Corticosteroid/Long-Acting Beta$_2$-Agonist Combinations (ICS/LABA Combinations)	
Fluticasone propionate/salmeterol –	
Advair Diskus[5] (GSK)	100, 250, 500 mcg/50 mcg/blister
Advair HFA[3]	45, 115, 230 mcg/21 mcg/inh
AirDuo Respiclick[3] (Teva)	55, 113, 232 mcg/14 mcg/inh
Fluticasone furoate/vilanterol –	
Breo Ellipta[6] (GSK)	100, 200 mcg/25 mcg/inh
Budesonide/formoterol –	
Symbicort[7] (AstraZeneca)	80, 160 mcg/4.5 mcg/inh

DPI = dry powder inhaler; ER = extended-release; HFA = hydrofluoroalkane; inh = inhalation; ISI = inhalation spray inhaler; MDI = metered-dose inhaler

1. All patients should be assessed for proper inhalation technique.
2. Approximate WAC for 30 days' treatment at the lowest usual adult dosage. WAC = wholesaler acquisition cost or manufacturer's published price to wholesalers; WAC represents a published catalogue or list price and may not represent an actual transactional price. Source: AnalySource® Monthly. March 5, 2017. Reprinted with permission by First Databank, Inc. All rights reserved. ©2017. www.fdbhealth.com/policies/drug-pricing-policy.
3. Not FDA-approved for treatment of COPD. Inhaled corticosteroid monotherapy is not recommended for treatment of COPD.

Delivery Device[1]	Usual Adult Dosage	Cost[2]
HFA MDI (120 inh/unit)	40-320 mcg bid	$156.70
HFA MDI[3a] (120 inh/unit)	40-320 mcg bid	169.30[3b]
DPI (60, 120 inh/unit)	180-720 mcg bid	216.50
HFA MDI (60 inh/unit)	80-320 mcg bid	228.90
HFA MDI (60, 120 inh/unit)	160-320 mcg bid	196.10
DPI (14, 30 inh/unit)	100-200 mcg once/d	159.00
DPI (28, 60 inh/unit)	100-1000 mcg bid	171.40
HFA MDI (120 inh/unit)	88-880 mcg bid	171.40
DPI (60 inh/unit)	55-232 mcg bid	169.30[3b]
HFA MDI (120 inh/unit)	200-400 mcg bid	178.80
DPI (30, 60, 120 inh/unit)	220-880 mcg once/d in evening or 220 mcg bid	179.00
DPI (28, 60 inh/unit)	250/50 mcg bid	361.40
HFA MDI (60, 120 inh/unit)	2 inh bid	290.90
DPI (60 inh/unit)	1 inh bid	302.10[3b]
DPI (14, 30 inh/unit)	1 inh once/d	321.70
HFA MDI (60, 120 inh/unit)	2 inh bid	308.70

3a. The *Redihaler* is a breath-actuated MDI that does not require coordination of inhalation with hand-actuation.
3b. Approximate WAC for 30 days' treatment at the lowest usual adult dosage. Source: AnalySource® Monthly. February 5, 2018.
4. Budesonide is also available as a suspension for nebulization (*Pulmicort Respules*, and generics) that is FDA-approved only for treatment of asthma in children 1-8 years old.
5. Only the 250/50 mcg dose is FDA-approved for use in COPD.
6. Only the 100/25 mcg dose is FDA-approved for use in COPD.
7. Only the 160/4.5 mcg dose is FDA-approved for use in COPD.

Continued on next page

Table 3. Some Inhaled Corticosteroids and Other Drugs for COPD (continued)	
Drug	**Some Available Formulations**
Inhaled Corticosteroid/Long-Acting Antimuscarinic Agent/Long-Acting Beta$_2$-Agonist Combination (ICS/LAMA/LABA Combination)	
Fluticasone furoate/umeclidinium/ vilanterol – *Trelegy Ellipta* (GSK)	100 mcg/62.5 mcg/25 mcg/inh
Phosphodiesterase-4 (PDE4) Inhibitor	
Roflumilast – *Daliresp* (AstraZeneca)	500 mcg tabs
Methylxanthine	
Theophylline[8,9] – generic	100, 200, 300, 400, 450, 600 mg ER tabs; 80 mg/15 mL soln
Elixophyllin (Nostrum Labs)	80 mg/15 mL soln
Theo-24 (Auxilium)	100, 200, 300, 400 mg ER caps
Theochron (Caraco)	100, 200, 300 mg ER tabs

DPI = dry powder inhaler
8. Extended-release formulations may not be interchangeable.
9. Periodic monitoring is recommended to maintain peak serum concentrations between 8 and 12 mcg/mL.

tions and a longer time to the first exacerbation than those receiving the ICS/LABA combination. The rates of mortality and adverse effects were similar between the two treatments.[25]

TRIPLE-THERAPY REGIMENS — Some studies have found that adding a LAMA to a LABA/ICS regimen can reduce exacerbations and improve lung function, symptoms, and quality of life.[26-29] Whether adding an ICS to a LABA/LAMA combination provides similar benefits remains to be established. In September 2017, the FDA approved *Trelegy Ellipta*,[40] a fixed-dose combination of the ICS fluticasone furoate, the LAMA umeclidinium, and the LABA vilanterol.

THEOPHYLLINE — Theophylline can be tried in patients with persistent symptoms despite treatment with inhaled triple-therapy. Its primary mechanism of action is bronchodilation; at low concentrations,

Delivery Device[1]	Usual Adult Dosage	Cost[2]
DPI (14, 30 inh/unit)	1 inh once/d	$530.00[3b]
none	500 mcg PO once/d	199.00
none	300-600 mg PO once/d or divided bid	15.90
	300-600 mg/d PO divided tid-qid	1261.30
	300-600 mg PO once/d[10]	86.50
	300-600 mg PO once/d	15.10

10. *Theo-24* should not be taken <1 hr before a high-fat content meal; the entire 24-hour dose can be released in a 4-hour period, resulting in toxicity.

it may have anti-inflammatory effects.[30] Theophylline has a narrow therapeutic index; monitoring is warranted periodically to maintain peak serum concentrations between 8 and 12 mcg/mL.

Adverse Effects – Dose-related adverse effects of theophylline include nausea, nervousness, headache, and insomnia. Vomiting, hypokalemia, hyperglycemia, tachycardia, cardiac arrhythmias, tremors, neuromuscular irritability, and seizures can occur at supratherapeutic serum concentrations. Theophylline is metabolized hepatically, primarily by CYP1A2 and CYP3A4; any drug that inhibits or induces these enzymes can affect theophylline serum concentrations.[31]

ROFLUMILAST — Roflumilast *(Daliresp)* is an oral phosphodiesterase-4 (PDE4) inhibitor approved for use in patients with severe COPD associated with chronic bronchitis and a history of exacerbations. It

Table 4. Treatment of COPD[1-3]

Occasional Dyspnea or Few Symptoms; $\leq$1 exacerbation[4]	
	Inhaled ipratropium as needed
	or Inhaled short-acting beta$_2$-agonist as needed
	or LAMA
	or LABA
Moderate to Severe Dyspnea or Symptoms; $\leq$1 exacerbation[4]	
Initial	LAMA
	or LABA
Persistent or Severe Symptoms	LAMA + LABA
Occasional Dyspnea or Few Symptoms; $\geq$1 exacerbation[5]	
Initial	LAMA (preferred)
	or LABA
Further Exacerbations	LAMA + LABA (preferred)
	or LABA + ICS
Moderate to Severe Dyspnea or Symptoms; $\geq$1 exacerbation[5]	
Initial	LABA + LAMA
Further Exacerbations	ICS + LABA + LAMA
	or ICS + LABA[6]
	or ICS + LABA + LAMA + roflumilast[7]
	or ICS + LABA + LAMA + azithromycin[8]

ICS = inhaled corticosteroid; LABA = inhaled long-acting beta$_2$-agonist; LAMA = inhaled long-acting antimuscarinic agent

1. Adapted from the Global Strategy for the Diagnosis, Management, and Prevention of COPD, Global Initiative for Chronic Obstructive Pulmonary Disease (GOLD) 2017. Available at: http://goldcopd.org. Accessed March 30, 2017. Dyspnea and symptoms should be assessed using mMRC (Modified British Medical Research Council) and CAT (COPD Assessment Test), respectively.
2. Short-acting anticholinergics and beta$_2$-agonists can be added to any regimen for acute relief.
3. Theophylline may be used if other long-acting bronchodilators are unavailable or unaffordable.
4. Exacerbation that did not lead to hospital admission.
5. $\geq$1 exacerbation leading to hospital admission or $\geq$2 exacerbations.
6. An ICS/LABA combination may be considered a first choice for patients with asthma/COPD overlap or high blood eosinophil levels.
7. In patients with FEV_1 <50% predicted and chronic bronchitis.
8. Or another macrolide. Consider use in former smokers.

reduces inflammation by increasing intracellular levels of cAMP; it does not cause bronchodilation.[32] Once-daily treatment can modestly improve lung function and reduce the frequency of exacerbations, but it does not appear to improve symptoms or quality of life.[33,34] Common adverse effects include nausea and diarrhea. Significant weight loss and changes in mood and behavior have been reported.

AZITHROMYCIN — Macrolide antibiotics have anti-inflammatory effects. Once-daily or three times a week off-label use of azithromycin (*Zithromax*, and generics) has been shown to reduce the risk of an exacerbation over one year and improve quality of life in patients with COPD at increased risk of exacerbation, but use of the drug has been associated with hearing loss and development of antimicrobial resistance.[35,36] Efficacy and safety data beyond one year of use are not available.

OXYGEN THERAPY — For patients with severe hypoxemia, use of long-term supplemental oxygen therapy has been shown to increase survival and may improve quality of life.[37] In a recent study, long-term oxygen therapy did not lead to reduced mortality or longer time to first hospitalization in patients with mild to moderate hypoxemia.[38]

PULMONARY REHABILITATION — The benefits of pulmonary rehabilitation programs for patients with COPD are well established. Pulmonary rehabilitation can improve dyspnea, functional capacity, and quality of life, and reduce the number of hospitalizations.[39]

1. Gold 2017 global strategy for the diagnosis, management and prevention of COPD. Available at: www.goldcopd.org. Accessed March 30, 2017.
2. A Qaseem et al. Diagnosis and management of stable chronic obstructive pulmonary disease: a clinical practice guideline update from the American College of Physicians, American College of Chest Physicians, American Thoracic Society, and European Respiratory Society. Ann Intern Med 2011; 155:179.
3. Drugs for tobacco dependence. Med Lett Drugs Ther 2016; 58:27.
4. CF Koegelenberg et al. Efficacy of varenicline combined with nicotine replacement therapy vs varenicline alone for smoking cessation: a randomized clinical trial. JAMA 2014; 312:155.

5. JO Ebbert et al. Combination varenicline and bupropion SR for tobacco-dependence treatment in cigarette smokers: a randomized trial. JAMA 2014; 311:155.
6. J Nichols. Combination inhaled bronchodilator therapy in the management of chronic obstructive pulmonary disease. Pharmacotherapy 2007; 27:447.
7. C Vogelmeier et al. Tiotropium versus salmeterol for the prevention of exacerbations of COPD. N Engl J Med 2011; 364:1093.
8. ML Decramer et al. Once-daily indacaterol versus tiotropium for patients with severe chronic obstructive pulmonary disease (INVIGORATE): a randomised, blinded, parallel-group study. Lancet Respir Med 2013; 1:524.
9. A Gershon et al. Comparison of inhaled long-acting ß-agonist and anticholinergic effectiveness in older patients with chronic obstructive pulmonary disease: a cohort study. Ann Intern Med 2011; 154:583.
10. JA Wedzicha. Choice of bronchodilator therapy for patients with COPD. N Engl J Med 2011; 364:1167.
11. KM Kew et al. Long-acting beta2-agonists for chronic obstructive pulmonary disease. Cochrane Database Syst Rev 2013; 10:CD010177.
12. DP Tashkin et al. A 4-year trial of tiotropium in chronic obstructive pulmonary disease. N Engl J Med 2008; 359:1543.
13. M Decramer et al. Effect of tiotropium on outcomes in patients with moderate chronic obstructive pulmonary disease (UPLIFT): a prespecified subgroup analysis of a randomised controlled trial. Lancet 2009; 374:1171.
14. Aclidinium bromide (Tudorza Pressair) for COPD. Med Lett Drugs Ther 2012; 54:99.
15. Seebri Neohaler and Utibron Neohaler for COPD. Med Lett Drugs Ther 2016; 58:39.
16. Umeclidinium (Incruse Ellipta) for COPD. Med Lett Drugs Ther 2015; 57:63.
17. T van der Molen and M Cazzola. Beyond lung function in COPD management: effectiveness of LABA/LAMA combination therapy on patient-centred outcomes. Prim Care Respir J 2012; 21:101.
18. HA Farne and CJ Cates. Long-acting beta2-agonist in addition to tiotropium versus either tiotropium or long-acting beta2-agonist alone for chronic obstructive pulmonary disease. Cochrane Database Syst Rev 2015; 10:CD008989.
19. PM Calverley et al. Salmeterol and fluticasone propionate and survival in chronic obstructive pulmonary disease. N Engl J Med 2007; 356:775.
20. LJ Nannini et al. Combined corticosteroid and long-acting beta(2)-agonist in one inhaler versus long-acting beta(2)-agonists for chronic obstructive pulmonary disease. Cochrane Database Syst Rev 2012; 9:CD006829.
21. JB Morjaria et al. Inhaled corticosteroid use and the risk of pneumonia and COPD exacerbations in the UPLIFT study. Lung 2017 March 3 (epub).
22. H Magnussen et al. Withdrawal of inhaled glucocorticoids and exacerbations of COPD. N Engl J Med 2014; 371:1285.
23. H Watz et al. Blood eosinophil count and exacerbations in severe chronic obstructive pulmonary disease after withdrawal of inhaled corticosteroids: a post-hoc analysis of the WISDOM trial. Lancet Respir Med 2016; 4:390.
24. N Horita et al. Long-acting muscarinic antagonist (LAMA) plus long-acting beta-agonist (LABA) versus LABA plus inhaled corticosteroid (ICS) for stable chronic obstructive pulmonary disease (COPD). Cochrane Database Syst Rev 2017; 10:CD012066.

25. JA Wedzicha et al. Indacaterol-glycopyrronium versus salmeterol-fluticasone for COPD. N Engl J Med 2016; 374:2222.
26. PA Frith et al. Glycopyrronium once-daily significantly improves lung function and health status when combined with salmeterol/fluticasone in patients with COPD: the GLISTEN study, a randomised controlled trial. Thorax 2015; 70:519.
27. D Singh et al. Superiority of "triple" therapy with salmeterol/fluticasone propionate and tiotropium bromide versus individual components in moderate to severe COPD. Thorax 2008; 63:592.
28. TM Siler et al. Efficacy and safety of umeclidinium added to fluticasone propionate/salmeterol in patients with COPD: results of two randomized, double-blind studies. COPD 2016; 13:1.
29. D Singh et al. Single inhaler triple therapy versus inhaled corticosteroid plus long-acting β2-agonist therapy for chronic obstructive pulmonary disease (TRILOGY): a double-blind, parallel group, randomised controlled trial. Lancet 2016; 388:963.
30. PJ Barnes. Theophylline. Am J Respir Crit Care Med 2013; 188:901.
31. Inhibitors and inducers of CYP enzymes and P-glycoprotein. Med Lett Drugs Ther 2017; 59:e56. Updated March 2, 2017. Available at: www.medicalletter.org/TML-article-1517f. Accessed March 30, 2017.
32. Roflumilast (Daliresp) for COPD. Med Lett Drugs Ther 2011; 53:59.
33. PM Calverley et al. Roflumilast in symptomatic chronic obstructive pulmonary disease: two randomised clinical trials. Lancet 2009; 374:685.
34. J Chong et al. Phosphodiesterase 4 inhibitors for chronic obstructive pulmonary disease. Cochrane Database Syst Rev 2013; 11:CD002309.
35. RK Albert et al. Azithromycin for prevention of exacerbations of COPD. N Engl J Med 2011; 365:689.
36. S Uzun et al. Azithromycin maintenance treatment in patients with frequent exacerbations of chronic obstructive pulmonary disease (COLUMBUS): a randomised, double-blind, placebo-controlled trial. Lancet Respir Med 2014; 2:361.
37. JK Stoller et al. Oxygen therapy for patients with COPD: current evidence and the long-term oxygen treatment trial. CHEST 2010; 138:179.
38. Long-Term Oxygen Treatment Trial Research Group et al. A randomized trial of long-term oxygen for COPD with moderate desaturation. N Engl J Med 2016; 375:1617.
39. B McCarthy et al. Pulmonary rehabilitation for chronic obstructive pulmonary disease. Cochrane Database Syst Rev 2015; 2:CD003793.
40. Trelegy Ellipta–a three-drug inhaler for COPD. Med Lett Drugs Ther 2018; 60:86.

DRUGS FOR Cognitive Loss and Dementia

Original publication date – September 2017

Alzheimer's disease (AD) is the most common cause of dementia, but cognitive loss is also associated with other neurological conditions such as Parkinson's disease, dementia with Lewy bodies, vascular dementia, and frontotemporal dementia.

Mild cognitive impairment (MCI) is generally defined as cognitive decline that is greater than expected for an individual's age and education, but does not interfere with activities of daily living (ADLs); it may be a transitional state between the cognitive changes of normal aging and dementia. No drugs are approved for treatment of MCI.

Treatment of reversible dementia due to drug toxicity, infection, or metabolic disorders is not included here.

NONPHARMACOLOGIC INTERVENTIONS

Patients with AD should be provided with a stable, nonconfrontational environment, a level of stimulation and autonomy commensurate with their stage of disease, and frequent reminders and orientation cues. Behavioral and psychiatric symptoms such as sleep disturbances, wandering, and agitation should be managed by addressing the causative personal or environmental factors when possible.[1,2] Other interventions such as light, music, aroma, acupuncture, or massage therapy can also be tried.[3] Education and support of caregivers has been shown to improve their skill and quality of life and to delay patient institutionalization.[4]

ACETYLCHOLINESTERASE INHIBITORS

Cognitive loss in AD is associated with depletion of acetylcholine, which is involved in learning and memory.[5] Acetylcholinesterase inhibitors increase acetylcholine concentrations in the brain and have been shown to produce modest improvements in dementia symptoms, but they do not slow, stop, or reverse progression of AD.

All three of the acetylcholinesterase inhibitors in Table 1 (p. 98) are FDA-approved for treatment of AD dementia, but few trials have been conducted in patients >85 years old, and data on their use for >1 year are lacking.[6] Rivastigmine is the only acetylcholinesterase inhibitor approved for treatment of mild to moderate dementia associated with Parkinson's disease. None of these drugs are approved for treatment of vascular dementia.

Gastrointestinal (GI) adverse effects are common with these agents, particularly during drug initiation and dose escalation. Bradycardia and syncope can occur, and an increased incidence of falls and hip fractures has been reported in elderly patients taking these drugs. They should be used with caution in patients who are at an increased risk for peptic ulcers and/or GI bleeding and in those with asthma or COPD.

Concurrent use of drugs with anticholinergic effects, including first-generation antihistamines such as diphenhydramine (*Benadryl*, and others), drugs for overactive bladder such as oxybutynin (*Ditropan*, and others), and tricyclic antidepressants such as imipramine (*Tofranil*, and others) might decrease the efficacy of acetylcholinesterase inhibitors.

DONEPEZIL — Donepezil (*Aricept,* and generics) is a centrally active, reversible inhibitor of acetylcholinesterase.[7] It is FDA-approved for treatment of mild, moderate, and severe AD dementia.

Recommendations for Treatment of Alzheimer's Disease
► Currently available drugs for treatment of Alzheimer's disease (AD) and other dementias do not slow, stop, or reverse the underlying neurodegenerative process. ► The acetylcholinesterase inhibitors donepezil, rivastigmine, and galantamine can modestly improve symptoms of dementia. Transdermal rivastigmine causes fewer gastrointestinal adverse effects than the oral formulation. ► The NMDA-receptor antagonist memantine may provide some modest benefit in patients with moderate to severe AD. It causes fewer adverse effects than acetylcholinesterase inhibitors. ► Whether adding memantine to an acetylcholinesterase inhibitor is more effective than an acetylcholinesterase inhibitor alone remains to be established.

Pharmacokinetics – Donepezil is rapidly absorbed from the gastrointestinal (GI) tract, reaching peak plasma concentrations in 3-4 hours with the 10-mg tablet and in ~8 hours with the 23-mg tablet. Donepezil has a half-life of about 70 hours. It is metabolized primarily by CYP2D6 and 3A4 and is excreted in urine.

Clinical Studies – In a randomized, double-blind, 3-year trial comparing donepezil 10 mg/day, vitamin E 2000 IU/day, and placebo in 769 patients with **MCI**, there were no significant differences in the probability of progression to AD at 3 years. The donepezil group had a significantly lower rate of progression during the first year of the study.[8]

In short-term, randomized, double-blind trials in patients with **mild to moderate AD dementia**, donepezil 5 or 10 mg/day improved scores on neuropsychological tests, assessments of behavior and ADLs, and patient-, clinician-, and caregiver-rated measures of global change.[9,10] In one randomized, double-blind, placebo-controlled trial, however, in 565 patients with mild to moderate AD dementia, donepezil had no effect on institutionalization or progression of disability at 3 years.[11]

FDA approval of donepezil for treatment of **severe AD dementia** was based on the results of two clinical trials. In one, a randomized, double-blind, placebo-controlled, 24-week trial in 248 nursing-home patients with severe AD dementia, donepezil improved ADLs, cognition, and global function, but not behavior.[12] In the other, a randomized, double-blind, 24-week trial in 343 ambulatory outpatients with severe AD dementia, donepezil was more effective than placebo in improving measures of cognition and global function.[13] In a trial in patients with **moderate to severe AD dementia**, those who continued taking donepezil had slightly higher mental status scores than those who stopped taking it.[14]

The results of some small, short-term (10-26 weeks), placebo-controlled trials have suggested a modest improvement in cognition, global function, and ADLs with donepezil in patients with **dementia associated with PD** and in those with **dementia associated with Lewy bodies**.[15-17] There is no evidence that donepezil improves cognition or global functioning in patients with **vascular dementia**.

Dosage – The recommended starting dosage of donepezil is 5 mg once daily. After 4-6 weeks, the dose can be increased to 10 mg daily. If treatment is interrupted for several days, donepezil should be restarted at the lowest daily dose. The drug is also available in 23-mg tablets for patients with a suboptimal response to lower doses, but the larger dose has marginal benefits at best and causes substantially more GI adverse effects.[18,19]

Adverse Effects – The most common adverse effects of donepezil have been nausea, vomiting, and diarrhea, particularly with drug initiation or dose escalation. Urinary incontinence, vivid dreams, bradycardia, and syncope have also occurred. Fatigue and muscle cramps have been reported. Higher plasma levels of the drug and possibly a higher incidence of adverse effects might occur in CYP2D6 poor metabolizers.

Drug Interactions – In addition to interactions with drugs that have cholinergic or anticholinergic effects, donepezil may interact with inhibitors of CYP3A4 or 2D6, or with inducers of CYP3A4.[20]

GALANTAMINE — Galantamine (*Razadyne, Razadyne ER,* and generics) is a reversible, competitive inhibitor of acetylcholinesterase. It also acts on nicotinic acetylcholine receptors; the clinical significance of its nicotinic activity remains to be established. Galantamine is FDA-approved for treatment of mild to moderate AD dementia.

Pharmacokinetics – Galantamine is rapidly absorbed from the GI tract. Serum concentrations of the immediate-release (IR) formulation peak in about 1 hour when taken without food and in about 2.5 hours with food. With the extended-release (ER) formulation, serum concentrations peak 4.5-5 hours after administration. Galantamine has a half-life of about 7 hours. It is metabolized in the liver by CYP2D6 and 3A4 to metabolites that have little anticholinesterase activity.

Clinical Studies – In two randomized, 2-year trials in a total of 2048 patients with **MCI**, there was no difference in the rate of progression to AD dementia between galantamine- and placebo-treated patients.[21]

In short-term (4-6 months) trials in patients with **mild to moderate AD dementia**, galantamine modestly improved cognitive and clinical global measures compared to placebo.[22,23] In a randomized, placebo-controlled, 2-year trial in 2045 patients with mild to moderate AD dementia or mixed AD/vascular dementia, patients taking background memantine did not benefit from addition of galantamine. Among 1549 patients not taking memantine, mortality rates were lower and there was less cognitive and functional loss with galantamine than with placebo.[24]

Several trials (6-12 months) in AD dementia patients with **cerebrovascular disease** have shown significant improvements in cognition, behavior, and ADLs with galantamine treatment.[25,26]

Dosage – The recommended starting dosage of galantamine is 8 mg daily (4 mg twice daily with the IR formulation or 8 mg once daily with the ER formulation) taken with food. The daily dose can be increased to 16 mg

Table 1. Dosage and Cost of Drugs for Alzheimer's Disease

Drugs	Formulations
Acetylcholinesterase Inhibitors	
Donepezil – generic	5, 10, 23 mg tabs[2]
Aricept (Eisai)	
orally disintegrating – generic	5, 10 mg orally disintegrating tabs
Galantamine – generic	4, 8, 12 mg tabs; 4 mg/mL soln[3]
Razadyne (Janssen)	
extended-release – generic	8, 16, 24 mg ER caps
Razadyne ER	
Rivastigmine – generic	1.5, 3, 4.5, 6 mg caps
transdermal – generic	4.6 mg/24 hrs, 9.5 mg/24 hrs,
Exelon Patch (Novartis)	13.3 mg/24 hrs patches
NMDA-Receptor Antagonist	
Memantine – generic	5, 10 mg tabs; 2 mg/mL soln[3]
Namenda (Allergan)	
extended-release –	
Namenda XR	7, 14, 21, 28 mg ER caps[7]
NMDA-Receptor Antagonist/Acetylcholinesterase Inhibitor	
Memantine/donepezil –	7/10, 14/10, 21/10, 28/10 mg ER caps[7]
Namzaric (Allergan)[8]	

ER = extended-release

1. Approximate WAC for 30 days' treatment at the lowest usual dosage. WAC = wholesaler acquisition cost or manufacturer's published price to wholesalers; WAC represents a published catalogue or list price and may not represent an actual transactional price. Source: AnalySource® Monthly. September 5, 2017. Reprinted with permission by First Databank, Inc. All rights reserved. ©2017. www.fdbhealth.com/policies/drug-pricing-policy.
2. The 23-mg tablet should not be split, crushed, or chewed.
3. The oral solution is only available generically.
4. In patients with CrCl 9-59 mL/min or moderate hepatic impairment, dosage should not exceed 16 mg/day. Patients with CrCl <9 mL/min or severe hepatic impairment should not take galantamine.
5. Every 4 weeks for dementia associated with Parkinson's disease.
6. In patients with severe renal impairment (CrCl 5-29 mL/min), the target dosage is 5 mg bid for immediate-release formulation and 14 mg once/day for the extended-release formulation.

Usual Dosage	Starting Dosage/Titration	Cost[1]
5-10 mg once/d in the evening	5 mg once/d; after 4-6 wks increase to 10 mg once/d; after an additional 3 months, can increase to 23 mg once/d	$5.50 506.10 31.80
8-12 mg bid, preferably with meals[4]	4 mg bid; after 4 wks increase to 8 mg bid; after an additional 4 wks can increase to 12 mg bid	135.10 320.20
16-24 mg once/d, preferably with the AM meal	8 mg once/d; after 4 wks increase to 16 mg once/d; after an additional 4 wks can increase to 24 mg once/d	140.00 320.20
4.5-6 mg bid with meals	1.5 mg bid; increase in increments of 1.5 mg bid every 2 wks[5] to 6 mg bid	105.30
9.5 mg or 13.3 mg once/d	4.6 mg once/d; after 4 wks increase to 9.5 mg once/d; after an additional 4 wks can increase to 13.3 mg once/d	372.90 593.70
10 mg bid[6]	5 mg once/d; increase in increments of 5 mg/wk to 10 mg bid	25.80 406.20
28 mg once/d[6]	7 mg once/d; increase in increments of 7 mg/wk to 28 mg once/d	387.60
28/10 mg once/d in the evening[9]	See footnote 10	385.90

7. Contents of capsules can be sprinkled on applesauce and consumed immediately. Capsules should not be divided, crushed, or chewed.
8. Approved for patients previously stabilized on donepezil 10 mg once/d.
9. The recommended dosage of *Namzaric* is 14/10 mg once/day for patients with severe renal impairment (CrCl 5-29 mL/min) previously stabilized on memantine 5 mg bid or 14 mg once/day and donepezil 10 mg once/day.
10. For patients who were taking donepezil 10 mg once/d without memantine, the recommended starting dosage is 7/10 mg once/d in the evening; the memantine daily dose can be increased in increments of 7 mg/week. For patients previously stabilized on donepezil 10 mg once/d and memantine 10 mg bid or 28 mg once/d, the recommended starting dosage is 28/10 mg once/d in the evening.

after 4 weeks and then to 24 mg after another 4 weeks. The maximum daily dose is 16 mg in patients with moderate hepatic or renal impairment; the drug should not be used in patients with severe hepatic or renal impairment. If treatment is interrupted for several days, galantamine should be restarted at the lowest daily dose.

Adverse Effects – Nausea, vomiting, diarrhea, dizziness, anorexia, and weight loss are common with rapid dose escalation of galantamine, and less common during maintenance treatment. Bradycardia and syncope can occur. Depression, fatigue, and somnolence have been reported. Higher plasma levels of the drug and possibly a higher incidence of adverse effects may occur in CYP2D6 poor metabolizers.

Drug Interactions – In addition to interactions with drugs that have anticholinergic or cholinergic effects, galantamine may interact with drugs that inhibit CYP3A4 or 2D6 or induce CYP3A4.[20]

RIVASTIGMINE — Rivastigmine is a carbamate-based, slowly reversible, noncompetitive cholinesterase inhibitor with good CNS penetration.[27] It is FDA-approved for treatment of mild to moderate dementia associated with AD or Parkinson's disease. The transdermal patch (*Exelon Patch*, and generics) is also approved for use in patients with severe AD dementia.

Pharmacokinetics – The oral formulation of rivastigmine is rapidly absorbed from the GI tract, reaching peak plasma concentrations in about 1 hour without food and in about 2.5 hours with food. The drug binds weakly to plasma proteins and has a short half-life in plasma (1.5 hours), but it has a half-life for cholinesterase inhibition in the CNS of about 10 hours. Rivastigmine is metabolized mainly through hydrolysis by esterases and is excreted in urine.

Clinical Studies – In a randomized, double-blind trial of up to 48 months in 1018 patients with **MCI**, there was no significant difference between rivastigmine and placebo in cognitive function or rate of progression to AD.[28]

A review of 13 randomized, double-blind, placebo-controlled, 12- to 52-week trials involving 4775 patients with **mild to moderate AD dementia** found that oral and transdermal rivastigmine slowed the rate of cognitive function decline and improved ADLs, but the effects were small and the clinical significance was unclear. The transdermal patches were better tolerated than the oral formulation.[29]

In a 24-week trial in 1195 patients with **severe AD dementia**, transdermal rivastigmine (9.5 mg/24 hours) was as effective as oral rivastigmine (12 mg/day), and the incidence of nausea and vomiting was about two-thirds lower with the patch.[30] In another 24-week trial, 716 patients with severe AD dementia were randomized to receive rivastigmine patches containing 4.6 or 13.3 mg/24 hours; at the end of the study, the mean decline from baseline on assessments of cognition and overall function was significantly less with the 13.3-mg patch.[31]

In a randomized, double-blind, placebo-controlled, 24-week trial in 541 patients with **dementia associated with PD**, rivastigmine produced statistically significant improvements in attention and cognition.[32] In a double-blind, 20-week trial in 120 patients with **dementia with Lewy bodies**, rivastigmine produced significant improvement in behavior compared to placebo.[33] In a randomized, double-blind, 24-week trial in 710 patients with **vascular dementia**, oral rivastigmine significantly improved performance on measures of cognition compared to placebo, but not global impression of change or ADLs.[34]

Dosage – The recommended starting dosage of **oral** rivastigmine is 1.5 mg twice daily with food. The daily dose can be increased in 1.5-mg increments at 2-week intervals, up to a maximum dose of 12 mg. If treatment is interrupted for several days, rivastigmine should be restarted at the lowest daily dose.

The **transdermal** patch may be a more reliable method of administration in patients with dementia.[35] The initial dose is one 4.6 mg/24 hours patch, placed on the back, chest, or upper arm; the application site should be rotated daily. After one month, the dose can be increased to 9.5 mg/24 hours; subsequent escalation 4 weeks later to a 13.3 mg/24 hours patch may provide additional benefit.[36] If treatment is interrupted for >3 days, it should be restarted with the lowest-dose patch.

Adverse Effects – Oral rivastigmine commonly causes nausea, vomiting, and diarrhea; GI tolerability can be improved if titration is slow and the drug is taken with food. These effects appear to be substantially less frequent with the transdermal formulation. Bradycardia and syncope can occur with either formulation of the drug.

Drug Interactions – Except for interactions with drugs that have anticholinergic or cholinergic effects, rivastigmine has no well-documented drug interactions.

CHOICE OF DRUG — Donepezil, galantamine, and rivastigmine appear to be similar in efficacy and safety in patients with AD dementia, but comparative trials are lacking. Transdermal rivastigmine may be better tolerated than the oral formulation. Both donepezil and rivastigmine have documented efficacy in dementia associated with Parkinson's disease and with Lewy body disease. Rivastigmine has improved cognitive performance in patients with vascular dementia.

AN NMDA-RECEPTOR ANTAGONIST

MEMANTINE — An *N*-methyl-D-aspartate (NMDA)-receptor antagonist, memantine (*Namenda*, and generics) is approved by the FDA for oral treatment of moderate to severe AD dementia.[37] Its mechanism of action in AD is unclear; it may reduce glutamatergic overstimulation at the NMDA receptor, which could have symptomatic benefits.[38]

Pharmacokinetics – Memantine is well absorbed from the GI tract, reaching peak plasma concentrations in about 3-7 hours with the IR formulation and about 9-12 hours with the ER formulation. The terminal elimination half-life is 60-80 hours. Memantine is excreted primarily in urine.

Clinical Studies – Memantine is approved only for treatment of moderate to severe AD dementia.

In a double-blind, 28-week trial in 252 patients with **moderate to severe AD dementia**, memantine treatment produced modest, but statistically significant benefits in global, functional, and cognitive scores, compared to placebo.[39]

In one randomized trial in patients with **moderate to severe AD dementia taking donepezil**, addition of memantine led to significantly better outcomes on measures of cognition, behavior, ADLs, and global improvement, compared to addition of placebo.[40] In another randomized trial, however, in 295 patients with moderate to severe AD dementia taking donepezil, addition of memantine did not significantly improve measures of cognition and ADLs compared to addition of placebo.[14]

There is no acceptable evidence that memantine is effective in **mild AD**. In a prospective, double-blind, 24-week study in 433 patients with **mild to moderate AD dementia taking a cholinesterase inhibitor**, addition of memantine was no more effective than addition of placebo.[41]

Memantine is available in an extended-release, fixed-dose combination with donepezil *(Namzaric)* that is approved for once-daily treatment of moderate to severe AD; its efficacy is unclear and it is expensive.[42]

Memantine has been reported to improve cognition in patients with mild to moderate **vascular dementia**.[43,44] It has not been shown to be effective in **dementia associated with PD** or **Lewy bodies**.[45]

Dosage – The recommended starting dosage of IR memantine is 5 mg once daily. The daily dose can be increased in weekly increments of 5 mg to a total of 20 mg, usually divided twice daily. The initial dosage of ER memantine is 7 mg once daily; the dose can be increased in weekly increments of 7 mg to a target dose of 28 mg. The maximum recommended dosage in patients with severe renal impairment is 5 mg of the IR formulation twice daily or one 14-mg ER tablet daily.

Adverse Effects – Memantine is usually well tolerated. Confusion and agitation can occur. Other adverse effects have included dizziness, insomnia, hallucinations, and delusions.

Drug Interactions – Memantine does not affect the activity of acetylcholinesterase inhibitors. Amantadine, which is used to treat Parkinson's disease, is also an NMDA-receptor antagonist and could theoretically have undesirable additive effects if taken with memantine.

ANTIPSYCHOTICS

Antipsychotic drugs are widely used off-label to treat agitation and other behavioral symptoms in elderly patients, especially those with dementia.[46] Second-generation antipsychotics used in low doses have generally been preferred because they have fewer extrapyramidal effects than first-generation drugs.

Efficacy in AD Dementia – Although many clinicians believe that use of second-generation antipsychotics such as quetiapine (*Seroquel*, and generics) to calm agitated or aggressive patients with dementia is beneficial, controlled-trial evidence for the efficacy of antipsychotic medications in dementia is limited. In one placebo-controlled, 36-week trial in 421 outpatients with AD dementia, antipsychotic treatment produced modest improvement in behavioral symptoms such as anger, aggression, and paranoid ideation, but did not improve functioning, care needs, or quality of life.[47]

Adverse Effects – Common adverse effects of antipsychotic drugs include somnolence and gait changes. Extrapyramidal effects can occur and may be more severe in patients also taking an acetylcholinesterase inhibitor.[48] In one study in 421 patients with AD dementia, cognitive function declined more in patients taking an antipsychotic than in those taking placebo.[49]

Risk of Death – The FDA requires manufacturers of all antipsychotic drugs to include a warning in the labeling about an increased risk of death among elderly patients with dementia treated with antipsychotics. In randomized trials, elderly patients with dementia taking second-generation antipsychotics had a higher mortality rate than those taking placebo (4.5% vs 2.6% in a typical 10-week controlled trial); most of the deaths were due to cardiovascular or infectious causes. The mortality risk with first-generation antipsychotics has not been adequately evaluated, and may be higher than the risk with second-generation drugs.

ANTIDEPRESSANTS

In addition to treating depression, antidepressants are used off-label to treat agitation and other behavioral symptoms in patients with dementia. A review of 9 trials in a total of 692 patients with dementia found that the selective serotonin reuptake inhibitors (SSRIs) sertraline (*Zoloft*, and generics) and citalopram (*Celexa*, and generics) significantly improved agitation, but not other behavioral symptoms.[50] In a randomized, double-blind, 9-week trial in 186 patients with AD dementia and clinically significant agitation, citalopram significantly improved measures of agitation compared to placebo, but was also associated with worsening of cognition and QT interval prolongation.[51]

OTHER DRUGS

Dextromethorphan/quinidine *(Nuedexta)* is FDA-approved for pseudobulbar affect, which occurs in a range of neurological disorders.[52] Quinidine is a strong CYP2D6 inhibitor[20]; it boosts serum concentrations of the CYP2D6 substrate dextromethorphan. In a randomized, placebo-controlled trial in 194 patients with Alzheimer's-related agitation, measures of agitation and aggression were modestly but significantly improved in those receiving the combination. Adverse effects were infrequent, but included dizziness, falls, diarrhea, and urinary tract infection.[53]

A randomized, placebo-controlled trial in 613 patients with mild to moderate AD compared 2000 IU/d of **vitamin E**, 20 mg of memantine, a combination of both vitamin E and memantine, and placebo. Functional decline was significantly slower, compared to placebo, with vitamin E, but not with memantine or the combination of vitamin E and memantine.[54]

The dietary supplement ***Ginkgo biloba*** is heavily promoted in the US for memory support. In several randomized, double-blind trials, it was not effective in preventing or treating dementia or for preventing cognitive decline in older adults.[55-58]

1. CH Sadowsky and JE Galvin. Guidelines for the management of cognitive and behavioral problems in dementia. J Am Board Fam Med 2012; 25:350.
2. LN Gitlin et al. Nonpharmacologic management of behavioral symptoms in dementia. JAMA 2012; 308:2020.
3. ME O'Neil et al. A systematic evidence review of non-pharmacological interventions for behavioral symptoms of dementia [internet]. VA Evidence-based Synthesis Program Reports. 2011 March (epub).
4. MS Mittelman and SJ Bartels. Translating research into practice: case study of a community-based dementia caregiver intervention. Health Aff (Millwood) 2014; 33:587.
5. TH Ferreira-Vieira et al. Alzheimer's disease: targeting the cholinergic system. Curr Neuropharmacol 2016; 14:101.
6. JS Buckley and SR Salpeter. A risk-benefit assessment of dementia medications: systematic review of the evidence. Drugs Aging 2015; 32:453.
7. Donepezil (Aricept) for Alzheimer's disease. Med Lett Drugs Ther 1997; 39:53.
8. RC Petersen et al. Vitamin E and donepezil for the treatment of mild cognitive impairment. N Engl J Med 2005; 352:2379.
9. SL Rogers et al. A 24-week, double-blind, placebo-controlled trial of donepezil in patients with Alzheimer's disease. Donepezil Study Group. Neurology 1998; 50:136.
10. SL Rogers and LT Friedhoff. The efficacy and safety of donepezil in patients with Alzheimer's disease: results of a US multicentre, randomized, double-blind, placebo-controlled trial. The Donepezil Study Group. Dementia 1996; 7:293.
11. C Courtney et al. Long-term donepezil treatment in 565 patients with Alzheimer's disease (AD2000): randomised double-blind trial. Lancet 2004; 363:2105.

12. B Winblad et al. Donepezil in patients with severe Alzheimer's disease: double-blind, parallel-group, placebo-controlled study. Lancet 2006; 367:1057.
13. SE Black et al. Donepezil preserves cognition and global function in patients with severe Alzheimer disease. Neurology 2007; 69:459.
14. RJ Howard et al. Donepezil and memantine for moderate-to-severe Alzheimer's disease. N Engl J Med 2012; 366:893.
15. M Rolinski et al. Cholinesterase inhibitors for dementia with Lewy bodies, Parkinson's disease dementia and cognitive impairment in Parkinson's disease. Cochrane Database Syst Rev 2012; 3:CD006504.
16. M Ikeda et al. Donepezil for dementia with Lewy bodies: a randomized, placebo-controlled, confirmatory phase III trial. Alzheimers Res Ther 2015; 7:4.
17. E Mori et al. Long-term donepezil use for dementia with Lewy bodies: results from an open-label extension of phase III trial. Alzheimers Res Ther 2015; 7:5.
18. MR Farlow et al. Effectiveness and tolerability of high-dose (23 mg/d) versus standard-dose (10 mg/d) donepezil in moderate to severe Alzheimer's disease: a 24-week, randomized, double-blind study. Clin Ther 2010; 32:1234.
19. DS Knopman. Donepezil 23 mg: an empty suit. Neurol Clin Pract 2012; 2:352.
20. Inhibitors and inducers of CYP enzymes and p-glycoprotein. Med Lett Drugs Ther 2017 May 18 (epub). Available at: medicalletter.org/downloads/CYP_PGP_Tables.pdf. Accessed September 13, 2017.
21. B Winblad et al. Safety and efficacy of galantamine in subjects with mild cognitive impairment. Neurology 2008; 70:2024.
22. Galantamine (Reminyl) for Alzheimer's disease. Med Lett Drugs Ther 2001; 43:53.
23. K Rockwood et al. Attainment of treatment goals by people with Alzheimer's disease receiving galantamine: a randomized controlled trial. CMAJ 2006; 174:1099.
24. K Hager et al. Effect of concomitant use of memantine on mortality and efficacy outcomes of galantamine-treated patients with Alzheimer's disease: post-hoc analysis of a randomized placebo-controlled study. Alzheimers Res Ther 2016; 8:47.
25. T Erkinjuntti et al. Efficacy of galantamine in probable vascular dementia and Alzheimer's disease combined with cerebrovascular disease: a randomised trial. Lancet 2002; 359:1283.
26. R Bullock et al. Management of patients with Alzheimer's disease plus cerebrovascular disease: 12-month treatment with galantamine. Dement Geriatr Cogn Disord 2004; 17:29.
27. Rivastigmine (Exelon) for Alzheimer's disease. Med Lett Drugs Ther 2000; 42:93.
28. HH Feldman et al. Effect of rivastigmine on delay to diagnosis of Alzheimer's disease from mild cognitive impairment: the InDDEx study. Lancet Neurol 2007; 6:501.
29. JS Birks and J Grimley Evans. Rivastigmine for Alzheimer's disease. Cochrane Database Syst Rev 2015; 4:CD001191.
30. B Winblad et al. A six-month double-blind, randomized, placebo-controlled study of a transdermal patch in Alzheimer's disease – rivastigmine patch versus capsule. Int J Geriatr Psychiatry 2007; 22:456.
31. MR Farlow et al. A 24-week, randomized, controlled trial of rivastigmine patch 13.3 mg/24 h versus 4.6 mg/24 h in severe Alzheimer's dementia. CNS Neurosci Ther 2013; 19:745.

32. E Mamikonyan et al. Rivastigmine for mild cognitive impairment in Parkinson disease: a placebo-controlled study. Mov Disord 2015; 30:912.
33. I McKeith et al. Efficacy of rivastigmine in dementia with Lewy bodies: a randomised, double-blind, placebo-controlled international study. Lancet 2000; 356:2031.
34. C Ballard et al. Efficacy, safety and tolerability of rivastigmine capsules in patients with probable vascular dementia: the VantagE study. Curr Med Res Opin 2008; 24:2561.
35. A Wentrup et al. Once-daily transdermal rivastigmine in the treatment of Alzheimer's disease. Drug Des Devel Ther 2009; 2:245.
36. J Cummings et al. Randomized, double-blind, parallel-group, 48-week study for efficacy and safety of a higher-dose rivastigmine patch (15 vs. 10 cm^2) in Alzheimer's disease. Dement Geriatr Cogn Disord 2012; 33:341.
37. Memantine for Alzheimer's disease. Med Lett Drugs Ther 2003; 45:73.
38. PT Francis et al. Rationale for combining glutamatergic and cholinergic approaches in the symptomatic treatment of Alzheimer's disease. Expert Rev Neurother 2012; 12:1351.
39. B Reisberg et al. Memantine in moderate-to-severe Alzheimer's disease. N Engl J Med 2003; 348:1333.
40. PN Tariot et al. Memantine treatment in patients with moderate to severe Alzheimer disease already receiving donepezil: a randomized controlled trial. JAMA 2004; 291:317.
41. AP Porsteinsson et al. Memantine treatment in patients with mild to moderate Alzheimer's disease already receiving a cholinesterase inhibitor: a randomized, double-blind, placebo-controlled trial. Curr Alzheimer Res 2008; 5:83.
42. Namzaric – a combination of 2 old drugs for Alzheimer's disease. Med Lett Drugs Ther 2015; 57:105.
43. JM Orgogozo et al. Efficacy and safety of memantine in patients with mild to moderate vascular dementia: a randomized, placebo-controlled trial (MMM 300). Stroke 2002; 33:1834.
44. G Wilcock et al. A double-blind, placebo-controlled multicentre study of memantine in mild to moderate vascular dementia (MMM500). Int Clin Psychopharmacol 2002; 17:297.
45. HF Wang et al. Efficacy and safety of cholinesterase inhibitors and memantine in cognitive impairment in Parkinson's disease, Parkinson's disease dementia, and dementia with Lewy bodies: systematic review with meta-analysis and trial sequential analysis. J Neurol Neurosurg Psychiatry 2015; 86:135.
46. VI Reus et al. The American Psychiatric Association practice guideline on the use of antipsychotics to treat agitation or psychosis in patients with dementia. Am J Psychiatry 2016; 173:543.
47. DL Sultzer et al. Clinical symptom responses to atypical antipsychotic medications in Alzheimer's disease: phase 1 outcomes from the CATIE-AD effectiveness trial. Am J Psychiatry 2008; 165:844.
48. HC Liu et al. Extrapyramidal side-effect due to drug combination of risperidone and donepezil. Psychiatry Clin Neurosci 2002; 56:479.
49. CL Vigen et al. Cognitive effects of atypical antipsychotic medications in patients with Alzheimer's disease: outcomes from CATIE-AD. Am J Psychiatry 2011; 168:831.

50. DP Seitz et al. Antidepressants for agitation and psychosis in dementia. Cochrane Database Syst Rev 2011; 2:CD008191.
51. AP Porsteinsson et al. Effect of citalopram on agitation in Alzheimer disease: the CitAD randomized clinical trial. JAMA 2014; 311:682.
52. Dextromethorphan/quinidine (Nuedexta) for pseudobulbar affect. Med Lett Drugs Ther 2011; 53:46.
53. JL Cummings et al. Effect of dextromethorphan-quinidine on agitation in patients with Alzheimer disease dementia: a randomized clinical trial. JAMA 2015; 314:1242.
54. MW Dysken et al. Effect of vitamin E and memantine on functional decline in Alzheimer disease: the TEAM-AD VA cooperative randomized trial. JAMA 2014; 311:33.
55. ST DeKosky et al. Ginkgo biloba for prevention of dementia: a randomized controlled trial. JAMA 2008; 300:2253.
56. LS Schneider et al. A randomized, double-blind, placebo-controlled trial of two doses of Ginkgo biloba extract in dementia of the Alzheimer's type. Curr Alzheimer Res 2005; 2:541.
57. BE Snitz et al. Ginkgo biloba for preventing cognitive decline in older adults: a randomized trial. JAMA 2009; 302:2663.
58. B Vellas et al. Long-term use of standardised Ginkgo biloba extract for the prevention of Alzheimer's disease (GuidAge): a randomised placebo-controlled trial. Lancet Neurol 2012; 11:851.

DRUGS FOR Type 2 Diabetes

Original publication date – January 2017 (revised March 2018)

The goal of drug therapy for type 2 diabetes is to achieve and maintain a near-normal glycated hemoglobin (A1C) concentration without inducing hypoglycemia; the target is generally an A1C of <7%.[1] Treating to this target has been shown to prevent microvascular complications (retinopathy, nephropathy, and neuropathy), but whether it prevents macrovascular outcomes is unclear. An A1C target of <8% may be appropriate for older patients and those with underlying cardiovascular disease, a history of severe hypoglycemia, diabetes-related complications or comorbidities, or a long duration of disease.[2,3]

LIFESTYLE MODIFICATIONS — Diet, exercise, and weight loss can improve glycemic control and are recommended for all patients, but most patients with type 2 diabetes ultimately require drug therapy. In a 10-year randomized controlled trial in 5145 overweight or obese patients with type 2 diabetes, an intensive lifestyle modification program reduced weight, lowered A1C, and improved cardiovascular risk factors, but did not reduce the incidence of cardiovascular events.[4]

METFORMIN — The oral biguanide metformin (*Glucophage*, and others) is the drug of choice for initial treatment of type 2 diabetes for most patients.[1,3,5] Its mechanism of action is complex.[6,7] Metformin decreases hepatic glucose production and increases secretion of glucagon-like peptide-1 (GLP-1). It may also reduce intestinal absorption of glucose and

Recommendations for Treatment of Type 2 Diabetes
► For most patients, the target of drug therapy is an A1C of <7%.
► Oral antihyperglycemic drugs lower A1C by 0.5-1.5%.
► Metformin is generally the drug of choice for initial treatment of type 2 diabetes.
► If metformin alone does not achieve the desired A1C goal, a second drug is usually added. Most patients with type 2 diabetes eventually require multi-drug therapy to maintain glycemic control.
► Reasonable second-line agents include a sulfonylurea, GLP-1 receptor agonist, DPP-4 inhibitor, or SGLT2 inhibitor.
► If maximum doses of two drugs prove insufficient, adding insulin may be appropriate to achieve glycemic control.
► Some diabetes experts favor early use of insulin if A1C remains poorly controlled on maximal-dose single-drug therapy.

(to a lesser extent) increase peripheral glucose uptake. A meta-analysis of 177 trials comparing use of metformin to either a sulfonylurea, a thiazolidinedione, a DPP-4 inhibitor, or an alpha-glucosidase inhibitor found that metformin was more effective than all the other drugs in achieving A1C goals.[8] Metformin produces about the same reduction in A1C as a sulfonylurea (1-1.5%), but metformin-induced reductions are more durable and metformin does not cause weight gain and rarely causes hypoglycemia.

Cardiovascular Benefits – Metformin has been associated with decreases in both microvascular and macrovascular complications. In a 10-year follow-up of the United Kingdom Prospective Diabetes Study (UKPDS), use of metformin reduced the risk of myocardial infarction by 33% and death from any cause by 27%, compared to dietary restriction alone.[9]

Renal Impairment – The FDA has removed earlier restrictions on use of metformin in patients with mild to moderate chronic kidney disease because recent studies indicate that it does not increase the risk of lactic acidosis in such patients.[10] Metformin is now contraindicated in patients with an eGFR <30 mL/min/1.73 m^2, and starting treatment with the drug in patients with an eGFR between 30 and 45 mL/min/1.73 m^2 is not recommended.[11]

SULFONYLUREAS — The sulfonylureas **glimepiride** (*Amaryl*, and generics), **glipizide** (*Glucotrol*, and others), and **glyburide** reduce A1C by 1-1.5%. They interact with ATP-sensitive potassium channels in the beta-cell membrane to increase secretion of insulin. In a 10-year follow-up of the United Kingdom Prospective Diabetes Study (UKPDS), use of a sulfonylurea or insulin reduced the risk of myocardial infarction by 15%, microvascular disease by 24%, and death from any cause by 13%, compared to dietary restriction alone.[9] Hypoglycemia and weight gain are the main deterrents to use of sulfonylureas.

Cardiovascular Effects – A review of the Nurses' Health Study, which followed 4902 women with diabetes and no cardiovascular disease, found an association between duration of sulfonylurea use and increased risk of coronary heart disease, but not stroke.[12] However, a meta-analysis of 47 randomized controlled trials found no increase in the risk of myocardial infarction, stroke, or cardiovascular or all-cause mortality with use of sulfonylureas, and long-term trials found that sulfonylureas reduced both microvascular and macrovascular complications of diabetes.[13] In the 10-year follow-up of the UKPDS trial, use of a sulfonylurea (glipizide [*Glucotrol*, and others] or glyburide) or insulin in the original trial was associated with a 15% lower risk of MI, a 24% lower risk of microvascular disease, and a 13% lower risk of death from any cause, compared to dietary restriction alone.[9]

GLP-1 RECEPTOR AGONISTS — Glucagon-like peptide-1 (GLP-1) receptor agonists potentiate glucose-dependent secretion of insulin, suppress glucagon secretion, slow gastric emptying, and promote satiety. They lower A1C by 1-1.5% and have been associated with weight loss.

Exenatide is injected subcutaneously twice daily *(Byetta)*[14] or once weekly *(Bydureon)*.[15] Immediate-release exenatide can be used with basal insulin; use of once-weekly exenatide with basal insulin has not been studied. In patients with or without cardiovascular disease, addition of once-weekly exenatide to standard therapy was not superior to addition of placebo in reducing the risk of the composite endpoint of death from cardiovascular causes, nonfatal myocardial infarction, or nonfatal stroke.[66]

Liraglutide *(Victoza)* is injected subcutaneously once daily and can be used with basal insulin. Liraglutide is also available in combination with insulin degludec *(Xultophy)*. In patients with type 2 diabetes and high cardiovascular risk, addition of liraglutide to standard therapy has been shown to reduce the rates of major cardiovascular events and death from cardiovascular causes compared to addition of placebo.[16] In August 2017, the FDA approved use of liraglutide to reduce the risk of major cardiovascular events (cardiovascular death, nonfatal myocardial infarction, or nonfatal stroke) in adults with type 2 diabetes and established cardiovascular disease.

Dulaglutide *(Trulicity)* and **albiglutide** *(Tanzeum)* are injected subcutaneously once weekly. Dulaglutide has reduced A1C by 0.8-1.6% when added to metformin alone, to metformin plus pioglitazone or glimepiride, or to prandial insulin. Albiglutide has reduced A1C by 0.6-0.8% when added to metformin alone, to metformin plus pioglitazone or a sulfonylurea, or to basal insulin glargine. It causes less weight loss than dulaglutide and more injection-site reactions.[17] A systematic review and meta-analysis of 34 randomized controlled trials found that extended-release exenatide and dulaglutide were more effective than albiglutide in reducing A1C and body weight, without increasing hypoglycemia.[18]

Meta-analyses have found no increase in the risk of major adverse cardiovascular events with use of albiglutide or dulaglutide.[67,68] The manufacturer of albiglutide has decided to withdraw the drug from the market; the commercial supply is expected to be depleted by May 2018.

Lixisenatide *(Adlyxin)* is injected subcutaneously once daily.[19] It is also available in combination with insulin glargine *(Soliqua)*. Lixisenatide has reduced A1C by 0.6-1% when added to metformin, a sulfonylurea, pioglitazone, or basal insulin (or a combination of these agents) and reduced weight by 0.2-2.8 kg.

In patients who had a recent acute coronary event, addition of lixisenatide to standard therapy was shown to be noninferior, but not superior, to addition of placebo in reducing the rate of major cardiovascular events.[20]

Semaglutide *(Ozempic)* is injected once weekly. It has reduced AIC by 1.2-1.7% when added to metformin, a sulfonylurea, a thiazolidinedione, or basal insulin (or a combination of these agents) and reduced weight by 3.2-6 kg.[69-73] In a randomized, open-label, 56-week trial (SUSTAIN-3) in patients inadequately controlled on metformin with or without a sulfonylurea, addition of once-weekly semaglutide was superior to addition of once-weekly exenatide in reducing A1C (-1.4% vs -0.9%) and weight (-4.8 kg vs -1.9 kg).[71]

In a 40-week trial (SUSTAIN-7) in patients taking metformin, addition of once-weekly semaglutide 0.5 mg was superior to addition of once-weekly dulaglutide 0.75 mg in reducing A1C (-1.5% vs -1.1%) and weight (-4.6 kg vs -2.3 kg), and addition of once-weekly semaglutide 1.0 mg was superior to addition of once-weekly dulaglutide 1.5 mg (-1.8% vs -1.4% and -6.5 kg vs -3.0 kg).[74]

In a randomized, double-blind, 109-week trial (SUSTAIN-6) in 3297 patients with poorly controlled type 2 diabetes who were at high cardiovascular risk, addition of once-weekly semaglutide 0.5 mg or 1.0 mg to standard therapy was noninferior to addition of placebo in reducing the incidence of the composite endpoint of cardiovascular death, nonfatal MI, or nonfatal stroke (6.6% vs 8.9%). This difference was statistically significant, but the trial was not designed to determine superiority.[75]

A meta-analysis of four placebo-controlled trials of cardiovascular outcomes with liraglutide, lixisenatide, exenatide, and semaglutide found that these GLP-1 receptor agonists significantly reduced the risk of cardiovascular mortality (by 13%), all-cause mortality (by 12%), and the composite endpoint of cardiovascular death, nonfatal myocardial infarction, or nonfatal stroke (by 10%).[76]

Table 1. Advantages and Adverse Effects

Drug Class (A1C Reduction[1])	Some Advantages
Biguanide (1-1.5%)	
Metformin	Inexpensive; durable A1C lowering; weight neutral or weight loss (2-3 kg); hypoglycemia is rare when used as monotherapy; reduction in micro- and macrovascular events
Sulfonylureas[5] (1-1.5%)	
Glimepiride, glipizide, glyburide	Inexpensive; long-term reduction in micro- and macrovascular complications
GLP-1 Receptor Agonists (1-1.5%)	
Albiglutide, dulaglutide, exenatide, liraglutide, lixisenatide, semaglutide[8]	Weight loss (1.5-2.8 kg); no hypoglycemia when used as monotherapy; albiglutide, dulaglutide, and extended-release exenatide *(Bydureon)* are administered once weekly; decrease in cardiovascular events with liraglutide in high-risk patients
DPP-4 Inhibitors (0.5-1%)	
Alogliptin, linagliptin, saxagliptin, sitagliptin	Weight neutral; hypoglycemia is rare when used as monotherapy[12]

1. When used as monotherapy.
2. Gastrointestinal adverse effects usually decrease over time and can be avoided by starting with a low dose. Use of extended-release formulations may also reduce GI adverse effects.
3. VR Aroda et al. J Clin Endocrinol Metab 2016; 101:1754.
4. Occurs rarely. Metformin should be not be administered for 48 hours after an iodinated contrast imaging procedure in patients with an eGFR <60 mL/min/1.73 m^2 or a history of liver disease, alcoholism, or decompensated heart failure, or in those receiving intra-arterial contrast, and eGFR should be re-evaluated before treatment is restarted.
5. First-generation sulfonylureas, such as tolbutamide and chlorpropamide, have been associated with an increased risk of cardiovascular mortality.
6. Because of its adverse effects, many experts no longer recommend use of glyburide (MC Riddle. J Clin Endocrinol Metab 2010; 95:4867).

Some Adverse Effects
GI effects (metallic taste, nausea, diarrhea, abdominal pain)[2]; vitamin B12 deficiency[3]; lactic acidosis[4]; decrease in hemoglobin and hematocrit (first year of treatment)
Hypoglycemia; weight gain; possible aggravation of myocardial ischemia; glyburide has a higher incidence of hypoglycemia and mortality than glimepiride or glipizide[6]; increased risk of hip and other fractures[7]
Nausea[9]; vomiting; diarrhea; renal insufficiency and acute renal failure with nausea and vomiting[10]; possible risk of acute pancreatitis; thyroid C-cell carcinomas have been reported in animals and thyroid C-cell hyperplasia has been reported in humans (liraglutide and extended-release exenatide)[11]
Hypersensitivity reactions (urticaria, angioedema, anaphylaxis, Stevens-Johnson syndrome, and vasculitis); possible risk of acute pancreatitis; fatal hepatic failure; higher rate of hospitalization for heart failure in one study with saxagliptin; possible severe and disabling joint pain

7. J Starup-Linde et al. Bone 2016; 95:136.
8. Albiglutide and extended-release exenatide (*Bydureon* and *Bydureon BCise*) must be reconstituted before use.
9. Titrating the dose over one week for liraglutide and over one month for exenatide can help reduce nausea.
10. In patients with pre-existing kidney disease or taking other nephrotoxic drugs (TD Filippatos and MS Elisaf. World J Diabetes 2013; 4:190).
11. Albiglutide, dulaglutide, liraglutide, and extended-release exenatide should not be used in patients with or who have a family history of medullary thyroid carcinoma or multiple endocrine neoplasia syndrome type 2.
12. The risk of hypoglycemic events increases significantly when taken with a sulfonylurea (AR Chacra et al. Int J Clin Pract 2009; 63:1395) or insulin.

Continued on next page

Table 1. Advantages and Adverse Effects (continued)	
Drug Class (A1C Reduction[1])	**Some Advantages**
SGLT2 Inhibitors (0.5-1%)	
Canagliflozin, dapagliflozin, empagliflozin, ertugliflozin	Weight loss (0.1-4 kg); risk of hypoglycemia comparable to placebo[13]; reduction in blood pressure, cardiovascular mortality and risk of nephropathy with empagliflozin[14]
Meglitinides (0.5-1%)	
Nateglinide, repaglinide	Short-acting
Thiazolidinediones (1-1.5%)	
Pioglitazone, rosiglitazone	Durable A1C lowering; low risk of hypoglycemia
Alpha-Glucosidase Inhibitors (0.5-1%)	
Acarbose, miglitol	No hypoglycemia when used as monotherapy[20]
Others (0.5%)	
Pramlintide	Weight loss; reduces postprandial glucose excursions
Colesevelam	No hypoglycemia; decreased LDL cholesterol
Bromocriptine	No hypoglycemia; may reduce risk of cardio-vascular events

13. WT Cefalu et al. Lancet 2013; 382:941.
14. B Zinman et al. N Engl J Med 2015; 373:2117; C Wanner et al. N Engl J Med 2016; 375:323.
15. Weight gain can be greater if used in combination with insulin.
16. Contraindicated in patients with NYHA class III or IV heart failure.
17. CB Maxwell and AT Jenkins. Am J Health Syst Pharm 2011; 68:1791.
18. YK Loke et al. CMAJ 2009; 180:32.

Some Adverse Effects
Genital mycotic infections in men and women; recurrent urinary tract infections; volume depletion; increased urinary frequency and volume; hypotension; ketoacidosis; increased serum creatinine and decreased eGFR; hyperphosphatemia with canagliflozin and dapagliflozin; hyperkalemia and hypermagnesemia with canagliflozin; fractures; increase in LDL-cholesterol; increase in hemoglobin and/or hematocrit; possible increased risk of bladder cancer with dapagliflozin
Hypoglycemia; weight gain; increased risk of hypoglycemia in patients with severe renal impairment taking nateglinide
Weight gain (2-3 kg over 6-12 months)[15]; peripheral edema; anemia; increased risk of heart failure[16,17]; macular edema; possible decrease in bone mineral density and increased incidence of fractures, especially in women[18]; hepatic failure; pioglitazone has been associated with an increased risk of bladder cancer[19]
Abdominal pain, diarrhea, and flatulence[21]; acarbose can cause transaminase elevations
Nausea; vomiting; headache; anorexia; severe hypoglycemia (when taken with insulin)
Constipation; nausea; dyspepsia; increased serum triglyceride concentrations
Nausea, vomiting, fatigue, headache, and dizziness (more common during titration and lasting for a median of 14 days); somnolence; orthostatic hypotension; syncope, especially in patients taking antihypertensives; lowers prolactin levels

19. FDA safety communication. Available at: www.fda.gov/Safety/MedWatch/SafetyInformation/SafetyAlertsforHumanMedicalProducts/ucm532772.htm.
20. If hypoglycemia occurs, it should be treated with oral glucose because these drugs interfere with the breakdown of sucrose.
21. Slow titration can minimize these effects.

Pancreatitis – GLP-1 receptor agonists have been associated with acute pancreatitis (see next page).[21]

DPP-4 INHIBITORS — The oral dipeptidyl peptidase-4 (DPP-4) inhibitors **alogliptin** *(Nesina)*,[22] **linagliptin** *(Tradjenta)*,[23] **saxagliptin** *(Onglyza)*,[24] and **sitagliptin** *(Januvia)*[25] potentiate glucose-dependent secretion of insulin and suppress glucagon secretion. They produce small reductions in A1C (0.5-1%) when used as monotherapy.

Cardiovascular Safety – **Saxagliptin** neither increased nor decreased the risk of ischemic events compared to placebo in 16,492 patients with type 2 diabetes who either had a history of cardiovascular disease or were at risk for cardiovascular events, but more patients taking saxagliptin were hospitalized for heart failure (3.5% vs 2.8%).[26] In 5380 patients with type 2 diabetes who had a recent acute coronary syndrome, **alogliptin** did not increase the incidence of cardiovascular death, nonfatal myocardial infarction, or nonfatal stroke, compared to placebo.[27] There was a nonsignificant trend towards more hospitalizations for heart failure in patients taking alogliptin, compared to those taking placebo.[28] In 14,671 patients with type 2 diabetes and established cardiovascular disease, addition of **sitagliptin** to standard therapy did not increase the risk of major cardiovascular events (cardiovascular death, nonfatal myocardial infarction, nonfatal stroke, or hospitalization for unstable angina) or hospitalization for heart failure, compared to placebo.[29] A meta-analysis of these three trials concluded that use of DPP-4 inhibitors did not significantly increase the risk of hospitalization for heart failure.[30] A pooled analysis of 19 trials including 9459 patients found that **linagliptin** did not increase the composite endpoint of cardiovascular death, nonfatal myocardial infarction, nonfatal stroke, or hospitalization for unstable angina, compared to placebo or active comparators.[31]

In a case-control analysis of 29,741 patients with diabetes who were hospitalized for heart failure, there was no increase in hospitalization rates with use of either DPP-4 inhibitors or GLP-1 receptor agonists, compared to use of other oral antidiabetic medications, among those with or without a history of heart failure.[32]

Pancreatitis – Incretin-based drugs (GLP-1 receptor agonists and DPP-4 inhibitors) have been associated with acute pancreatitis.[21] After adjustment for confounding variables, a population-based case-control study of 12,868 patients with acute pancreatitis and 128,680 matched controls concluded that use of incretin-based drugs did not appear to be associated with an increased risk of acute pancreatitis.[33] A review of data by the FDA and the European Medicines Agency did not find a causal link between use of these drugs and pancreatic disease, but both agencies will continue to consider pancreatitis a risk associated with these drugs until more data become available.[34]

SGLT2 INHIBITORS — SGLT2 (sodium-glucose co-transporter 2), a membrane protein expressed in the kidney, transports filtered glucose from the proximal renal tubule into tubular epithelial cells. The SGLT2 inhibitors **canagliflozin** *(Invokana),*[35] **dapagliflozin** *(Farxiga),*[36] **empagliflozin** *(Jardiance)*[37], and **ertugliflozin** *(Steglatro)*[78] decrease renal glucose reabsorption and increase urinary glucose excretion, reducing fasting and prandial blood glucose levels, and achieving a 0.5-1% reduction in A1C when used as monotherapy or in addition to other drugs. Other beneficial effects include a 3-6 mm Hg reduction in systolic blood pressure and weight loss of about 0.1-4 kg.

In a randomized double-blind trial in 7020 patients with type 2 diabetes and established cardiovascular disease, addition of empagliflozin to standard care reduced the incidence of pooled cardiovascular events (cardiovascular death, nonfatal myocardial infarction, or nonfatal stroke), as well as hospitalizations for heart failure, cardiovascular death, and death from any cause, compared to addition of placebo.[38] Based on the results of this study, the FDA has approved use of empagliflozin to reduce the risk of cardiovascular death in adults with type 2 diabetes and established cardiovascular disease. Empagliflozin has also reduced the risk of nephropathy compared to placebo.[39,40]

In two randomized, double-blind trials with a median follow-up of 126.1 weeks in a total of 10,142 patients with type 2 diabetes and high cardio-

Table 2. Formulations, Dosage, and Cost	
Drug	**Some Available Formulations**
Biguanide	
Metformin[2] – generic	500, 850, 1000 mg tabs
Glucophage (BMS)	
liquid – *Riomet* (Ranbaxy)	500 mg/5 mL soln (4, 16 oz)
extended-release – generic	500, 750, 1000 mg ER tabs
Glucophage XR (BMS)	500, 750 mg ER tabs
Glumetza (Salix)	500, 1000 mg ER tabs
Fortamet (Shionogi)	500, 1000 mg ER tabs
Sulfonylureas	
Glimepiride – generic	1, 2, 4 mg tabs
Amaryl (Sanofi)	
Glipizide – generic	5, 10 mg tabs
Glucotrol (Pfizer)	
extended-release – generic	2.5, 5, 10 mg tabs
Glucotrol XL	
Glyburide[8] – generic	1.25, 2.5, 5 mg tabs
micronized tablets – generic	1.5, 3, 6 mg tabs
Glynase Prestab (Pfizer)	
GLP-1 Receptor Agonists	
Albiglutide – *Tanzeum* (GSK)[9,9a]	30, 50 mg single-dose pens[10]
Dulaglutide – *Trulicity* (Lilly)[9]	0.75 mg/0.5 mL, 1.5 mg/0.5 mL single-dose pens or syringes
Exenatide – immediate-release	
Byetta (BMS/AstraZeneca)	250 mcg/mL (1.2, 2.4 mL) prefilled pens

ER = extended release; soln = solution

1. Approximate WAC for 4 weeks' or 30 days' treatment with the lowest usual adult dosage. WAC = wholesaler acquisition cost or manufacturer's published price to wholesalers; WAC represents a published catalogue or list price and may not represent an actual transactional price. Source: AnalySource® Monthly. December 5, 2016. Reprinted with permission by First Databank, Inc. All rights reserved. ©2016. www.fdbhealth.com/policies/drug-pricing-policy.
2. Metformin is contraindicated in patients with an eGFR <30 mL/min/1.73 m^2. Starting metformin therapy in patients with an eGFR between 30 and 45 mL/min/1.73 m^2 is not recommended. If the eGFR falls below 45 mL/min/1.73 m^2 in patients already taking metformin, the benefits and risks of continuing treatment should be assessed.
3. Taken with meals.
4. Cost of one 16-ounce bottle.
5. Taken with the evening meal.

Usual Adult Dosage	Cost[1]
1500-2550 mg/d PO divided bid-tid[3]	$9.10
	88.20
1500-2550 mg/d PO divided bid-tid[3]	615.90[4]
1500-2000 mg PO once/d[5]	35.00
	30.00
	1544.40
	1990.90
1-4 mg PO once/d[6]	6.30
	39.60
10-20 mg PO once/d[6] or divided bid[7]	2.70
	70.50
5-20 mg PO once/d[6]	8.70
	37.60
5-20 mg PO once/d[6] or divided bid[3]	7.40
0.75-12 mg PO once/d[6] or divided bid[3]	2.30
	20.40
30 or 50 mg SC once/wk	478.90
0.75 or 1.5 mg SC once/wk	626.00
5 or 10 mcg SC bid[11,12]	607.50[13]

6. Taken with breakfast or first meal of the day.
7. Doses >15 mg/day should be divided and given before meals of adequate caloric content.
8. Because of its adverse effects, many experts no longer recommend use of glyburide (MC Riddle. J Clin Endocrinol Metab 2010; 95:4867).
9. Contraindicated in patients with or who have a family history of medullary thyroid carcinoma, and in patients with multiple endocrine neoplasia syndrome type 2.

9a. The manufacturer of albiglutide has decided to withdraw the drug from the market; the commercial supply is expected to be depleted by May 2018.

10. Must be reconstituted before administration.
11. Starting dose is 5 mcg twice daily, up to an hour before the morning and evening meals. After one month, the dose can be increased to 10 mcg twice daily.
12. Not recommended for patients with a CrCl <30 mL/min.
13. Cost of one 1.2-mL prefilled pen.

Continued on next page

Table 2. Formulations, Dosage, and Cost (continued)

Drug	Some Available Formulations
GLP-1 Receptor Agonists (continued)	
Exenatide (continued)	
extended-release	
Bydureon (BMS/AstraZeneca)[9]	2 mg single-dose pen or powder for injectable suspension[10]
Bydureon BCise[9]	2 mg/0.85 mL single-dose auto-injector[10]
Liraglutide – *Victoza* (Novo Nordisk)[9]	6 mg/mL (3 mL) prefilled pens
Lixisenatide – *Adlyxin* (Sanofi)	50 mcg/mL, 100 mcg/mL (3 mL prefilled pen)
Semaglutide – *Ozempic* (Novo Nordisk)[9]	1.34 mg/mL (1.5 mL) prefilled pen
DPP-4 Inhibitors	
Alogliptin – generic	6.25, 12.5, 25 mg tabs
Nesina (Takeda)	
Linagliptin – *Tradjenta* (Boehringer Ingelheim)	5 mg tabs
Saxagliptin – *Onglyza* (AstraZeneca)	2.5, 5 mg tabs
Sitagliptin – *Januvia* (Merck)	25, 50, 100 mg tabs
SGLT2 Inhibitors	
Canagliflozin – *Invokana* (Janssen)	100, 300 mg tabs
Dapagliflozin – *Farxiga* (AstraZeneca)	5, 10 mg tabs
Empagliflozin – *Jardiance* (Boehringer Ingelheim/Lilly)	10, 25 mg tabs
Ertugliflozin – *Steglatro* (Merck)	5, 15 mg tabs
Meglitinides	
Nateglinide – generic	60, 120 mg tabs
Starlix (Novartis)	
Repaglinide – generic	0.5, 1, 2 mg tabs
Prandin (Novo Nordisk)	

13a. Approximate WAC for 4 weeks' or 30 days' treatment with the lowest usual adult dosage. Source: AnalySource® Monthly. March 5, 2018.
14. Starting dosage is 0.6 mg once daily for 7 days, followed by 1.2 mg thereafter.
15. Cost of two 18 mg/3 mL pens.
16. Starting dosage is 10 mcg once daily, up to an hour before the morning meal, for 14 days, followed by 20 mcg thereafter.
16a. Starting dosage is 0.25 mg once weekly for 4 weeks.
17. The recommended dosage is 12.5 mg once daily for patients with a CrCl of 30 to 59 mL/min and 6.25 mg once daily for a CrCl <30 mL/min.
18. The recommended dosage is 2.5 mg once daily for patients with a CrCl ≤50 mL/min.

Usual Adult Dosage	Cost[1]
2 mg SC once/wk[12]	$576.70
2 mg SC once/wk[12]	660.20[13a]
1.2 or 1.8 mg SC once/d[14]	498.40[15]
20 mcg SC once/d[16]	557.20
0.5 or 1 mg SC once/wk[16a]	676.00[42]
25 mg PO once/d[17]	195.00
	363.40
5 mg PO once/d	357.10
2.5-5 mg PO once/d[18]	363.30
100 mg PO once/d[19]	363.40
100-300 mg PO once/d[6,20]	391.70
5-10 mg PO once/d[6,21]	391.70
10-25 mg PO once/d[6,22]	391.70
5-15 mg PO once/d[6,22a]	268.20[13a]
60-120 mg PO tid[23]	103.50
	283.00
1-4 mg PO tid[23,24]	118.50
	563.00

19. The recommended dosage is 50 mg once daily for patients with a CrCl of ≥30 to 49 mL/min and 25 mg once daily for a CrCl <30 mL/min.
20. Maximum dose is 100 mg in patients with moderate renal impairment (eGFR 45-59 mL/min/1.73 m^2). It should not be given to patients with an eGFR <45 mL/min/1.73 m^2.
21. Should not be started in patients with an eGFR <60 mL/min/1.73 m^2 or in those with active bladder cancer.
22. Should not be started in patients with an eGFR <45 mL/min/1.73 m^2.
22a. Should not be started in patients with an eGFR <60 mL/min/1.73 m^2.
23. Doses should be taken 15-30 minutes before meals. Should not be taken if meal is missed.
24. A starting dose of 0.5 mg tid with meals is recommended for patients with a CrCl 20-40 mL/min.

Continued on next page

Table 2. Formulations, Dosage, and Cost (continued)	
Drug	**Some Available Formulations**
Thiazolidinediones	
Pioglitazone – generic	15, 30, 45 mg tabs
Actos (Takeda)	
Rosiglitazone – *Avandia* (GSK)	2, 4 mg tabs
Alpha-Glucosidase Inhibitors	
Acarbose – generic	25, 50, 100 mg tabs
Precose (Bayer)	
Miglitol – generic	25, 50, 100 mg tabs
Glyset (Pfizer)	
Other	
Colesevelam – *Welchol* (Daiichi Sankyo)	625 mg tabs; 3.75 g/packet
Bromocriptine[29] – *Cycloset* (Valeant/VeroScience)	0.8 mg tabs
Pramlintide – *Symlin* (AstraZeneca)	1000 mcg/mL (1.5, 2.7 mL prefilled pen)
Combination Products	
Metformin/glipizide[2] – generic	250/2.5, 500/2.5, 500/5 mg tabs
Metformin/glyburide[2] – generic	250/1.25, 500/2.5, 500/5 mg tabs
Glucovance (BMS)	500/2.5, 500/5 mg tabs
Metformin/repaglinide[2] – generic	500/1 mg tabs
Metformin/pioglitazone[2] – generic	500/15, 850/15 mg tabs
Actoplus Met (Takeda)	
Actoplus Met XR	1000/15, 1000/30 mg ER tabs
Metformin/rosiglitazone[2] – *Avandamet* (GSK)	500/2, 500/4, 1000/2, 1000/4 mg tabs

25. Should not be started in patients with ALT >3 times upper limit of normal (ULN) with serum total bilirubin >2 times ULN. Contraindicated in patients with NYHA class III or IV heart failure.
26. The initial dose of pioglitazone is 15 mg once daily in patients with NYHA class I or II heart failure.
26a. Price from the manufacturer (May 2017).
27. Should not be started in patients with active liver disease or ALT >2.5 times ULN. Contraindicated in patients with NYHA class III or IV heart failure.

Usual Adult Dosage	Cost[1]
15-45 mg PO once/d[25,26]	$9.00
	388.57[26a]
4-8 mg PO once/d or divided bid[27]	148.10
50-100 mg PO tid[3,28]	47.70
	96.90
50-100 mg PO tid[3,28]	170.30
	207.30
3.75 g PO once/d or divided bid[3]	565.20
1.6-4.8 mg PO once/d[30]	199.70
60-120 mcg SC tid[31]	885.00
500/2.5 mg PO bid[3]	40.90
500/5 mg PO bid[3]	5.20
	77.90
500/1 mg PO bid-tid[23]	294.60
500/15 mg PO bid[3,25]	191.80
	573.20
1000/15 mg PO once/d[3,25]	310.40
500/2 mg PO bid[3,27]	137.80

28. Not recommended for patients with a serum creatinine >2 mg/dL.
29. Contraindicated in women who are breastfeeding.
30. Should be taken within 2 hours of waking in the morning.
31. Dose for patients with type 2 diabetes. Should be taken immediately before meals that contain ≥30 g of carbohydrate. Insulin dose should be reduced by 50%.

Continued on next page

Table 2. Formulations, Dosage, and Cost (continued)

Drug	Some Available Formulations
Combination Products (continued)	
Metformin/alogliptin[2] – generic *Kazano* (Takeda)	500/12.5, 1000/12.5 mg tabs
Metformin/linagliptin[2] – *Jentadueto* (Boehringer Ingelheim)	500/2.5, 850/2.5, 1000/2.5 mg tabs
Jentadueto XR	1000/2.5, 1000/5 mg ER tabs
Metformin/saxagliptin[2] – *Kombiglyze XR* (BMS)	500/5, 1000/2.5, 1000/5 mg ER tabs
Metformin/sitagliptin[2] – *Janumet* (Merck)	500/50, 1000/50 mg tabs
Janumet XR	500/50, 1000/50, 1000/100 mg ER tabs
Metformin/canagliflozin[2] – *Invokamet* (Janssen)	500/50, 1000/50, 500/150, 1000/150 mg tabs
Invokamet XR	500/50, 1000/50, 500/150, 1000/150 mg ER tabs
Metformin/dapagliflozin[2] – *Xigduo XR* (AstraZeneca)	500/5, 1000/5, 500/10, 1000/10 mg ER tabs
Metformin/empagliflozin[2] – *Synjardy* (Boehringer Ingelheim/Lilly)	500/5, 1000/5, 500/12.5, 1000/12.5 mg tabs
Metformin/ertugliflozin – *Segluromet* (Merck)	500/2.5, 500/7.5, 1000/2.5, 1000/7.5 mg tabs
Glimepiride/pioglitazone – *Duetact* (Takeda)	2/30, 4/30 mg tabs
Alogliptin/pioglitazone – generic *Oseni* (Takeda)	12.5/15, 12.5/30, 12.5/45, 25/15, 25/30, 25/45 mg tabs
Dapagliflozin/saxagliptin – *Qtern* (AstraZeneca)	10/5 mg tabs
Empagliflozin/linagliptin – *Glyxambi* (Boehringer Ingelheim)	10/5, 25/5 mg tabs
Ertugliflozin/sitagliptin – *Steglujan* (Merck)	5/100, 15/100 mg tabs

32. Patients who need 2000 mg/day of metformin should take two 1000/2.5 mg tablets once daily.
33. Maximum daily dose is 2000/300 mg in patients with an eGFR ≥60 mL/min/1.73 m². Patients with an eGFR 45 to <60 mL/min/1.73 m² should not receive more than 50 mg of canagliflozin bid.

Usual Adult Dosage	Cost[1]
500/12.5-1000/12.5 mg PO bid[3]	$195.00
	363.40
500/2.5-1000/2.5 mg PO bid[3]	357.10
1000/5-2000/5 mg PO once/d[3,32]	357.10
1000/5-2000/5 mg PO once/d[5]	363.30
500/50-1000/50 mg PO bid[3]	363.40
1000/100-2000/100 mg PO once/d[5]	363.40
500/50-500/150 mg PO bid[3,33]	391.70
1000/100-1000/300 mg PO once/d[6,33]	391.70
500/5-1000/10 mg PO once/d[6,21]	391.70
500/5-1000/12.5 mg PO bid[3,22]	391.70
500/2.5-1000/7.5 mg PO bid[3,21]	268.20[13a]
2/30-4/30 mg PO once/d[6,25]	576.50
25/15-25/45 mg PO once/d[25,34]	195.00
	363.40
10/5 PO once/d[6,22a]	464.50[13a]
10/5-25/5 mg PO once/d[6,22]	508.30
5/100-15/100 mg PO once/d[6,22a]	523.50[13a]

34. Limit the initial dose of pioglitazone to 15 mg once daily in patients with NYHA class I or II heart failure. Reduce the alogliptin dose to 12.5 mg/d in patients with a CrCl of 30-59 mL/min.

Continued on next page

Table 2. Formulations, Dosage, and Cost (continued)	
Drug	**Some Available Formulations**
Long-Acting Insulin/GLP-1 Receptor Agonist Combinations	
Insulin degludec/liraglutide – *Xultophy* 100/3.6 (Novo Nordisk)	3 mL prefilled pen[35]
Insulin glargine/lixisenatide – *Soliqua* 100/33 (Sanofi)	3 mL prefilled pen[36]

35. Contains 100 units/mL of insulin degludec and 3.6 mg/mL of liraglutide.
35a. Starting dosage is 16 units/0.58 mg; titrate up or down by 2 units every 3-4 days to achieve desired fasting plasma glucose. Should be given at the same time each day with or without food.
35b. Cost of 30 days' treatment for a patient using *Soliqua* 40 units/13.3 mcg daily or *Xultophy* 40 units/1.44 mg daily.

vascular risk, the rate of the composite of cardiovascular death, nonfatal MI, or nonfatal stroke was significantly lower with addition of canagliflozin to standard care, compared to addition of placebo (26.9 vs 31.5 per 1000 patient-years). However, the risk of toe, foot, or leg amputation was higher with the active drug (6.3 vs 3.4 per 1000 patient-years).[77]

There is no convincing evidence to date that dapagliflozin reduces the incidence of cardiovascular events.

Since SGLT2 inhibitors increase sodium excretion, they can cause hypovolemia and dehydration; acute renal injury can occur.

MEGLITINIDES — **Repaglinide** (*Prandin*, and generics) and **nateglinide** (*Starlix*, and generics), although structurally different from the sulfonylureas, also bind to ATP-sensitive potassium channels on beta cells and increase insulin release. Repaglinide is more effective than nateglinide in lowering A1C (1% vs 0.5%) and has the advantage of being safe for use in patients with renal failure.[41] Both are rapidly absorbed and cleared; plasma levels of insulin peak 30-60 minutes after each dose and multiple daily doses are required. These drugs permit more dosing flexibility than sulfonylureas, but they also cause hypo-

Usual Adult Dosage	Cost[1]
16-50 units SC once/d[35a]	$508.00[35b]
15-60 units SC once/d[37,38]	762.40[35b]

36. Contains 100 units/mL of insulin glargine and 33 mcg/mL of lixisenatide.
37. Within one hour before first meal of the day.
38. Starting dosage is 15 units/5 mcg in patients inadequately controlled on <30 units of basal insulin or on lixisenatide and is 30 units/10 mcg in those inadequately controlled on 30-60 units of basal insulin; titrate up or down by 2-4 units/week to achieve desired fasting plasma glucose.

glycemia and they have not been shown to reduce microvascular or macrovascular complications.

Meglitinides have not been shown to have an effect on cardiovascular outcomes in patients with type 2 diabetes.

THIAZOLIDINEDIONES (TZDs) — **Pioglitazone** (*Actos*, and generics) and **rosiglitazone** *(Avandia)* increase the insulin sensitivity of adipose tissue, skeletal muscle and the liver, and reduce hepatic glucose production. They reduce A1C by 1-1.5%. Whether the benefits of these agents outweigh their risks (weight gain, heart failure, anemia, increased fracture risk) remains unclear. They are FDA-approved for use as monotherapy or in combination with metformin, a sulfonylurea, or (only pioglitazone) insulin.

Cardiovascular Risk – Both pioglitazone and rosiglitazone have been associated with an increased risk of heart failure.[42] A meta-analysis found an increased risk of myocardial infarction with rosiglitazone,[43] but in an independent re-evaluation of data from a randomized controlled trial, there was no significant difference between rosiglitazone and metformin plus a sulfonylurea in the risk of cardiovascular death, myocardial infarction, or stroke.[44] Restrictions placed on rosiglitazone in 2010 because of concerns about its cardiovascular safety have been lifted.[45]

ALPHA-GLUCOSIDASE INHIBITORS — **Acarbose** (*Precose*, and generics) and **miglitol** (*Glyset*, and generics) inhibit the alpha-glucosidase enzymes that line the brush border of the small intestine, interfering with hydrolysis of carbohydrates and delaying absorption of glucose and other monosaccharides. They reduce A1C by 0.5-1%. To lower postprandial glucose concentrations, these drugs must be taken with each meal.

PRAMLINTIDE — The amylinomimetic agent pramlintide *(Symlin)* acts by slowing gastric emptying, increasing satiety, and suppressing postprandial plasma glucagon and hepatic glucose production. It is injected subcutaneously before meals and is approved for use in patients with type 2 diabetes on prandial insulin.[46] It reduces A1C by 0.5%. The dose of short-acting insulins, including premixed insulins, should be reduced by 50% when pramlintide is started, and frequent (including postprandial) glucose monitoring is recommended. To avoid hypoglycemia, pramlintide should not be given before meals that contain <30 g of carbohydrate.

COLESEVELAM — A bile-acid sequestrant used to lower LDL cholesterol, colesevelam *(Welchol)* is also FDA-approved as an adjunct to diet and exercise for treatment of type 2 diabetes.[47] Its mechanism of action remains unclear. It reduces A1C by 0.5%. Colesevelam is not recommended for use as monotherapy.

BROMOCRIPTINE — An immediate-release formulation of the ergot-derived dopamine agonist bromocriptine mesylate *(Cycloset)* is minimally effective in decreasing A1C (0.5%) in patients with type 2 diabetes,[48] but it may reduce the risk of cardiovascular events. In a randomized, placebo-controlled 52-week trial in 3070 patients with type 2 diabetes, addition of *Cycloset* reduced the risk of the composite end point of myocardial infarction, stroke, and hospitalization for unstable angina, heart failure, or revascularization surgery.[49]

REGULAR AND RAPID-ACTING INSULINS — Rapid-acting insulin analogs have a faster onset and shorter duration of action than regular insulin and are generally administered with or just before a meal. In general, **insulin aspart** *(Novolog)*, **insulin glulisine** *(Apidra)*, and **insulin lispro** *(Humalog)* are slightly more effective than regular insulin in decreasing A1C, with less hypoglycemia.[50]

Inhaled Insulin – *Afrezza* is an inhaled, rapid-acting, dry powder formulation of recombinant human insulin FDA-approved for use as a prandial insulin in adults with type 2 diabetes. Compared to insulin lispro, *Afrezza* has an earlier maximum effect (50 vs 120 minutes) and shorter duration of action (~3 vs ~4 hours). In one 24-week study, addition of *Afrezza* to metformin (alone or with other oral agents) was more effective in lowering A1C than addition of placebo (additional 0.4% reduction).[51] Cough has been the most common reason for discontinuation of the drug, and hypoglycemia can occur.

LONGER-ACTING INSULINS — **NPH**, an intermediate-acting insulin, can be used in combination with regular and rapid-acting insulins. It has a 16- to >24-hour duration of action with a peak effect at 4 to 8 hours. Alternatively, patients can use premixed combinations, which simplify administration of insulin, but dose titration is more difficult and hypoglycemia may be more frequent than with individual insulins.

Insulin glargine *(Lantus, Basaglar, Toujeo)*, a recombinant DNA analog of human insulin, forms microprecipitates in subcutaneous tissue, prolonging its duration of action. Insulin glargine has less peak-to-trough variation and causes less nocturnal hypoglycemia than NPH insulin. *Basaglar* is a "follow-on" insulin glargine product similar to *Lantus*; both contain 100 units/mL.[52] *Toujeo* is a concentrated formulation of insulin glargine (300 units/mL) that is absorbed more slowly from the subcutaneous depot, resulting in more even activity throughout the dosing period and a longer duration of action. A randomized trial of insulin glargine 300 units/mL versus glargine 100 units/mL in patients with type 2 diabetes using basal and prandial insulin found comparable reductions in A1C;

Table 3. Some Insulin Products

	Some Available Formulations[1]
Rapid-Acting	
Insulin aspart – *Fiasp* (Novo Nordisk)	10 mL vial; 3 mL *Flex Touch* pen
Novolog (Novo Nordisk)	10 mL vial; 3 mL cartridge; 3 mL *FlexPen*
Insulin glulisine – *Apidra* (Sanofi)	10 mL vial; 3 mL *Solostar* pen
Insulin lispro – *Humalog* (Lilly)	3, 10 mL vials; 3 mL *KwikPen*[3]
Admelog (Sanofi)	10 mL vial; 3 mL *Solostar* pen
Insulin inhalation powder – *Afrezza* (Mannkind)	4, 8 unit cartridges[4]
Regular Insulin	
Humulin R (Lilly)	3, 10 mL vials[6]
Novolin R (Novo Nordisk)	10 mL vial
Intermediate-Acting	
NPH – *Humulin N* (Lilly)	3, 10 mL vials; 3 mL *KwikPen*
Novolin N (Novo Nordisk)	10 mL vial
Long-Acting	
Insulin detemir – *Levemir* (Novo Nordisk)	10 mL vial; 3 mL *FlexTouch* pen
Insulin glargine – *Lantus* (Sanofi)	10 mL vial; 3 mL *SoloStar* pen
Toujeo (Sanofi)	1.5 mL *SoloStar* pen[7]
Basaglar[8] (Lilly/Boehringer Ingelheim)	3 mL *KwikPen*
Insulin degludec – *Tresiba* (Novo Nordisk)	3 mL *FlexTouch* pen[3]
Premixed	
Humalog Mix 50/50 (Lilly) (50% insulin lispro protamine susp and 50% insulin lispro)	3 mL *KwikPen*
Humalog Mix 75/25 (Lilly) (75% insulin lispro protamine susp and 25% insulin lispro)	3 mL *KwikPen*

susp = suspension
1. Available in a concentration of 100 units/mL.
2. Approximate WAC for one 10-mL vial of the lowest strength or one 3-mL pen if vial not available. WAC = wholesaler acquisition cost or manufacturer's published price to wholesalers; WAC represents a published catalogue or list price and may not represent an actual transactional price. Source: AnalySource® Monthly. December 5, 2016. Reprinted with permission by First Databank, Inc. All rights reserved. ©2016. www.fdbhealth.com/policies/drug-pricing-policy.
2a. Med Lett Drugs Ther 2018; 60:6.
2b. Approximate WAC for one 3 mL pen. Source: AnalySource® Monthly. January 5, 2018.

Onset	Peak	Duration	Cost[2]
10-30 min	30 min-3 hrs	3-5 hrs	
~5 min[2a]	~63 min	3-5 hrs	$106.40[2b]
			255.40
			255.10
			254.80
			233.50[2c]
10-30 min	12-15 min	~3 hrs	278.60[5]
30-60 min	2.5-5 hrs	4-12 hrs	
			137.90
			137.70
1-2 hrs	4-8 hrs	16-24+ hrs	
			137.90
			137.70
1-4 hrs	relatively flat	12-20 hrs	269.00
1-4 hrs	no peak	22-26 hrs	248.50
1-6 hrs	no peak	24-36 hrs	111.80
1-4 hrs	no peak	~24 hrs[9]	63.40
1-9 hrs	no peak	>42 hrs	88.80
15-30 min	50 min-5 hrs	14-24 hrs	98.40
15-30 min	1-6.5 hrs	14-24 hrs	98.40

2c. Source: AnalySource® Monthly. April 5, 2018.
3. Also available in a concentration of 200 units/mL.
4. Administered via inhaler.
5. Cost for one package containing 60 8-unit and 30 4-unit cartridges of *Afrezza* and two inhalers.
6. Also available in a concentration of 500 units/mL.
7. *Toujeo* contains 300 units/mL compared to 100 units/mL in *Lantus* and *Basaglar*.
8. *Basaglar* is a "follow on" insulin glargine product similar to *Lantus*.
9. H Linnebjerg et al. Diabetes Obes Metab 2016 Aug 3 (epub).

Continued on next page

Table 3. Some Insulin Products (continued)	
	Some Available Formulations[1]
Premixed (continued)	
Humulin 70/30 (Lilly) (70% insulin aspart protamine susp and 30% insulin aspart)	10 mL vial; 3 mL *KwikPen*
Novolin 70/30 (Novo Nordisk) (70% NPH, human insulin isophane susp and 30% regular human insulin)	10 mL vial
Novolog Mix 70/30 (Novo Nordisk) (70% insulin aspart protamine susp and 30% insulin aspart)	10 mL vial; 3 mL *FlexPen*
Long-Acting Insulin/GLP-1 Receptor Agonist Combinations	
Insulin degludec/liraglutide – *Xultophy* 100/3.6 (Novo Nordisk)	3 mL prefilled pen[10]
Insulin glargine/lixisenatide – *Soliqua* 100/33 (Sanofi)	3 mL prefilled pen[13]

10. Contains 100 units/mL of insulin degludec and 3.6 mg/mL of liraglutide.
11. Onset of insulin component only.

rates of nocturnal hypoglycemia were lower with glargine 300 units/mL.[53] Initial recommendations for switching from glargine 100 units/mL to glargine 300 units/mL are for a 1:1 transition by units, but patients may ultimately require about 10-15% more basal insulin per day.[54]

Insulin detemir *(Levemir)* has both delayed absorption from subcutaneous tissue and, due to reversible binding to albumin, delayed clearance from the circulation. Like insulin glargine, insulin detemir causes less nocturnal hypoglycemia than NPH. Since its effectiveness appears to decrease after 12 hours, insulin detemir is more effective when used twice daily.[55]

Insulin degludec *(Tresiba)*, a recombinant insulin analog that forms multihexamers in subcutaneous tissue, has delayed absorption and elimination that prolongs its duration of action to >42 hours. Compared to other long-acting insulins, it causes similar reductions in A1C with sim-

Onset	Peak	Duration	Cost[2]
30-60 min	2-12 hrs	18-24 hrs	$137.90
30-60 min	2-12 hrs	18-24 hrs	137.70
10-20 min	1-4 hrs	18-24 hrs	264.90
1-9 hrs[11]	no peak	See footnote 12	190.60
1-4 hrs[11]	no peak	See footnote 12	127.00

12. Refer to individual components alone.
13. Contains 100 units/mL of insulin glargine and 33 mcg/mL of lixisenatide.

ilar rates of hypoglycemia and, in some studies, causes less nocturnal hypoglycemia, especially when compared to insulin glargine.[56-58] In a randomized trial in 7637 patients, insulin degludec was noninferior to insulin glargine for the composite endpoint of cardiovascular death, nonfatal myocardial infarction, or nonfatal stroke in patients with type 2 diabetes at high risk of cardiovascular events, and was associated with a significantly lower risk of hypoglycemia.[59]

Adverse Effects – All insulins, including long-acting and inhaled formulations, can cause hypoglycemia and weight gain. Inhaled insulin can cause bronchospasm, cough, and reductions in forced expiratory volume in one second (FEV_1); it is not recommended for patients with chronic lung disease or active smokers. Until more long-term safety data become available, injectable prandial insulin is preferred over inhaled insulin. Some observational studies have found an increased risk of cancer, in particular breast cancer, in patients using insulin glargine, but a randomized controlled trial in >12,000 patients found no increase in cancer compared to standard-of-care diabetes therapy.[60]

LONG-ACTING INSULIN/GLP-1 RECEPTOR AGONIST COMBINATIONS — *Xultophy*, a combination of insulin degludec and liraglutide, and *Soliqua*, a combination of insulin glargine and lixisenatide, have been approved for patients with type 2 diabetes who are inadequately controlled on basal insulin, or on liraglutide or lixisenatide, respectively. *Xultophy* reduced A1C more than its individual components when added to either metformin, pioglitazone, or a sulfonylurea.[61,62] When added to metformin, *Soliqua* reduced A1C significantly more than insulin glargine alone (1.1% vs 0.6%).[63]

ADDITION OF INSULIN — When insulin is added to oral agents, it is usually given either as a single dose in the evening or at bedtime. In general, 10 units (or 0.2-0.5 units/kg) of NPH, insulin detemir, or insulin glargine at bedtime can be added initially. The dose can then be increased to achieve fasting plasma glucose concentrations between 70-130 mg/dL. Given the increased risk of hypoglycemia and reduced dosing flexibility, premixed insulin combinations are not recommended for insulin-naive patients.

A premixed insulin (30% rapid-acting insulin aspart/70% intermediate-acting protaminated insulin aspart) given twice daily, prandial insulin aspart given before meals three times daily, and basal insulin detemir given at bedtime or twice daily have been compared for initial insulin therapy in patients with type 2 diabetes and suboptimal glycemic control (mean A1C 8.5%) while taking metformin and a sulfonylurea. All regimens achieved similar A1C levels (6.8-7.1%), with the most weight gain and hypoglycemia occurring in the prandial group and the least in the basal group.[64]

PREGNANCY — Insulin is the drug of choice for treatment of pregestational type 2 diabetes that is not adequately controlled with diet, exercise, and metformin.[65]

1. American Diabetes Association. Professional practice committee for the standards of medical care in diabetes – 2016. Diabetes Care 2016; 39(Suppl 1).
2. SE Inzucchi et al. Management of hyperglycemia in type 2 diabetes, 2015: a patient-centered approach: update to a position statement of the American Diabetes Association and the European Association for the Study of Diabetes. Diabetes Care 2015; 38:140.
3. AJ Garber et al. Consensus statement by the American Association of Clinical Endocrinologists and American College of Endocrinology on the comprehensive type 2 diabetes management algorithm–2016 executive summary. Endocr Pract 2016; 22:84.
4. Look AHEAD Research Group et al. Cardiovascular effects of intensive lifestyle intervention in type 2 diabetes. N Engl J Med 2013; 369:145.
5. A Qaseem et al. Oral pharmacologic treatment of type 2 diabetes mellitus: a clinical practice guideline from the American College of Physicians. Ann Intern Med 2017 January 3 (epub).
6. E Ferrannini. The target of metformin in type 2 diabetes. N Engl J Med 2014; 371:1547.
7. JB Buse et al. The primary glucose-lowering effect of metformin resides in the gut, not the circulation: results from short-term pharmacokinetic and 12-week dose-ranging studies. Diabetes Care 2016; 39:198.
8. SC Palmer et al. Comparison of clinical outcomes and adverse events associated with glucose-lowering drugs in patients with type 2 diabetes. a meta-analysis. JAMA 2016; 316:313.
9. RR Holman et al. 10-year follow-up of intensive glucose control in type 2 diabetes. N Engl J Med 2008; 359:1577.
10. SE Inzucchi et al. Metformin in patients with type 2 diabetes and kidney disease: a systematic review. JAMA 2014; 312:2668.
11. FDA Drug Safety Communication: FDA revises warnings regarding use of the diabetes medicine metformin in certain patients with reduced kidney function. Available at: www.fda.gov/drugs/drugsafety/ucm493244.htm. Accessed January 5, 2017.
12 Y Li et al. Sulfonylurea use and incident cardiovascular disease among patients with type 2 diabetes: prospective cohort study among women. Diabetes Care 2014; 37:3106.
13. D Varvaki Rados et al. The association between sulfonylurea use and all-cause and cardiovascular mortality: a meta-analysis with trial sequential analysis of randomized clinical trials. PLoS Med 2016; 13:e1001992.
14. Exenatide (Byetta) for type 2 diabetes. Med Lett Drugs Ther 2005; 47:45.
15. Extended-release exenatide (Bydureon) for type 2 diabetes. Med Lett Drugs Ther 2012; 54:21.
16. SP Marso et al. Liraglutide and cardiovascular outcomes in type 2 diabetes. N Engl J Med 2016; 375:311.
17. Two new GLP-1 receptor agonists for diabetes. Med Lett Drugs Ther 2014; 56:109.
18. F Zaccardi et al. Benefits and harms of once-weekly glucagon-like peptide-1 receptor agonist treatments: a systematic review and network meta-analysis. Ann Intern Med 2016; 164:102.
19. Lixisenatide for type 2 diabetes. Med Lett Drugs Ther 2017; 59:19.
20. MA Pfeffer et al. Lixisenatide in patients with type 2 diabetes and acute coronary syndrome. N Engl J Med 2015; 373:2247.
21. PC Butler et al. A critical analysis of the clinical use of incretin-based therapies: are the GLP-1 therapies safe? Diabetes Care 2013; 36:2118.

22. Alogliptin (Nesina) for type 2 diabetes. Med Lett Drugs Ther 2013; 55:41.
23. Linagliptin (Tradjenta) – a new DPP-4 inhibitor for type 2 diabetes. Med Lett Drugs Ther 2011; 53:49.
24. Saxagliptin (Onglyza) for type 2 diabetes. Med Lett Drugs Ther 2009; 51:85.
25. Sitagliptin (Januvia) for type 2 diabetes. Med Lett Drugs Ther 2007; 49:1.
26. BM Scirica et al. Saxagliptin and cardiovascular outcomes in patients with type 2 diabetes mellitus. N Engl J Med 2013; 369:1317.
27. WB White et al. Alogliptin after acute coronary syndrome in patients with type 2 diabetes. N Engl J Med 2013; 369:1327.
28. VP Sanon et al. Play of chance versus concerns regarding dipeptidyl peptidase-4 inhibitors: heart failure and diabetes. Clin Diabetes 2014; 32:121.
29. JB Green et al. Effect of sitagliptin on cardiovascular outcomes in type 2 diabetes. N Engl J Med 2015; 373:232.
30. KB Filion and S Suissa. DPP-4 inhibitors and heart failure: some reassurance, some uncertainty. Diabetes Care 2016; 39:735.
31. J Rosenstock et al. Cardiovascular safety of linagliptin in type 2 diabetes: a comprehensive patient-level pooled analysis of prospectively adjudicated cardiovascular events. Cardiovasc Diabetol 2015; 14:57.
32. KB Filion et al. A multicenter observational study of incretin-based drugs and heart failure. N Engl J Med 2016: 374:1145.
33. RW Thomsen et al. Incretin-based therapy and risk of acute pancreatitis: a nationwide population-based case-control study. Diabetes Care 2015; 38:1089.
34. AG Egan et al. Pancreatic safety of incretin-based drugs–FDA and EMA assessment. N Engl J Med 2014; 370:794.
35. Canagliflozin (Invokana) for type 2 diabetes. Med Lett Drugs Ther 2013; 55:37.
36. Dapagliflozin (Farxiga) for type 2 diabetes. Med Lett Drugs Ther 2014; 56:13.
37. Empagliflozin (Jardiance) for diabetes. Med Lett Drugs Ther 2014; 56:99.
38. B Zinman et al. Empagliflozin, cardiovascular outcomes, and mortality in type 2 diabetes. N Engl J Med 2015; 373:2117.
39. C Wanner et al. Empagliflozin and progression of kidney disease in type 2 diabetes. N Engl J Med 2016; 375:323.
40. SGLT2 inhibitors and renal function. Med Lett Drugs Ther 2016; 58:91.
41. DM Nathan. Diabetes: advances in diagnosis and treatment. JAMA 2015; 314:1052.
42. AV Hernandez et al. Thiazolidinediones and risk of heart failure in patients with or at high risk of type 2 diabetes mellitus: a meta-analysis and meta-regression analysis of placebo-controlled randomized clinical trials. Am J Cardiovasc Drugs 2011; 11:115.
43. SE Nissen and K Wolski. Effect of rosiglitazone on the risk of myocardial infarction and death from cardiovascular causes. N Engl J Med 2007; 356:2457.
44. KW Mahaffey et al. Results of a reevaluation of cardiovascular outcomes in the RECORD trial. Am Heart J 2013; 166:240.
45. In brief: Rosiglitazone (Avandia) unbound. Med Lett Drugs Ther 2014; 56:12.
46. Pramlintide (Symlin) for diabetes. Med Lett Drugs Ther 2005; 47:43.
47. In brief: a new indication for colesevelam (Welchol). Med Lett Drugs Ther 2008; 50:33.

48. Bromocriptine (Cycloset) for type 2 diabetes. Med Lett Drugs Ther 2010; 52:97.
49. JM Gaziano et al. Effect of bromocriptine-QR (a quick-release formulation of bromocriptine mesylate) on major adverse cardiovascular events in type 2 diabetes subjects. J Am Heart Assoc 2012; 1:e002279.
50. Rapid-acting insulin analogues. Med Lett Drugs Ther 2009; 51:98.
51. An inhaled insulin (Afrezza). Med Lett Drugs Ther 2015; 57:34.
52. Another insulin glargine (Basaglar) for diabetes. Med Lett Drugs Ther 2017; 59:3.
53. MC Riddle et al. One-year sustained glycaemic control and less hypoglycaemia with new insulin glargine 300 U/ml compared with 100 U/ml in people with type 2 diabetes using basal plus meal-time insulin: the EDITION 1 12-month randomized trial, including 6-month extension. Diabetes Obes Metab 2015; 17:835.
54. Concentrate insulin glargine (Toujeo) for diabetes. Med Lett Drugs Ther 2015; 57:69.
55. Insulin detemir (Levemir), a new long-acting insulin. Med Lett Drugs Ther 2006; 48:54.
56. P Hollander et al. Insulin degludec improves long-term glycaemic control similarly to insulin glargine but with fewer hypoglycaemic episodes in patients with advanced type 2 diabetes on basal-bolus insulin therapy. Diabetes Obes Metab 2015; 17:202.
57. B Zinman et al. Insulin degludec versus insulin glargine in insulin-naive patients with type 2 diabetes: a 1-year, randomized, treat-to-target trial (BEGIN Once Long). Diabetes Care 2012; 35:2464.
58. Insulin degludec (Tresiba) – a new long-acting insulin for diabetes. Med Lett Drugs Ther 2015; 57:163.
59. SP Marso et al. Design of DEVOTE (trial comparing cardiovascular safety of insulin degludec vs insulin glargine in patients with type 2 diabetes at high risk of cardiovascular events) - DEVOTE 1. Am Heart J 2016; 179:175.
60. ORIGIN Trial Investigators et al. Basal insulin and cardiovascular and other outcomes in dysglycemia. N Engl J Med 2012; 367:319.
61. HW Rodbard et al. Safety and efficacy of insulin degludec/liraglutide (IDegLira) added to sulphonylurea alone or to sulphonylurea and metformin in insulin-naive people with type 2 diabetes: the DUAL IV trial. Diabet Med 2016 Sep 2 (epub).
62. VR Aroda et al. Effect of adding insulin degludec to treatment in patients with type 2 diabetes inadequately controlled with metformin and liraglutide: a double-blind randomized controlled trial (BEGIN: ADD TO GLP-1 Study). Diabetes Obes Metab 2016; 18:663.
63. VR Aroda et al. Efficacy and safety of LixiLan, a titratable fixed-ratio combination of insulin glargine plus lixisenatide in type 2 diabetes inadequately controlled on basal insulin and metformin: the LixiLan-L randomized trial. Diabetes Care 2016; 39:1972.
64. RR Holman et al. Three-year efficacy of complex insulin regimens in type 2 diabetes. N Engl J Med 2009; 361:1736.
65. American Diabetes Association. Professional practice committee for the standards of medical care in diabetes - 2016. Management of diabetes in pregnancy. Diabetes Care 2016; 39(Suppl 1):S94.
66. RR Holman et al. Effects of once-weekly exenatide on cardio-vascular outcomes in type 2 diabetes. N Engl J Med 2017; 377:1228.
67. M Fisher et al. Cardiovascular safety of albiglutide in the Harmony programme: a meta-analysis. Lancet Diabetes Edocrinol 2015; 3:697.

68. KC Ferdinand et al. Cardiovascular safety for once-weekly dulaglutide in type 2 diabetes: a pre-specified meta-analysis of prospectively adjudicated cardiovascular events. Cardiovasc Diabetol 2016; 15:38.
69. C Sorli et al. Lancet diabetes efficacy and safety of once-weekly semaglutide monotherapy versus placebo in patients with type 2 diabetes (SUSTAIN 1): a double-blind, randomised, placebo-controlled, parallel-group, multinational multicentre phase 3a trial. Endocrinol 2017; 5:251.
70. B Ahrén et al. Efficacy and safety of once-weekly semaglutide versus once-daily sitagliptin as an add-on to metformin, thiazolidinediones, or both, in patients with type 2 diabetes (SUSTAIN 2): a 56-week, double-blind, phase 3a, randomised trial. Lancet Diabetes Endocrinol 2017; 5:341.
71. AJ Ahmann et al. Efficacy and safety of once-weekly semaglutide versus exenatide ER in subjects with type 2 diabetes (SUSTAIN 3): a 56-week, open-label, randomized clinical trial. Diabetes Care 2018; 41:258.
72. VR Aroda et al. Efficacy and safety of once-weekly semaglutide versus once-daily insulin glargine as add-on to metformin (with or without sulfonylureas) in insulin-naive patients with type 2 diabetes (SUSTAIN 4): a randomised, open-label, parallel-group, multicentre, multinational, phase 3a trial. Lancet Diabetes Endocrinol 2017; 5:355.
73. H Rodbard et al. Efficacy and safety of semaglutide once-weekly vs placebo as add-on to basal insulin alone or in combination with metformin in subjects with type 2 diabetes (SUSTAIN 5). Diabetologia 2016; 59:S364 suppl. Abstract 766.
74. RE Pratleyet et al. Semaglutide versus dulaglutide once weekly in patients with type 2 diabetes (SUSTAIN 7): a randomized, open-label, phase 3b trial. Lancet Diabetes Endocrinol 2018 Jan 31 (epub).
75. SP Marso et al. Semaglutide and cardiovascular outcomes in patients with type 2 diabetes. N Engl J Med 2016; 375:1834.
76. MA Bethel et al. Cardiovascular outcomes with glucagon-like peptide-1 receptor agonists in patients with type 2 diabetes: a meta-analysis. Lancet Diabetes Endocrinol 2017; 6:105.
77. B Neal et al. Canagliflozin and cardiovascular and renal events in type 2 diabetes. N Engl J Med 2017; 377:644.
78. Ertugliflozin for type 2 diabetes. Med Lett Drugs Ther 2018; 60:70.

DRUGS FOR Epilepsy

Original publication date – July 2017

Treatment of epilepsy should begin with a single antiepileptic drug (AED), increasing its dosage gradually until seizures are controlled or adverse effects become intolerable. If seizures persist, specialists generally recommend trying at least one and sometimes a second alternative drug as monotherapy before considering use of two drugs concurrently. When used for the appropriate seizure type, AEDs are roughly equivalent in efficacy. Drug choice is usually based on factors such as ease of use, adverse effects, drug interactions, presence of comorbidities, and cost.

Newer AEDs are often initially approved by the FDA only as adjunctive therapy for partial seizures, but they are commonly used off-label for treatment of other types of seizures and as monotherapy.

NEW TERMINOLOGY — In the revised International League Against Epilepsy (ILAE) classification of seizure types, "partial" is replaced with "focal" and "primary generalized" with "bilateral tonic-clonic."[1]

BRIVARACETAM — Brivaracetam *(Briviact),* an analog of levetiracetam, is FDA-approved for treatment of partial seizures in patients ≥16 years old.[2] Like levetiracetam, it may also prove to be effective for treatment of primary generalized, absence, and myoclonic seizures, but more studies are needed.[3]

Table 1. Treatment of Epilepsy[1]

Drugs of Choice	Some Alternatives
Partial, Including Secondarily Generalized Seizures[2]	
Drugs of Choice:	**Some Alternatives:**
Carbamazepine	Brivaracetam
Lamotrigine	Clobazam
Levetiracetam	Eslicarbazepine
Oxcarbazepine	Gabapentin
	Lacosamide
	Perampanel
	Phenytoin
	Pregabalin
	Topiramate
	Valproate
	Zonisamide
Primary Generalized Tonic-Clonic Seizures[2]	
Drugs of Choice:	**Some Alternatives:**
Lamotrigine	Perampanel
Levetiracetam	Topiramate
Valproate	Zonisamide
Absence Seizures	
Drugs of Choice:	**Some Alternatives:**
Ethosuximide	Clonazepam
Valproate	Lamotrigine
	Levetiracetam
	Zonisamide
Atypical Absence, Myoclonic, Atonic Seizures	
Drugs of Choice:	**Some Alternatives:**
Lamotrigine	Clobazam
Levetiracetam	Clonazepam
Valproate	Felbamate
	Rufinamide
	Topiramate
	Zonisamide

1. Some of the drugs listed here have not been approved by the FDA for such use. Approved indications can be found in the text.
2. In the revised International League Against Epilepsy (ILAE) classification of seizure types, "partial" is replaced with "focal" and "primary generalized" with "bilateral tonic-clonic." Fisher et al. Epilepsia 2017; 58:531.

Adverse Effects – In clinical trials, the most common adverse effects of brivaracetam were somnolence, dizziness, fatigue, and nausea/vomiting. Psychiatric adverse effects (mainly anxiety and depression) have occurred; whether they occur at a similar rate as with levetiracetam is unclear.

Drug Interactions – Coadministration of rifampin (*Rifadin*, and generics) decreases serum concentrations of brivaracetam; the dose of brivaracetam may need to be increased by up to 100%. Brivaracetam increases serum concentrations of phenytoin and an active metabolite of carbamazepine; dosage reductions may be needed. Brivaracetam is a substrate of CYP2C19; patients who are CYP2C19 poor metabolizers or are taking CYP2C19 inhibitors may require reductions in the dosage of brivaracetam.[4]

CARBAMAZEPINE — Carbamazepine (*Tegretol*, and generics) is an older AED with broad indications for use as an anticonvulsant. It is particularly effective for treatment of partial and secondarily generalized tonic-clonic seizures, but it may worsen absence or myoclonic seizures. Carbamazepine induces its own metabolism; serum concentrations often fall after a few weeks of treatment. Storing carbamazepine tablets (both brand and generic) in humid conditions can cause concretion of the tablets, resulting in poor bioavailability and therapeutic failure. Carbamazepine is generally administered as an extended-release formulation (*Tegretol XR*, and generics), which allows for twice-daily dosing. It is also available in an IV formulation *(Carnexiv)*.

Other Uses – Oral carbamazepine is FDA-approved for treatment of pain due to trigeminal neuralgia. *Equetro* is also approved for treatment of acute manic or mixed episodes of bipolar I disorder.

Adverse Effects – Carbamazepine can cause drowsiness, impaired cognition, blurred vision, diplopia, headache, dizziness, ataxia, nausea, and vomiting. Use of an extended-release formulation has been associated with fewer CNS adverse effects.

Table 2. Some Oral Antiepileptic Drugs

Drug	Some Oral Formulations
Brivaracetam – *Briviact* (UCB)	10, 25, 50, 75, 100 mg tabs; 10 mg/mL, 50 mg/5 mL oral soln
Carbamazepine – generic	200 mg tabs; 100 mg chewable tabs;
Tegretol (Novartis)	100 mg/5 mL susp
extended release – generic	100, 200 mg ER caps and tabs; 300 mg ER caps, 400 mg ER tabs
Tegretol XR	100, 200, 400 mg ER tabs
Carbatrol (Shire)	100, 200, 300 mg ER caps
Equetro (Validus)	100, 200, 300 mg ER caps
Clobazam – *Onfi* (Lundbeck)	10, 20 mg tabs; 2.5 mg/mL susp
Clonazepam – generic	0.5, 1, 2 mg tabs; 0.125, 0.25, 0.5, 1, 2 mg ODTs
Klonopin (Genentech)	0.5, 1, 2 mg tabs
Eslicarbazepine – *Aptiom* (Sunovion)	200, 400, 600, 800 mg tabs
Ethosuximide – generic	250 mg caps; 250 mg/5 mL syrup
Zarontin (Pfizer)	
Felbamate – generic	400, 600 mg tabs; 600 mg/5 mL susp
Felbatol (Meda)	
Gabapentin – generic	100, 300, 400 mg caps; 600, 800 mg tabs;
Neurontin (Pfizer)	250 mg/5 mL soln

ER = extended-release; ODT = orally disintegrating tablet

1. Most antiepileptic drugs (AEDs) are started at a low dose and slowly titrated over a period of weeks. The usual dosage may vary depending on whether the drug is prescribed as monotherapy or adjunctive therapy, or is used concomitantly with one or more interacting drugs. Dosage may also need to be adjusted for renal or hepatic impairment.
2. Approximate WAC for 30 days' treatment at the lowest usual adult maintenance dosage using the smallest whole number of dosage units. WAC = wholesaler acquisition cost or manufacturer's published price to wholesalers; WAC represents a published catalogue or list price and may not represent an actual transactional price. Source: AnalySource® Monthly. July 5, 2017. Reprinted with permission by First Databank, Inc. All rights reserved. ©2017. www.fdbhealth.com/policies/drug-pricing-policy.

Usual Adult Maintenance Dosage[1]	Usual Pediatric Maintenance Dosage[1]	Cost[2]
50-200 mg/d in 2 divided doses	Not approved for patients <16 years old	$1000.10
800-1600 mg/d in 2 or 3 divided doses[3] 800-1600 mg/d in 2 divided doses[3]	<6 yrs: 20-35 mg/kg/d in 3 or 4 divided doses[3] 6-12 yrs: 400-1000 mg/d in 3 or 4 divided doses (2 doses if ER)[3]	100.00 263.20 273.80 281.00 212.70 435.80
10-60 mg once/d or in 2 divided doses	5-20 mg once/d or in 2 divided doses	949.40
1.5-8 mg/d in 2 or 3 divided doses	<10 yrs or <30 kg: 0.1-0.2 mg/kg/d in 2 or 3 divided doses	3.90 161.30
800 mg once/d	≥4 yrs: 11-21 kg: 400-600 mg/d 22-31 kg: 500-800 mg/d 32-38 kg: 600-900 mg/d >38 kg: 800-1200 mg/d	834.90
750-1250 mg/d in 2 divided doses	20-30 mg/kg/d in 2 or 3 divided doses	118.50 304.20
2400-3600 mg/d in 3 or 4 divided doses[4]	2-14 yrs: 30-45 mg/kg/d in 3 or 4 divided doses[4,5]	586.50 1500.00
1800-3600 mg/d in 3 divided doses	3-4 yrs: 40 mg/kg/d in 3 divided doses 5-11 yrs: 25-35 mg/kg/d in 3 divided doses	47.80 830.20

3. Measurement of serum concentrations may be useful to guide therapy. Some usual therapeutic serum concentrations are: carbamazepine 4-12 mcg/mL, phenobarbital 10-40 mcg/mL, phenytoin 10-20 mcg/mL, valproate 50-100 mcg/mL. Some patients achieve complete seizure control at lower concentrations, and some may need higher concentrations.
4. When felbamate is added as adjunctive therapy, the doses of other antiepileptic drugs should be reduced by 20%.
5. In children 2-14 years old, only FDA-approved for adjunctive treatment of Lennox-Gastaut syndrome.

Continued on next page

Table 2. Some Oral Antiepileptic Drugs (continued)	
Drug	**Some Oral Formulations**
Lacosamide – *Vimpat* (UCB)	50, 100, 150, 200 mg tabs; 10 mg/mL soln
Lamotrigine – generic *Lamictal* (GSK) extended release – generic *Lamictal XR*	25, 100, 150, 200, 250 mg tabs; 2, 5, 25 mg chewable tabs; 25, 50, 100, 200 mg ODTs 25, 50, 100, 200, 250, 300 mg ER tabs
Levetiracetam – generic *Keppra* (UCB) *Spritam* (Aprecia) extended release – generic *Keppra XR*	250, 500, 750, 1000 mg tabs; 100 mg/mL soln 250, 500, 750, 1000 mg tabs 500, 750 mg ER tabs
Oxcarbazepine – generic *Trileptal* (Novartis)	150, 300, 600 mg tabs; 300 mg/5 mL susp
extended release – *Oxtellar XR* (Supernus)	150, 300, 600 mg ER tabs
Perampanel – *Fycompa* (Eisai)	2, 4, 6, 8, 10, 12 mg tabs; 0.5 mg/mL oral susp
Phenobarbital – generic	15, 30, 60, 100 mg tabs; 20 mg/5 mL elixir
Phenytoin – generic *Dilantin* (Pfizer) *Phenytek* (Mylan)	30, 100, 200, 300 mg caps; 125 mg/5 mL susp; 50 mg chewable tabs 30, 100 mg caps; 125 mg/5 mL susp; 50 mg chewable tabs 200, 300 mg caps

ER = extended-release; ODT = orally disintegrating tablet

6. Maximum 300 mg/d. The recommended dosage for patients taking valproate is 1-5 mg/kg once daily or in 2 divided doses (maximum 200 mg/d; 1-3 mg/kg/d for patients taking lamotrigine and valproate without other antiepileptic drugs). The recommended dosage for patients taking lamotrigine with carbamazepine, phenytoin, phenobarbital, or primidone, but not with valproate, is 5-15 mg/kg/d in 2 divided doses (maximum 400 mg/d).

Usual Adult Maintenance Dosage[1]	Usual Pediatric Maintenance Dosage[1]	Cost[2]
200-400 mg/d in 2 divided doses	Not approved for patients <17 years old	$830.50
100-500 mg/d in 2 divided doses	2-12 yrs: 4.5-7.5 mg/kg/d in 2 divided doses[6]	17.80 794.20
200-600 mg once/d	Not approved for patients <13 years old	301.80 698.50
500-1500 mg bid	4-<16 yrs: 30 mg/kg bid	22.50 458.30 463.70
1000-3000 mg once/d	Not approved for patients <12 years old	42.50 415.40
1200-2400 mg/d in 2 or 3 divided doses	2-<4 yrs: 30-60 mg/kg/d in 2 or 3 divided doses (max 600 mg/d) 4-16 yrs: 20-29 kg: 450 mg bid 30-39 kg: 600 mg bid 40-49 kg: 900 mg bid	72.10 833.00
1200-2400 mg once/d	≥6 yrs: 20-29 kg: 900 mg once/d 30-39 kg: 1200 mg once/d 40-49 kg: 1800 mg once/d	866.50
4-12 mg once/d	Not approved for patients <12 yrs old	742.50
90-150 mg/d in 2 or 3 divided doses[3]	3-6 mg/kg/d in 2 or 3 divided doses[3]	23.80
300-400 mg/d in 1-3 divided doses[3,7]	4-8 mg/kg/d in 2 or 3 divided doses (max 300 mg/d)[3]	54.10 101.60 60.20

7. Adjustments in maintenance dosage above 300 mg/day for adults should usually be made in 25- or 30-mg increments.

Continued on next page

Table 2. Some Oral Antiepileptic Drugs (continued)	
Drug	**Some Oral Formulations**
Pregabalin – *Lyrica* (Pfizer)	25, 50, 75, 100, 150, 200, 225, 300 mg caps
Primidone – generic *Mysoline* (Valeant)	50, 250 mg tabs
Rufinamide – *Banzel* (Eisai)	200, 400 mg tabs; 40 mg/mL susp
Topiramate – generic *Topamax* (Janssen) *Topamax Sprinkle* extended release – *Trokendi XR* (Supernus) *Qudexy XR* (Upsher-Smith)	15, 25 mg caps; 25, 50, 100, 200 mg tabs 25, 50, 100, 200 mg tabs 15, 25 mg caps 25, 50, 100, 200 mg ER caps 25, 50, 100, 150, 200 mg ER caps
Valproate Valproic acid – generic *Depakene* (Abbott) Divalproex sodium – generic *Depakote* (Abbott) *Depakote Sprinkle* extended release – generic *Depakote ER*	 250 mg caps; 250 mg/5 mL syrup 125, 250, 500 mg delayed-release tabs; 125 mg caps 125, 250, 500 mg delayed-release tabs 125 mg delayed-release caps 250, 500 mg ER tabs
Vigabatrin – *Sabril* (Lundbeck)	500 mg tabs; 500 mg powder for soln (50 mg/mL)
Zonisamide – generic *Zonegran* (Eisai)	25, 50, 100 mg caps 25, 100 mg caps

ER = extended-release

Mild leukopenia and hyponatremia are fairly common with use of carbamazepine. At high doses, thrombocytopenia can occur, but it is usually reversible with drug discontinuation. Aplastic anemia, agranulocytosis, cardiac toxicity, aseptic meningitis, intractable diarrhea, and hepatitis are rare. Circulating concentrations of thyroid hormones may be reduced even though thyroid stimulating hormone

Usual Adult Maintenance Dosage[1]	Usual Pediatric Maintenance Dosage[1]	Cost[2]
150-600 mg/d in 2 or 3 divided doses	Not approved for pediatric use	$413.20
750-1250 mg/d in 3 or 4 divided doses	<8 yrs: 125-250 mg tid or 10-25 mg/kg/d in divided doses	40.30 3689.40
3200 mg/d in 2 divided doses	45 mg/kg/d in 2 divided doses (max 3200 mg/d)	4776.00
100-400 mg/d in 2 divided doses	5-9 mg/kg/d in 2 divided doses	19.80 625.70 716.90
100-400 mg once/d	≥6 yrs: 5-9 mg/kg once/d	634.60 471.90
1000-3000 mg/d in 2-3 divided doses[3]	≥10 yrs: 20-60 mg/kg/d in 3 divided doses[3]	43.30 558.80 29.10
		361.10 506.80
1250-3500 mg once/d[3]	≥10 yrs: 20-60 mg/kg once/d[3]	253.50 469.80
3 g/d in 2 divided doses	10-16 yrs: 2 g/d in 2 divided doses[8]	21,776.60
100-400 mg once/d or in 2 divided doses	Not approved for patients <16 yrs old	20.50 426.70

8. Patients weighing >60 kg should receive the adult dosage.

(TSH) concentrations remain normal. Abnormal color perception can occur rarely.

Carbamazepine can cause rash, particularly with high starting doses or rapid dose escalation. Severe reactions such as Stevens-Johnson syndrome and toxic epidermal necrolysis have occurred rarely; the risk is significantly higher in patients with the human leukocyte antigen (HLA)-B*1502 allele.[5] The FDA recommends that Asian patients, who have a 10-fold higher incidence than non-Asians of carbamazepine-induced Stevens-Johnson syndrome and toxic epidermal necrolysis, be tested for this allele before starting treatment with carbamazepine.

Drug Interactions – Carbamazepine is a strong inducer of multiple hepatic enzymes; it can reduce serum concentrations and possibly the effectiveness of many other drugs, including oral contraceptives and other AEDs. Carbamazepine is metabolized by CYP3A4; drugs that induce or inhibit CYP3A4 could affect its serum concentrations.[4]

CLOBAZAM — The benzodiazepine clobazam *(Onfi)* is FDA-approved only for adjunctive treatment of seizures associated with Lennox-Gastaut syndrome in patients ≥2 years old,[6] but it has been widely used for years in Canada and other countries for treatment of anxiety and many other types of seizures.

Adverse Effects – The most common adverse effects of clobazam are somnolence, pyrexia, lethargy, drooling, and constipation. As with other benzodiazepines, anterograde amnesia, ataxia, withdrawal symptoms, and seizures can occur if the drug is stopped abruptly. Clobazam is classified as a schedule IV controlled substance.

Drug Interactions – Clobazam inhibits CYP2D6; it may be necessary to reduce the dosage of CYP2D6 substrates such as fluoxetine (*Prozac*, and generics) if they are taken concurrently. Clobazam is metabolized primarily by CYP3A4 to its active metabolite, which is further metabolized by CYP2C19. Concurrent use of moderate or strong inhibitors of CYP2C19 such as fluconazole (*Diflucan*, and generics) or omeprazole (*Prilosec*, and generics) can increase serum concentrations of the active metabolite.[4]

CLONAZEPAM — The benzodiazepine clonazepam (*Klonopin*, and generics) is FDA-approved for treatment of Lennox-Gastaut syndrome (petit mal variant) and myoclonic and atonic seizures. It is also used to treat absence seizures resistant to other AEDs, but it is generally less effective than ethosuximide or valproate for this indication, and development of tolerance to its effects is common.

Other Uses – Clonazepam is FDA-approved for treatment of panic disorder and is used to treat other types of anxiety disorders.

Adverse Effects – Clonazepam can cause drowsiness, ataxia, and behavior disorders. As with other benzodiazepines, anterograde amnesia, ataxia, withdrawal symptoms, and seizures can occur if the drug is stopped abruptly. Clonazepam is classified as a schedule IV controlled substance.

Drug Interactions – Clonazepam is partially metabolized by CYP3A4; inducers of CYP3A4 such as carbamazepine and phenytoin may decrease serum concentrations of clonazepam, and strong inhibitors such as clarithromycin (*Biaxin*, and generics) can increase them.[4]

ESLICARBAZEPINE — Eslicarbazepine acetate *(Aptiom)*[7] is FDA-approved as monotherapy and adjunctive therapy for partial-onset seizures in patients ≥4 years old.[8] It is rapidly converted to eslicarbazepine, the S-isomer of the active metabolite of oxcarbazepine, which is chemically similar to carbamazepine. The three drugs have similar mechanisms of action, but differ pharmacokinetically and pharmacodynamically.[9]

Adverse Effects – The most common adverse effects of eslicarbazepine are dizziness, somnolence, nausea, headache, diplopia, and tremor. Hyponatremia and serious dermatological reactions including Stevens-Johnson syndrome have been reported; whether these are more or less common than with carbamazepine or oxcarbazepine is unclear.

Drug Interactions – Eslicarbazepine can induce CYP3A4 and inhibit CYP2C19; it can increase serum concentrations of CYP2C19 substrates such as clobazam, and decrease serum concentrations of CYP3A4 substrates such as simvastatin (*Zocor,* and generics) and oral contraceptives.

The INR should be closely monitored in patients taking warfarin (*Coumadin,* and others) concomitantly. Enzyme-inducing drugs, such as carbamazepine, can reduce serum levels of eslicarbazepine. Eslicarbazepine should not be administered concomitantly with oxcarbazepine.

ETHOSUXIMIDE — Ethosuximide (*Zarontin*, and generics) is FDA-approved for treatment of absence seizures and is generally well tolerated.[10] It is not effective for treatment of generalized tonic-clonic or partial seizures.

Adverse Effects – Ethosuximide can cause nausea, vomiting, lethargy, hiccups, headache, and behavioral changes. Psychotic behavior can occur. Hematologic abnormalities, erythema multiforme, Stevens-Johnson syndrome, and systemic lupus erythematosus have been reported.

Drug Interactions – Ethosuximide is partially metabolized by CYP3A4; inducers of CYP3A4 such as carbamazepine and phenytoin may decrease serum concentrations of ethosuximide, and strong inhibitors such as clarithromycin can increase them.[4]

GABAPENTIN — Gabapentin (*Neurontin*, and generics) is FDA-approved for adjunctive treatment of partial seizures with and without secondary generalization in patients ≥3 years old. It is also effective as monotherapy for these seizure types. Like carbamazepine, gabapentin can exacerbate myoclonic seizures. The percentage of gabapentin absorbed from the GI tract decreases at higher doses.

Other Uses – Gabapentin is also FDA-approved for treatment of neuropathic pain. A once-daily formulation *(Gralise)* is approved for treatment of postherpetic neuralgia.[11] Gabapentin enacarbil *(Horizant)*, a prodrug, is approved for restless legs syndrome.[12]

Adverse Effects – Gabapentin can cause somnolence, dizziness, ataxia, fatigue, nystagmus, blurred vision, and confusion. Edema, weight gain, and movement disorders have been reported. Behavioral changes have occurred in children, especially those with underlying behavioral or developmental problems.

Drug Interactions – Unlike some other AEDs, gabapentin does not induce or inhibit CYP isozymes, and is not appreciably metabolized.

LACOSAMIDE — Oral lacosamide (*Vimpat*, and generics) is FDA-approved as monotherapy or adjunctive therapy for adults with partial onset seizures.[13] Lacosamide is also available in an IV formulation for short-term use.

Adverse Effects – The most common adverse effects of oral lacosamide have been dizziness, headache, nausea, vomiting, fatigue, ataxia, diplopia, somnolence, and tremor. Lacosamide is classified as a schedule V controlled substance because of reports of euphoria.

Drug Interactions – Lacosamide is a substrate and inhibitor of CYP2C19, but no clinically significant drug interactions have been reported. The drug can cause a small, dose-dependent increase in the PR interval; caution is advised in patients with cardiac conduction abnormalities and in those taking other drugs that may prolong the PR interval, such as beta blockers or calcium channel blockers.

LAMOTRIGINE — Lamotrigine (*Lamictal*, and generics) is FDA-approved for adjunctive treatment of patients ≥2 years old with partial seizures, primary generalized tonic-clonic seizures, or generalized seizures of Lennox-Gastaut syndrome. It is commonly used for secondarily generalized seizures, primary generalized tonic-clonic seizures, and atypical absence, myoclonic, and atonic seizures. In elderly patients with newly diagnosed partial or generalized seizures, lamotrigine has been as effective as carbamazepine and better tolerated.[14] Although generally effective for treatment of myoclonic seizures, some reports suggest that lamotrigine can make myoclonus worse, particularly in severe myoclonic epilepsy of infancy. Lamotrigine may be less effective than ethosuximide or valproate for treatment of absence seizures in children, but some clinicians use it as first-line treatment because of its tolerability.[15]

Adverse Effects – The most common adverse effects of lamotrigine have been dizziness, ataxia, somnolence, headache, diplopia, nausea, vomiting, rash, insomnia, and incoordination. Lamotrigine causes fewer adverse cognitive effects than carbamazepine or topiramate. Acute hepatitis and aseptic meningitis have been reported. Life-threatening rashes including Stevens-Johnson syndrome have occurred rarely, usually during the first two months of use. The risk may be increased by high starting doses, rapid increases in dosage, or coadministration with valproate. The manufacturer recommends discontinuing lamotrigine at the first sign of rash.

Drug Interactions – Lamotrigine does not induce or inhibit CYP isozymes. Enzyme-inducing drugs, such as carbamazepine reduce lamotrigine serum concentrations by about 40%. Valproate increases lamotrigine concentrations more than 2-fold.

LEVETIRACETAM — Oral levetiracetam (*Keppra*, and generics) is FDA-approved as adjunctive therapy for patients ≥1 month old with partial seizures, patients ≥6 years old with primary generalized tonic-clonic seizures, and patients ≥12 years old with myoclonic seizures. It is commonly used, however, as monotherapy for partial and generalized seizures and may also be effective in absence seizures and in Lennox-Gastaut syndrome. A rapidly-disintegrating oral levetiracetam tablet *(Spritam)* is approved for the same indications, except that in partial seizures it is only approved for use in patients ≥4 years old.[16] Levetiracetam is also available in an IV formulation.

Adverse Effects – Dizziness, somnolence, and weakness occur commonly. Behavioral changes such as agitation, hostility and irritability, hallucinations, and psychosis have also occurred, especially in patients with underlying psychiatric disorders. Coordination difficulties and serious dermatological reactions, including Stevens-Johnson syndrome and toxic epidermal necrolysis, have been reported. Mild decreases in white blood cell count and hematocrit, which do not require discontinuation of the drug, occur rarely. Levetiracetam appears to have a low incidence of adverse cognitive effects.

Drug Interactions – Levetiracetam does not induce or inhibit CYP isozymes, and is not appreciably metabolized. No clinically significant drug interactions have been reported.

OXCARBAZEPINE — Oxcarbazepine (*Trileptal*, and generics) is FDA-approved as monotherapy or adjunctive therapy for partial seizures in patients ≥4 years old, and as adjunctive therapy in children 2-3 years old. The extended-release formulation *(Oxtellar XR)* is approved for adjunctive treatment of partial seizures in patients ≥6 years old. Oxcarbazepine is chemically similar to carbamazepine, but it causes less induction of hepatic enzymes and does not induce its own metabolism. Its clinical effect is mostly due to its 10-monohydroxy (MHD) metabolite, which has a half-life of 8-10 hours. Like carbamazepine, oxcarbazepine is effective for treatment of secondarily generalized seizures, but may worsen myoclonic and absence seizures. Oxcarbazepine has been as effective as carbamazepine for treatment of partial seizures and may be better tolerated.

Other Uses – Oxcarbazepine is used off-label for treatment of bipolar disorder and neuropathic pain.

Adverse Effects – Common adverse effects of oxcarbazepine are somnolence, dizziness, diplopia, ataxia, nausea, and vomiting. Taking the extended-release formulation with food increases peak concentrations of the drug and the likelihood of adverse effects. Stevens-Johnson syndrome and toxic epidermal necrolysis have occurred, and multi-organ hypersensitivity reactions have been reported. Cross-reactivity with carbamazepine hypersensitivity occurs in 20-30% of patients. Hyponatremia is more common with oxcarbazepine than with carbamazepine.

Drug Interactions – Oxcarbazepine induces CYP3A4/5 and inhibits CYP2C19.[4] It can increase phenytoin levels by up to 40%. Levels of its active metabolite are reduced in the presence of enzyme-inducing drugs such as phenobarbital or phenytoin. Oxcarbazepine should not be administered concomitantly with eslicarbazepine.

PERAMPANEL — Perampanel *(Fycompa)* is FDA-approved for adjunctive treatment of partial seizures and primary generalized tonic-clonic seizures in patients ≥12 years old.[17-19]

Adverse Effects – The most common adverse effects of perampanel are dizziness and drowsiness. Weight gain, ataxia, dysarthria, diplopia, vertigo, nausea, and fatigue have also been reported. Serious psychiatric and behavioral reactions, including irritability, aggression, anger, mood changes, and anxiety can occur.

Drug Interactions – Perampanel is partially metabolized by CYP3A; inhibitors of CYP3A such as clarithromycin may increase serum concentrations of perampanel, and CYP3A inducers such as carbamazepine can decrease them.[4]

PHENYTOIN — Phenytoin (*Dilantin*, and generics) is as effective as carbamazepine for treatment of partial and secondarily generalized tonic-clonic seizures, but it is no longer considered a drug of choice because of its complicated pharmacokinetics, adverse effects, and many drug interactions. Different formulations of phenytoin may not be bioequivalent, especially at higher doses. Fosphenytoin (*Cerebyx*, and generics) is a water-soluble prodrug of phenytoin available for IV and IM use.

Adverse Effects – Nystagmus may occur with therapeutic serum concentrations of phenytoin and is usually present at higher concentrations. Drowsiness, ataxia, and diplopia are more likely to occur at serum concentrations >20 mcg/mL, but can also occur at lower levels, particularly in patients with low serum albumin levels and in the elderly. Phenytoin may interfere with cognitive function. Cerebellar atrophy has been reported with long-term use and after acute intoxication.

A morbilliform or scarlatiniform rash may occur, usually in the first four weeks of treatment, sometimes with hepatitis, fever, and lymphadenopathy; rarely, it progresses to exfoliative dermatitis or Stevens-Johnson syndrome. Asian patients who test positive for the HLA-B*1502 allele may have an increased risk of serious skin reactions with phenytoin or fosphenytoin. Patients who develop hypersensitivity reactions to phenytoin are often susceptible to developing similar reactions with carbamazepine and phenobarbital.

Less common adverse effects include megaloblastic anemia, a lupus-like syndrome, peripheral neuropathy, nephritis, and hepatitis leading rarely to fatal hepatic necrosis. Osteopenia, gingival hyperplasia, coarsening of facial features, and hirsutism can occur with long-term use. Serum folic acid, thyroxine, and vitamin K concentrations may decrease with long-term therapy. Fosphenytoin is less likely to cause soft-tissue injury than older IV formulations, but rapid infusion can cause transient paresthesias and pruritus.

Drug Interactions – Phenytoin is metabolized by CYP2C9 and CYP2C19; inducers and inhibitors of these enzymes may affect its serum concentrations.[4] Like carbamazepine, phenytoin is a strong enzyme inducer; it can reduce serum concentrations and possibly the effectiveness of many other drugs, including oral contraceptives and other AEDs. Phenytoin may initially cause an increase in response to warfarin, followed by a reduction in its anticoagulant effect.

PREGABALIN — Pregabalin *(Lyrica)* is FDA-approved for adjunctive treatment of partial seizures in adults.[20] Its mechanism of action is similar to that of gabapentin, suggesting it will not be useful in the treatment of myoclonic seizures. A randomized trial comparing pregabalin and gabapentin in patients with refractory focal seizures suggested similar efficacy.[21]

Other Uses – Pregabalin is also FDA-approved for treatment of neuropathic pain and fibromyalgia.[22] It has been used off-label for treatment of generalized anxiety disorder; the drug is approved in Europe for this indication.

Adverse Effects – Pregabalin can cause somnolence, dizziness, ataxia, weight gain, dry mouth, blurred vision, peripheral edema, and confusion. Myoclonus has developed in patients with epilepsy taking pregabalin. Pregabalin is classified as a schedule V controlled substance because of reports of euphoria.

Drug Interactions – Like gabapentin, pregabalin does not induce or inhibit CYP isozymes, and is not appreciably metabolized.

RUFINAMIDE — Rufinamide (*Banzel,* and generics) is FDA-approved for adjunctive treatment of Lennox-Gastaut syndrome in patients ≥1 year old.[23] It appears to be particularly effective for treatment of tonic-atonic seizures.[24] There is also evidence that adjunctive treatment with rufinamide reduces the frequency of partial seizures.[25]

Adverse Effects – The most frequent adverse effects of rufinamide have been somnolence and vomiting. Headache, dizziness, fatigue, nausea, diplopia, and tremor have been reported. Rufinamide can shorten the QT interval in some patients; it should not be used in patients with short QT syndrome or in those taking other drugs known to shorten the QT interval, such as digoxin (*Lanoxin*, and others) and magnesium.

Drug Interactions – Rufinamide is a mild inducer of CYP3A4. It has been shown to reduce ethinyl estradiol, norethindrone, and triazolam (*Halcion*, and generics) serum concentrations, and could have a similar effect on other drugs metabolized by CYP3A4.

TOPIRAMATE — Topiramate (*Topamax*, and generics; *Qudexy XR*[26]; *Trokendi XR*) is FDA-approved as monotherapy or adjunctive therapy for partial and primary generalized tonic-clonic seizures in patients ≥2 years old. It is also approved for adjunctive treatment of children ≥2 years old with Lennox-Gastaut syndrome and is effective for treatment of atonic seizures in children.[27] *Trokendi XR* is approved for the same indications in patients ≥6 years old.[28]

Other Uses – Topiramate (*Topamax,* and generics) is also FDA-approved for migraine prophylaxis,[29] and is available in a fixed-dose combination with phentermine *(Qsymia)* for chronic weight management.[30]

Adverse Effects – The most common adverse effects of topiramate are drowsiness, dizziness, headache, and ataxia. Nervousness, confusion, paresthesias, weight loss, and diplopia can occur. Psychomotor slowing, word-finding difficulty, impaired concentration, and interference with memory are common, particularly with rapid dose escalation and higher maintenance doses, and may require dosage reduction or drug discontinuation. Acute myopia associated with secondary angle-closure glaucoma, which is infrequent but severe, typically occurs within one month of starting the drug. Hepatic failure, oligohidrosis, hyperthermia, and heat stroke have been reported. Topiramate is a mild carbonic anhydrase inhibitor and can cause metabolic acidosis, which increases the risk of symptomatic renal stones.

Drug Interactions – Topiramate is a mild inducer of CYP3A and an inhibitor of CYP2C19. It can increase serum lithium levels, particularly at high doses. Carbamazepine and phenytoin decrease topiramate serum concentrations. Coadministration of valproic acid and topiramate has been associated with hyperammonemia and hypothermia. Use of topiramate with other carbonic anhydrase inhibitors such as zonisamide or acetazolamide could increase the severity of metabolic acidosis.

VALPROATE — Valproic acid (*Depakene*, and generics) and divalproex sodium (*Depakote*, and generics) dissociate to valproate in the GI tract. Valproate products are FDA-approved as monotherapy or adjunctive therapy for complex partial seizures and absence seizures and as adjunctive therapy for multiple seizure types that involve absence. Because valproate is effective and usually well tolerated, it is widely used to treat myoclonic and atonic seizures and is considered a drug of choice for primary generalized tonic-clonic seizures. It is highly effective in treating photosensitive epilepsy and juvenile myoclonic epilepsy. Valproate is less effective than carbamazepine in controlling complex partial seizures, but equally effective in controlling secondarily generalized seizures.

A once-daily extended-release formulation of divalproex sodium (*Depakote ER*, and generics) is as effective as *Depakote*. It is not bioequivalent to other formulations; when switching from valproate capsules or delayed-release tablets to *Depakote ER*, the daily dose should be increased by 8-20%. Valproate is also available in an IV formulation (*Depacon,* and generics).

Other Uses – Valproate is FDA-approved for migraine prophylaxis and divalproex sodium is approved for treatment of manic episodes of bipolar disorder.

Adverse Effects – Drowsiness caused by valproate is usually mild and transient, and adverse cognitive effects are generally minimal. Nausea and vomiting can be minimized by using the enteric-coated formulation (*Depakote*, and generics), by taking the drug with food, and by slow titration to an optimal dose. Weight gain is common. Use of valproate has been associated with polycystic ovary syndrome, hyperinsulinemia, lipid abnormalities, hirsutism, and menstrual disturbances in women, and with increased serum androgen concentrations in men. Dose-related tremor, transient hair thinning and loss, decreased platelet function, and thrombocytopenia can also occur.

Serious adverse effects of valproate are uncommon, but fatal liver failure has occurred, particularly in children <2 years old taking valproate in combination with other AEDs and in patients with developmental delays and/or metabolic disorders; liver failure has also been reported in older children and adults taking valproate alone. Valproate can interfere with conversion of ammonia to urea, causing lethargy associated with hyperammonemia. Fatal hyperammonemic encephalopathy has occurred in patients with genetic defects in urea metabolism; the drug is contraindicated in these patients. Life-threatening pancreatitis, interstitial nephritis, reversible parkinsonism, and edema requiring diuretics have occurred rarely.

Drug Interactions – Valproate interacts with fewer drugs than carbamazepine or phenytoin. Enzyme-inducing AEDs increase valproate clearance. Carbapenem antibiotics such as imipenem may significantly reduce valproate serum concentrations. Valproate is a weak enzyme inhibitor; it can increase serum concentrations of some other AEDs, including carbamazepine, phenytoin, phenobarbital, ethosuximide, lamotrigine, and rufinamide, and of tricyclic antidepressants.

ZONISAMIDE — Zonisamide (*Zonegran*, and others) is FDA-approved for adjunctive treatment of partial seizures in adults. It appears to have a broad spectrum of activity (infantile spasms, myoclonic, generalized, and atypical absence seizures), and there is considerable experience worldwide with its use as monotherapy for various seizure types and in children.

Other Uses – Zonisamide also appears to be effective for migraine prophylaxis and for weight loss in obese patients, but it is not FDA-approved for these indications.[31,32]

Adverse Effects – Adverse effects of zonisamide include somnolence, dizziness, confusion, anorexia, nausea, diarrhea, weight loss, agitation, irritability, and rash. Fatal Stevens-Johnson syndrome and toxic epidermal necrolysis have been reported. Oligohidrosis, hyperthermia, and heat stroke have occurred in children. Psychosis, psychomotor slowing, word-finding difficulty, and impaired concentration can occur. Aplastic anemia and agranulocytosis have been reported. Slow titration and taking the drug with food may decrease the incidence of adverse effects. Zonisamide is a mild carbonic anhydrase inhibitor and can cause metabolic acidosis, which increases the risk of symptomatic renal stones.

Drug Interactions – Zonisamide is metabolized by CYP3A4; drugs that induce or inhibit CYP3A4 could affect its serum concentrations.[4] Zonisamide does not inhibit CYP isozymes. Use of zonisamde with other carbonic anhydrase inhibitors such as topiramate could increase the risk of renal stone formation.

OTHER DRUGS — **Felbamate** (*Felbatol,* and generics) is FDA-approved as monotherapy and adjunctive therapy for partial and secondarily generalized seizures, and for adjunctive treatment of seizures associated with Lennox-Gastaut syndrome in patients whose disease has not responded to other drugs. Aplastic anemia and hepatic failure have occurred rarely.

Phenobarbital and **primidone** (*Mysoline*, and generics) are effective for treatment of partial and secondarily generalized tonic-clonic seizures, but they have a higher incidence of sedation than other drugs.

Tiagabine (*Gabitril,* and generics) is FDA-approved for adjunctive treatment of partial seizures. It has GI and CNS adverse effects. Off-label use for treatment of bipolar disorder, anxiety, and neuropathic pain in nonepileptic patients has been associated with development of new-onset seizures and status epilepticus.[33]

Vigabatrin *(Sabril)* is FDA-approved as monotherapy for infantile spasms and as adjunctive treatment for complex partial seizures refractory to several other AEDs.[34] It is only available through a restricted distribution program due to concerns about retinal toxicity and permanent visual field loss.

Diazepam rectal gel *(Diastat AcuDial)* is approved for intermittent treatment of increased seizure activity in patients taking other antiepileptic drugs. When given rectally, diazepam is rapidly and completely absorbed. At-home use of rectal diazepam in children may help terminate seizure activity and reduce emergency room visits.[35]

CANNABIS — Cannabidiol, a major cannabinoid found in cannabis, has been effective in reducing the frequency of drug-related seizures in children with Dravet syndrome.[36] Data are insufficient to recommend use of any cannabinoid for treatment of patients with more common types of epilepsy.

OTHER ISSUES — Suicidality – The results of a large cohort study in the US suggest that patients taking gabapentin, lamotrigine, oxcarbazepine, or tiagabine are at greater risk of suicidal acts than those taking topiramate or carbamazepine.[37] In a cohort study in the UK, use of AEDs in patients with epilepsy was not associated with an increased risk of suicide-related events, but an increased risk was seen in patients with depression taking AEDs.[38]

Bone Density – Prolonged use of AEDs, particularly those that induce hepatic enzymes (phenytoin, carbamazepine, phenobarbital, primidone), may increase the risk of osteoporosis. Valproate has also been associated with decreases in bone mineral density.

AEDs and Oral Contraceptives – Enzyme-inducing AEDs such as carbamazepine, phenytoin, primidone, and phenobarbital and, to a lesser extent, felbamate, topiramate, oxcarbazepine, eslicarbazepine, rufinamide, clobazam, and perampanel, may decrease serum concentrations of estrogens and/or progestins, possibly resulting in contraceptive failure.[39] Hormonal contraceptives may increase seizure frequency in some women with epilepsy.[40]

AEDs and Pregnancy – The risk to offspring from taking AEDs is generally considered to be less than the risk of seizures during pregnancy.[41] Most pregnant women exposed to AEDs deliver infants without birth defects, but fetal exposure to older AEDs, particularly valproate and phenobarbital, can cause congenital anomalies, including oral cleft, cardiac, urinary tract, and neural tube defects.[42] Exposure to valproate *in utero* has also been associated with lower IQ scores and an increased risk of autism.[43,44] Topiramate appears to increase the risk of oral cleft defects[45] and has been associated with hypospadias.

Pregnancy itself tends to induce the metabolism of AEDs, particularly lamotrigine; monitoring lamotrigine serum concentrations may improve seizure control.[46] Use of an enzyme-inducing AED such as phenytoin, carbamazepine, phenobarbital, or primidone may cause neonatal hemorrhage due to vitamin K deficiency; all newborns should receive vitamin K at delivery.[47] Vitamin K supplementation has been recommended for the mother in the final month of pregnancy, but whether it reduces the risk of hemorrhagic complications is unclear.

Generic Substitution – Many AEDs are available generically. Generic drugs must meet FDA standards for bioequivalence to their brand-name counterparts (pharmacokinetic parameters within 80-125%) and are usually less expensive. A meta-analysis of randomized controlled trials comparing use of brand-name and generic formulations of phenytoin, carbamazepine, and valproate found no difference in seizure control.[48] A double-blind, randomized, crossover trial of two generic lamotrigine products confirmed their bioequivalence and found no significant change in seizure frequency or adverse effects.[49] When switching to a different manufacturer, variations in the appearance of pills might concern some patients, but in one study, switching to a different manufacturer was not associated with an increased risk of seizures.[50]

1. RS Fisher et al. Instruction manual for the ILAE 2017 operational classification of seizure types. Epilepsia 2017; 58:531.
2. Brivaracetam (Briviact) for epilepsy. Med Lett Drugs Ther 2016; 58:95.
3. P Kwan et al. Adjunctive brivaracetam for uncontrolled focal and generalized epilepsies: results of a phase III, double-blind, randomized, placebo-controlled, flexible-dose trial. Epilepsia 2014: 55:38.
4. Inhibitors and inducers of CYP enzymes and p-glycoprotein. Med Lett Drugs Ther 2017 May 18 (epub). Available at: medicalletter.org/downloads/CYP_PGP_Tables.pdf. Accessed July 18, 2017.
5. P Chen et al. Carbamazepine-induced toxic effects and HLA-B*1502 screening in Taiwan. N Engl J Med 2011; 364:1126.
6. Clobazam (Onfi) for Lennox-Gastaut syndrome. Med Lett Drugs Ther 2012; 54:18.
7. Eslicarbazepine acetate (Aptiom) for epilepsy. Med Lett Drugs Ther 2014; 56:42.
8. MR Sperling et al. Conversion to eslicarbazepine acetate monotherapy: a pooled analysis of 2 phase III studies. Neurology 2016; 86:1095.
9. SD Shorvon et al. Eslicarbazepine acetate: its effectiveness as adjunctive therapy in clinical trials and open studies. J Neurol 2017; 264:421.

10. EP Vining. Ethosuximide in childhood absence epilepsy–older and better. N Engl J Med 2010; 362:843.
11. Once-daily gabapentin (Gralise) for postherpetic neuralgia. Med Lett Drugs Ther 2011; 53:94.
12. Gabapentin enacarbil (Horizant) for restless legs syndrome. Med Lett Drugs Ther 2011; 53:70.
13. Lacosamide for epilepsy. Med Lett Drugs Ther 2009; 51:50.
14. E Saetre et al. Antiepileptic drugs and quality of life in the elderly: results from a randomized double-blind trial of carbamazepine and lamotrigine in patients with onset of epilepsy in old age. Epilepsy Behav 2010; 17:395.
15. TA Glauser et al. Ethosuximide, valproic acid, and lamotrigine in childhood absence epilepsy: initial monotherapy outcomes at 12 months. Epilepsia 2013; 54:141.
16. Spritam – a new formulation of levetiracetam for epilepsy. Med Lett Drugs Ther 2016; 58:78.
17. GL Krauss et al. Randomized phase III study 306: adjunctive perampanel for refractory partial-onset seizures. Neurology 2012; 78:1408.
18. JA French et al. Adjunctive perampanel for refractory partial-onset seizures: randomized phase III study 304. Neurology 2012; 79:589.
19. JA French et al. Evaluation of adjunctive perampanel in patients with refractory partial-onset seizures: results of randomized global phase III study 305. Epilepsia 2013; 54:117.
20. Pregabalin (Lyrica) for neuropathic pain and epilepsy. Med Lett Drugs Ther 2005; 47:75.
21. J French et al. Adjunctive pregabalin vs gabapentin for focal seizures: interpretation of comparative outcomes. Neurology 2016; 87:1242.
22. Pregabalin (Lyrica) for fibromyalgia. Med Lett Drugs Ther 2007; 49:77.
23. Rufinamide (Banzel) for epilepsy. Med Lett Drugs Ther 2009; 51:18.
24. G Kluger et al. Adjunctive rufinamide in Lennox-Gastaut syndrome: a long-term, open-label extension study. Acta Neurol Scand 2010; 122:202.
25. V Biton et al. A randomized, double-blind, placebo-controlled, parallel-group study of rufinamide as adjunctive therapy for refractory partial-onset seizures. Epilepsia 2011; 52:234.
26. In brief: Topiramate extended-release capsules (Qudexy XR). Med Lett Drugs Ther 2014; 56:e126.
27. GD Montouris et al. The efficacy and tolerability of pharmacologic treatment options for Lennox-Gastaut syndrome. Epilepsia 2014; 55 Suppl 4:10.
28. Topiramate extended-release (Trokendi XR) for epilepsy. Med Lett Drugs Ther 2013; 55:87.
29. Topiramate (Topamax) for prevention of migraine. Med Lett Drugs Ther 2005; 47:9.
30. Two drugs for weight loss. Med Lett Drugs Ther 2012; 54:69.
31. SE Mohammadianinejad et al. Zonisamide versus topiramate in migraine prophylaxis: a double-blind randomized clinical trial. Clin Neuropharmacol 2011; 34:174.
32. KM Gadde et al. Zonisamide for weight reduction in obese adults: a 1-year randomized controlled trial. Arch Intern Med 2012; 172:1557.
33. CM Flowers et al. Seizure activity and off-label use of tiagabine. N Engl J Med 2006; 354:773.
34. Vigabatrin (Sabril) for epilepsy. Med Lett Drugs Ther 2010; 52:14.

35. C O'Dell et al. Rectal diazepam gel in the home management of seizures in children. Pediatr Neurol 2005; 33:166.
36. O Devinsky et al. Trial of cannabidiol for drug-resistant seizures in the Dravet syndrome. N Engl J Med 2017; 376:2011.
37. E Patorno et al. Anticonvulsant medications and the risk of suicide, attempted suicide, or violent death. JAMA 2010; 303:1401.
38. A Arana et al. Suicide-related events in patients treated with antiepileptic drugs. N Engl J Med 2010; 363:542.
39. DS Reddy. Clinical pharmacokinetic interactions between antiepileptic drugs and hormonal contraceptives. Expert Rev Clin Pharmacol 2010; 3:183.
40. DS Reddy. Do oral contraceptives increase epileptic seizures? Expert Rev of Neurother 2017; 17:129.
41. CL Harden et al. Practice parameter update: management issues for women with epilepsy–focus on pregnancy (an evidence-based review): teratogenesis and perinatal outcomes: report of the Quality Standards Subcommittee and Therapeutics and Technology Assessment Subcommittee of the American Academy of Neurology and American Epilepsy Society. Neurology 2009; 73:133.
42. J Jentink et al. Valproic acid monotherapy in pregnancy and major congenital malformations. N Engl J Med 2010; 362:2185.
43. KJ Meador et al. Effects of fetal antiepileptic drug exposure: outcomes at age 4.5 years. Neurology 2012; 78:1207.
44. J Christensen et al. Prenatal valproate exposure and risk of autism spectrum disorders and childhood autism. JAMA 2013; 309:1696.
45. S Hernández-Diaz et al. Comparative safety of antiepileptic drugs during pregnancy. Neurology 2012; 78:1692.
46. PB Pennell et al. Lamotrigine in pregnancy: clearance, therapeutic drug monitoring, and seizure frequency. Neurology 2008; 70:2130.
47. CL Harden et al. Practice parameter update: management issues for women with epilepsy–focus on pregnancy (an evidence-based review): vitamin K, folic acid, blood levels, and breastfeeding: report of the Quality Standards Subcommittee and Therapeutics and Technology Assessment Subcommittee of the American Academy of Neurology and American Epilepsy Society. Neurology 2009; 73:142.
48. AS Kesselheim et al. Seizure outcomes following the use of generic versus brand-name antiepileptic drugs: a systematic review and meta-analysis. Drugs 2010; 70:605.
49. MD Privitera et al. Generic-to-generic lamotrigine switches in people with epilepsy: the randomised controlled EQUIGEN trial. Lancet Neurol 2016; 15:365.
50. AS Kesselheim et al. Switching generic antiepileptic drug manufacturer not linked to seizures. Neurology 2016; 87:1796.

DRUGS FOR Hypertension

Original publication date – March 2017 (revised March 2018)

Drugs available for treatment of chronic hypertension in the US and their dosages, adverse effects, and costs are listed in the tables that begin on page 172. Treatment of hypertensive urgencies and emergencies is not discussed here.

GUIDELINES — New guidelines for the treatment of hypertension published in 2017[1] recommend that blood pressure-lowering medication be used for secondary prevention in patients with cardiovascular disease and an average systolic blood pressure (SBP) ≥130 mm Hg or diastolic blood pressure (DBP) ≥80 mm Hg, and for primary prevention in adults with an estimated 10-year atherosclerotic cardiovascular disease (ASCVD) risk[2] of ≥10% and an average SBP ≥130 mm Hg or DBP ≥80 mm Hg. A blood pressure target of <130/80 mm Hg is now recommended for such patients.

For patients with no history of cardiovascular disease and an estimated 10-year ASCVD risk of <10%, blood pressure-lowering medication is recommended for those with an average SBP ≥140 mm Hg or an average DBP ≥90 mm Hg. A blood pressure goal of <130/80 mm Hg[1] may be reasonable for those patients according to the new guideline.

The American Academy of Family Physicians recommends more conservative blood pressure goals for patients >60 years old: a target systolic

Table 1. Initial Monotherapy

General Population	
Non-black	THZD, ACE inhibitor, ARB, or CCB
Black	THZD or CCB
Chronic Kidney Disease (CKD)	
Non-black	ACE inhibitor or ARB
Black	ACE inhibitor or ARB
Diabetes	
Non-black	ACE inhibitor or ARB[1]
Black	THZD or CCB[2]

ACE = angiotensin-converting enzyme; ARB = angiotensin receptor blocker; CCB = calcium channel blocker; THZD = thiazide-like diuretic (chlorthalidone)
1. In the absence of albuminuria, a THZD or a CCB would also be a reasonable choice.
2. Black patients with both diabetes and CKD should receive an ACE inhibitor or an ARB.

blood pressure of <150 mm Hg for most and <140 mm Hg for those at high cardiovascular risk.[3,4]

DIURETICS — Thiazide and thiazide-like diuretics are often used for initial treatment of hypertension. Most positive studies used **chlorthalidone** or **indapamide** and found them to be at least as effective as other antihypertensive agents in reducing cardiovascular and renal risk and superior in preventing heart failure.[6] Chlorthalidone and indapamide have longer durations of action than **hydrochlorothiazide** that persist throughout the nighttime hours, and they have been shown to be more effective.[7] **Metolazone** may be effective in patients with impaired renal function when other thiazide or thiazide-like diuretics are not, but outcomes data are lacking.

Loop diuretics such as **furosemide** can be used instead of thiazide or thiazide-like diuretics to lower blood pressure in patients with moderate to severe renal impairment.[8] **Ethacrynic acid** can be used in patients allergic to sulfonamides (thiazide and loop diuretics other than ethacrynic acid contain sulfonamide moieties).

Recommendations for Treatment of Hypertension
► Guidelines recommend a thiazide-like diuretic (chlorthalidone is preferred), a calcium channel blocker, an angiotensin-converting enzyme (ACE) inhibitor, or an angiotensin receptor blocker (ARB) as initial therapy for the general population of hypertensive patients. ► For black patients, a thiazide-like diuretic or calcium channel blocker is recommended for initial therapy, except for those with chronic kidney disease or heart failure, who should receive an ACE inhibitor or an ARB. ► Beta blockers are only recommended as initial therapy for patients with another indication for a beta blocker, such as coronary heart disease or left ventricular dysfunction. ► Most experts would use an ACE inhibitor or an ARB for initial treatment of hypertension in non-black patients with diabetes. In the absence of albuminuria, a thiazide-like diuretic or a calcium channel blocker would also be a reasonable choice. ► Many patients with hypertension need more than one drug to control their blood pressure. If the first drug does not achieve blood pressure goals, adding a second drug with a different mechanism of action is generally more effective than increasing the dose of the first drug and often allows for use of lower, better tolerated doses of both drugs. ► If an ACE inhibitor or an ARB was used initially, it would be reasonable to add a thiazide-like diuretic such as chlorthalidone, or a calcium channel blocker. Two renin-angiotensin system inhibitors should not be used together. ► When baseline blood pressure is >20/10 mm Hg above goal, many experts would begin therapy with two drugs.

Potassium-sparing diuretics such as **amiloride** and **triamterene** are generally used with other diuretics to prevent or correct hypokalemia. They can cause hyperkalemia, particularly in patients with renal impairment and in those taking ACE inhibitors, ARBs, beta blockers, or aliskiren.

The aldosterone antagonists **spironolactone** and **eplerenone** have both been effective as add-on treatments in patients with refractory hypertension.[9,10] Both drugs are potassium sparing. Eplerenone is selective for the mineralocorticoid receptor; it is less likely than spironolactone to cause gynecomastia at high doses. Both spironolactone and eplerenone

Table 2. Diuretics

Drug	Some Available Oral Formulations
Thiazide and Thiazide-Like	
Chlorthalidone – generic	25, 50 mg tabs
Chlorothiazide – generic	250, 500 mg tabs
Diuril (Salix)	250 mg/5 mL susp
Hydrochlorothiazide – generic	12.5 mg caps; 12.5, 25, 50 mg tabs
Microzide (Allergan)	12.5 mg caps
Indapamide – generic	1.25, 2.5 mg tabs
Metolazone – generic	2.5, 5, 10 mg tabs
Loop	
Bumetanide[4] – generic	0.5, 1, 2 mg tabs
Ethacrynic acid[4] – generic	25 mg tabs
Edecrin (Valeant)	
Furosemide – generic	20, 40, 80 mg tabs; 10 mg/mL, 40 mg/5 mL soln
Lasix (Validus)	20, 40, 80 mg tabs
Torsemide – generic	5, 10, 20, 100 mg tabs
Demadex (Meda)	10, 20 mg tabs
Potassium-Sparing	
Amiloride – generic	5 mg tabs
Triamterene[4] – *Dyrenium* (Concordia)	50, 100 mg caps
Aldosterone Antagonists	
Eplerenone – generic	25, 50 mg tabs
Inspra (Pfizer)	
Spironolactone – generic	25, 50, 100 mg tabs
Aldactone (Pfizer)	
CaroSpir (CMP)	25 mg/5 mL susp

soln = solution; susp = suspension

1. Dosage may need to be adjusted for renal or hepatic impairment.
2. Class effects. Some adverse effects may not have been reported with every drug in the class. Antihypertensive drugs may also interact adversely with other drugs.
3. Approximate WAC for 30 days' treatment at the lowest usual dosage using the smallest whole number of dosage units. WAC = wholesaler acquisition cost or manufacturer's published price to wholesalers; WAC represents a published catalogue or list price and may not represent an actual transactional price. Source: AnalySource® Monthly. February 5, 2017. Reprinted with permission by First Databank, Inc. All rights reserved. ©2017. www.fdbhealth.com/policies/drug-pricing-policy.

Usual Adult Dosage[1]	Frequent or Severe Adverse Effects[2]	Cost[3]
12.5-25 mg once/d	Hyperuricemia, hypokalemia, hypomagnesemia, hyperglycemia, hyponatremia, hypercalcemia, hypercholesterolemia, hypertriglyceridemia, pancreatitis, rash and other allergic reactions, photosensitivity reactions	$43.20
500-1000 mg once/d		89.20
or divided bid		80.10
25-50 mg once/d		1.10
or divided bid		
		70.20
1.25-2.5 mg once/d		9.30
2.5-5 mg once/d		65.90
0.5-2 mg once/d	Dehydration, circulatory collapse, hypokalemia, hyponatremia, hypomagnesemia, hyperglycemia, metabolic alkalosis, hyperuricemia, blood dyscrasias, rash, hypercholesterolemia, hypertriglyceridemia	31.70
or divided bid		
50-200 mg once/d		1197.40
or divided bid		1345.50
20-80 mg once/d		1.20
or divided bid		
		17.90
5-10 mg once/d		8.60
		79.30
5-10 mg once/d	Hyperkalemia, GI disturbances, rash, headache	19.70
50-150 mg once/d or divided bid	Hyperkalemia, GI disturbances, nephrolithiasis	287.40
50 mg once/d or bid	Hyperkalemia, hyponatremia	104.10
		285.60
50-100 mg once/d	Hyperkalemia, hyponatremia, mastodynia, gynecomastia, menstrual abnormalities, GI disturbances, rash	13.90
or divided bid		111.80
		616.50[5]

4. Not FDA-approved for treatment of hypertension.
5. Approximate WAC for 30 days' treatment at the lowest usual dosage. Source: AnalySource® Monthly. January 5, 2018.

Table 3. Renin-Angiotensin System Inhibitors	
Drug	**Some Available Oral Formulations**
Angiotensin-Converting Enzyme (ACE) Inhibitors	
Benazepril – generic	5, 10, 20, 40 mg tabs
Lotensin (Validus)	20, 40 mg tabs
Captopril – generic	12.5, 25, 50, 100 mg tabs
Enalapril – generic	2.5, 5, 10, 20 mg tabs
Vasotec (Valeant)	
Epaned (Silvergate)	1 mg/mL soln
Fosinopril – generic	10, 20, 40 mg tabs
Lisinopril – generic	2.5, 5, 10, 20, 30, 40 mg tabs
Zestril (Almatica)	
Prinivil (Merck)	5, 10, 20 mg tabs
Qbrelis (Silvergate)	1 mg/mL soln
Moexipril – generic	7.5, 15 mg tabs
Perindopril – generic	2, 4, 8 mg tabs
Quinapril – generic	5, 10, 20, 40 mg tabs
Accupril (Pfizer)	
Ramipril – generic	1.25, 2.5, 5, 10 mg caps
Altace (Pfizer)	
Trandolapril – generic	1, 2, 4 mg tabs
Mavik (Abbvie)	1, 2 mg tabs

1. Dosage may need to be adjusted for renal or hepatic impairment.
2. Class effects. Some adverse effects may not have been reported with every drug in the class. Antihypertensive drugs may also interact adversely with other drugs.
3. Approximate WAC for 30 days' treatment at the lowest usual dosage using the smallest whole number of dosage units. WAC = wholesaler acquisition cost or manufacturer's published price to wholesalers; WAC represents a published catalogue or list price and may not represent an actual transactional price. Source: AnalySource® Monthly. February 5, 2017. Reprinted with permission by First Databank, Inc. All rights reserved. ©2017. www.fdbhealth.com/policies/drug-pricing-policy.

Usual Adult Dosage[1]	Frequent or Severe Adverse Effects[2]	Cost[3]
20-80 mg once/d		$8.90
or divided bid		57.40
50-100 mg bid		98.00
5-40 mg once/d		14.10
or divided bid		482.10
	Cough, hypotension (particularly with	492.00[4]
10-80 mg once/d	diuretic use or volume depletion), rash,	8.80
or divided bid	acute renal failure in patients with	
10-40 mg once/d	bilateral renal artery stenosis or ste-	1.80
	nosis of the artery to a solitary kidney,	381.60
	angioedema, hyperkalemia (particularly	46.80
	if also taking potassium supplements	988.00[4]
7.5-30 mg once/d	or potassium-sparing diuretics), mild to	27.10
or divided bid	moderate loss of taste, hepatotoxicity,	
4-8 mg once/d	pancreatitis, blood dyscrasias, and renal	16.40
or divided bid	damage (particularly in patients with	
10-80 mg once/d	renal dysfunction)	5.00
or divided bid		121.30
2.5-20 mg once/d		7.40
or divided bid		149.40
2-8 mg once/d		14.00
or divided bid		63.20

4. Approximate WAC for 30 days' treatment at the lowest usual dosage using the smallest whole number of dosage units. Source: AnalySource® Monthly. January 5, 2018.

Continued on next page

Table 3. Renin-Angiotensin System Inhibitors (continued)	
Drug	**Some Available Oral Formulations**
Angiotensin Receptor Blockers (ARBs)	
Azilsartan – *Edarbi* (Arbor)	40, 80 mg tabs
Candesartan – generic	4, 8, 16, 32 mg tabs
Atacand (AstraZeneca)	
Eprosartan – generic	600 mg tabs
Irbesartan – generic	75, 150, 300 mg tabs
Avapro (Sanofi)	
Losartan – generic	25, 50, 100 mg tabs
Cozaar (Merck)	
Olmesartan – generic	5, 20, 40 mg tabs
Benicar (Daiichi Sankyo)	
Telmisartan – generic	20, 40, 80 mg tabs
Micardis (Boehringer Ingelheim)	
Valsartan – generic	40, 80, 160, 320 mg tabs
Diovan (Novartis)	
Prexxartan (Medicure)	4 mg/mL soln
Direct Renin Inhibitor	
Aliskiren – *Tekturna* (Novartis)	150, 300 mg tabs

N.A. = cost not yet available

have been shown to reduce mortality when added to standard therapy in patients with heart failure.[11]

ACE INHIBITORS — Angiotensin-converting enzyme (ACE) inhibitors are effective in treating hypertension and are generally well tolerated. They are less effective in black patients unless they are combined with a thiazide-like diuretic or a calcium channel blocker. ACE inhibitors have been shown to prolong survival in heart failure patients with reduced ejection fraction and in patients with left ventricular dysfunction after a myocardial infarction, to reduce mortality in patients without heart failure or left ventricular dysfunction who are at high risk for cardiovascular events, and to reduce proteinuria in patients with either diabetic or non-diabetic nephropathy. Angioedema, a rare but potentially fatal

Usual Adult Dosage[1]	Frequent or Severe Adverse Effects[2]	Cost[3]
80 mg once/d		$181.00
8-32 mg once/d		86.20
or divided bid		97.00
600 mg once/d		82.20
150-300 mg once/d		10.70
		170.70
25-100 mg once/d	Similar to ACE inhibitors; rarely cause cough or angioedema	5.40
or divided bid		78.30
20-40 mg once/d		158.30
		192.00
40-80 mg once/d		105.20
		188.50
80-320 mg once/d		14.70
		203.90
		N.A.
150-300 mg once/d	Same as ARBs, but can also cause GI adverse effects such as diarrhea	165.10

adverse effect of ACE inhibitors, is significantly more common in black than in white patients. ACE inhibitors should not be used during pregnancy (see page 187).

ANGIOTENSIN RECEPTOR BLOCKERS (ARBs) — ARBs are as effective as ACE inhibitors in lowering blood pressure, and appear to be at least equally reno- and cardioprotective, with fewer adverse effects. Like ACE inhibitors, they are less effective in black patients unless they are combined with a thiazide-like diuretic or a calcium channel blocker. ARBs should not be used during pregnancy (see page 187).

DIRECT RENIN INHIBITOR — **Aliskiren**, a direct renin inhibitor, is FDA-approved for use alone or in combination with other antihypertensive

Table 4. Calcium Channel Blockers

Drug	Some Available Oral Formulations
Dihydropyridines	
Amlodipine[4] – generic	2.5, 5, 10 mg tabs
Norvasc (Pfizer)	
Felodipine – generic	2.5, 5, 10 mg ER tabs
Isradipine – generic	2.5, 5 mg caps
Nicardipine – generic	20, 30 mg caps
Nifedipine ER[5] – generic	30, 60, 90 mg ER tabs
Adalat CC (Almatica)	
Procardia XL (Pfizer)	
Nisoldipine – generic	8.5, 17, 20, 25.5, 30, 34, 40 mg ER tabs
Sular (Shionogi)	8.5, 17, 34 mg ER tabs
Nondihydropyridines	
Diltiazem[5] – generic (extended-release)	180, 240, 300, 360, 420 mg ER tabs
Cardizem LA[6] (Valeant)	
Matzim LA (Teva)	
generic (extended-release)	120, 180, 240, 300, 360 mg ER caps
Taztia XT (Actavis)	
Tiazac[7] (Valeant)	
generic (continuous-delivery)	120, 180, 240, 300, 360 mg ER caps
Cardizem CD (Valeant)	
Cartia XT[8] (Actavis)	
generic (degradable)	120, 180, 240 mg ER degradable caps
Dilt-XR (Apotex)	
Verapamil – generic	40, 80, 120 mg tabs
Calan (Pfizer)	
long-acting – generic	120, 180, 240 mg SR tabs
Calan SR (Pfizer)	
generic	120, 180, 240, 360 mg SR caps
Verelan (Kremers Urban)	
generic	100, 200, 300 mg ER caps
Verelan PM (Kremers Urban)	

ER = extended-release; SR = sustained-release
1. Dosage may need to be adjusted for renal or hepatic impairment.
2. Class effects. Some adverse effects may not have been reported with every drug in the class. Antihypertensive drugs may also interact adversely with other drugs.
3. Approximate WAC for 30 days' treatment at the lowest usual dosage using the smallest whole number of dosage units. WAC = wholesaler acquisition cost or manufacturer's published price to wholesalers; WAC represents a published catalogue or list price and may not represent an actual transactional price. Source: AnalySource® Monthly. February 5, 2017. Reprinted with permission by First Databank, Inc. All rights reserved. ©2017. www.fdbhealth.com/policies/drug-pricing-policy.

Usual Adult Dosage[1]	Frequent or Severe Adverse Effects[2]	Cost[3]
2.5-10 mg once/d	Dizziness, headache, peripheral edema (more than with verapamil and diltiazem, more common in women), flushing, tachycardia, rash, gingival hyperplasia	$2.10
		155.80
2.5-10 mg once/d		27.10
5-10 mg divided bid		70.60
60-120 mg divided tid		138.00
30-90 mg once/d		28.00
		50.30
		155.20
17-34 mg once/d		182.80
		565.30
240-360 mg once/d	Dizziness, headache, edema, constipation (especially verapamil), AV block, bradycardia, heart failure, lupus-like rash with diltiazem	80.00
		135.10
		80.00
		27.90
		37.90
		91.60
		39.00
		1276.30
		39.80
		24.70
		26.40
80-160 mg tid		6.40
		253.20
240-480 mg once/d		32.20
or divided bid		221.60
240-480 mg once/d		51.60
		227.00
200-400 mg once/d		59.10
		200.10

4. Amlodipine is also available in combination with atorvastatin (*Caduet*, and generics).
5. Immediate-release formulation is not recommended for treatment of hypertension.
6. *Cardizem LA* is also available in 120-mg ER tabs.
7. *Tiazac* is also available in 420-mg ER caps.
8. *Cartia XT* is not available in 360-mg ER caps.

Table 5. Beta-Adrenergic Blockers

Drug	Some Available Oral Formulations
Atenolol[4] – generic	25, 50, 100 mg tabs
Tenormin (Almatica)	
Betaxolol[4] – generic	10, 20 mg tabs
Bisoprolol[4] – generic	5, 10 mg tabs
Zebeta (Teva)	10 mg tabs
Metoprolol[4] – generic	25, 37.5, 50, 75, 100 mg tabs
Lopressor (Validus)	50, 100 mg tabs
extended-release – generic	25, 50, 100, 200 mg ER tabs
Toprol-XL (AstraZeneca)	
Nadolol – generic	20, 40, 80 mg tabs
Corgard (US Worldmeds)	
Propranolol – generic	10, 20, 40, 60, 80 mg tabs
extended-release – generic	60, 80, 120, 160 mg ER caps
Inderal LA (Ari)	
Inderal XL (Mist)	80, 120 mg ER caps
InnoPran XL (Akrimax)	80, 120 mg ER caps
Timolol – generic	5, 10, 20 mg tabs
Beta-Adrenergic Blockers with Intrinsic Sympathomimetic Activity	
Acebutolol[4] – generic	200, 400 mg caps
Penbutolol – *Levatol* (Auxilium)	20 mg tabs
Pindolol – generic	5, 10 mg tabs
Beta-Adrenergic Blockers with Alpha-Blocking Properties	
Carvedilol – generic	3.125, 6.25, 12.5, 25 mg tabs
Coreg (GSK)	
extended-release	
Coreg CR (GSK)	10, 20, 40, 80 mg ER caps
Labetalol – generic	100, 200, 300 mg tabs

ER = extended-release

1. Dosage may need to be adjusted for renal or hepatic impairment.
2. Class effects. Some adverse effects may not have been reported with every drug in the class. Antihypertensive drugs may also interact adversely with other drugs.
3. Approximate WAC for 30 days' treatment at the lowest usual dosage using the smallest whole number of dosage units. WAC = wholesaler acquisition cost or manufacturer's published price to wholesalers; WAC represents a published catalogue or list price and may not represent an actual transactional price. Source: AnalySource® Monthly. February 5, 2017. Reprinted with permission by First Databank, Inc. All rights reserved. ©2017. www.fdbhealth.com/policies/drug-pricing-policy.

Usual Adult Dosage[1]	Frequent or Severe Adverse Effects[2]	Cost[3]
50-100 mg once/d	Fatigue, depression, bradycardia, erectile dysfunction, decreased exercise tolerance, heart failure, worsening of peripheral arterial insufficiency, may aggravate allergic reactions, bronchospasm, may mask symptoms of and delay recovery from hypoglycemia, Raynaud's phenomenon, insomnia, vivid dreams or hallucinations, increased serum triglycerides, decreased HDL cholesterol, increased incidence of diabetes, sudden withdrawal may lead to exacerbation of angina and myocardial infarction or precipitate thyroid storm	$2.50
		381.60
10-20 mg once/d		21.20
5-20 mg once/d		24.80
		155.80
100-450 mg divided bid or tid		3.20
		115.20
25-400 mg once/d		23.00
		35.90
40-320 mg once/d		95.60
		147.20
80-240 mg divided bid		25.40
60-240 mg once/d		48.50
		530.50
80-120 mg once/d at hs		681.40
80-120 mg once/d at hs		681.40
20-60 mg divided bid		81.70
200-1200 mg once/d or divided bid	Similar to other beta-adrenergic blockers, but with less resting bradycardia and lipid changes; acebutolol has been associated with a positive antinuclear antibody test and occasional drug-induced lupus	12.50
10-80 mg once/d		101.70
10-60 mg divided bid		40.80
12.5-50 mg divided bid	Similar to other beta-adrenergic blockers, but more orthostatic hypotension; hepatotoxicity with labetalol	9.30
		274.10
20-80 mg once/d		275.30
200-1200 mg divided bid		22.00

4. Cardioselective.

Continued on next page

Table 5. Beta-Adrenergic Blockers (continued)	
Drug	**Some Available Oral Formulations**
Beta-Adrenergic Blocker with Nitric Oxide-Mediated Vasodilating Activity	
Nebivolol – *Bystolic* (Allergan)	2.5, 5, 10, 20 mg tabs

5. J Fongemie and E Felix-Getzik. A review of nebivolol pharmacology and clinical evidence. Drugs 2015; 75:1349.

drugs for treatment of hypertension.[12] It has not been shown to have any advantage over an ACE inhibitor or an ARB. Aliskiren should not be used with an ACE inhibitor or an ARB, or during pregnancy (see page 187).

CALCIUM CHANNEL BLOCKERS — The calcium channel blockers are structurally and functionally heterogeneous. They all cause vasodilation and decrease total peripheral resistance. The cardiac response to decreased vascular resistance is variable; some dihydropyridines (**felodipine**, **nicardipine**, and **nisoldipine**) usually cause an initial reflex tachycardia, but others (**isradipine**, **nifedipine**, and **amlodipine**) generally have a lesser effect on heart rate. The nondihydropyridines **verapamil** and **diltiazem** slow heart rate and can slow atrioventricular conduction; they should be used with caution in patients who are also taking a beta blocker.

In one meta-analysis, the risk of heart failure was higher in patients treated with a calcium channel blocker than in those treated with an ACE inhibitor, a beta blocker, or a diuretic.[13] In one large outcomes trial (ACCOMPLISH), however, the ACE inhibitor benazepril plus the calcium channel blocker amlodipine was more effective in reducing adverse cardiovascular outcomes than benazepril plus the diuretic hydrochlorothiazide.[14]

BETA-ADRENERGIC BLOCKERS — A beta blocker may be an acceptable choice for treatment of hypertension in patients with another indication for a beta blocker, such as migraine headache prophylaxis, certain cardiac arrhythmias, angina pectoris, myocardial infarction, or heart

Usual Adult Dosage[1]	Frequent or Severe Adverse Effects[2]	Cost[3]
5-40 mg once/d	Similar to other beta-adrenergic blockers, but may improve erectile dysfunction[5]	$119.50

failure, and possibly in younger patients (<60 years old) and in those with hyperkinetic circulation (palpitations, tachycardia, anxiety).[15] One meta-analysis of cardiovascular outcomes trials concluded that a beta blocker was less effective in preventing cardiovascular events (especially stroke) than an ACE inhibitor, an ARB, a calcium channel blocker, or a diuretic.[16] Like ACE inhibitors and ARBs, beta blockers are less effective in lowering blood pressure in black patients.

Acebutolol, **penbutolol**, and **pindolol** have intrinsic sympathomimetic activity (ISA). Beta blockers without ISA are preferred in patients with angina or a history of myocardial infarction.

Labetalol combines beta receptor blockade with alpha-adrenergic receptor blockade. **Carvedilol** is another beta blocker with alpha-blocking properties; compared to metoprolol, it may be less likely to interfere with glycemic control in patients with type 2 diabetes and hypertension.[17] **Nebivolol** does not have alpha-blocking properties at clinically relevant doses, but does have nitric oxide-mediated vasodilating activity.[18,19]

ALPHA-ADRENERGIC BLOCKERS — **Doxazosin**, **prazosin**, and **terazosin** cause less tachycardia than direct vasodilators, but they are more likely to cause postural hypotension, especially in the elderly and after the first dose. Treatment of essential hypertension with doxazosin, compared to treatment with chlorthalidone, has been associated with an increased incidence of heart failure, stroke, and combined cardiovascular disease

Table 6. Alpha-Adrenergic Blockers, Central Alpha-Adrenergic Agonists, and Direct Vasodilators

Drug	Some Available Oral Formulations
Alpha-Adrenergic Blockers	
Doxazosin – generic	1, 2, 4, 8 mg tabs
Cardura (Pfizer)	
extended-release – *Cardura XL*[4]	4, 8 mg ER tabs
Prazosin – generic	1, 2, 5 mg caps
Minipress (Pfizer)	
Terazosin – generic	1, 2, 5, 10 mg caps
Central Alpha-Adrenergic Agonists	
Clonidine – generic	0.1, 0.2, 0.3 mg tabs[5]
Catapres (Boehringer Ingelheim)	
Guanfacine – generic	1, 2 mg tabs
Methyldopa – generic	250, 500 mg tabs

ER = extended-release

1. Dosage may need to be adjusted for renal or hepatic impairment.
2. Class effects. Some adverse effects may not have been reported with every drug in the class. Antihypertensive drugs may also interact adversely with other drugs.
3. Approximate WAC for 30 days' treatment at the lowest usual dosage using the smallest whole number of dosage units. WAC = wholesaler acquisition cost or manufacturer's published price to wholesalers; WAC represents a published catalogue or list price and may not represent an actual transactional price. Source: AnalySource® Monthly. February 5, 2017. Reprinted with permission by First Databank, Inc. All rights reserved. ©2017. www.fdbhealth.com/policies/drug-pricing-policy.

Usual Adult Dosage[1]	Frequent or Severe Adverse Effects[2]	Cost[3]
1-16 mg once/d	Syncope with first dose (less likely with terazosin and doxazosin), dizziness and vertigo, headache, palpitations, fluid retention, drowsiness, weakness, anticholinergic effects, priapism, thrombocytopenia, atrial fibrillation	$19.30
		116.60
4-8 mg once/d		134.10
6-20 mg divided bid or tid		76.40
		260.70
1-20 mg once/d or divided bid		4.50
0.2-0.6 mg divided bid or tid	CNS reactions (similar to methyldopa, but more sedation and dry mouth), bradycardia, heart block, rebound hypertension (less likely with patch), contact dermatitis from patch	3.20
		142.30
1-3 mg once/d[6]	Similar to clonidine, but milder	8.10
500-2000 mg divided bid or qid	Sedation, fatigue, depression, dry mouth, orthostatic hypotension, bradycardia, heart block, autoimmune disorders (including colitis, hepatitis), hepatic necrosis, Coombs-positive lupus-like syndrome, thrombocytopenia, red cell aplasia, erectile dysfunction, hemolytic anemia	10.50

4. Not FDA-approved for treatment of hypertension.
5. Clonidine is also available as extended-release transdermal patches (*Catapres TTS*, and generics). The usual dosage is one patch (0.1, 0.2, or 0.3 mg/24 hrs) applied once every 7 days.
6. The first dose is 1 mg at bedtime; 1-mg doses of the drug provide all or most of its antihypertensive effect and are generally well tolerated.

Continued on next page

Table 6. Alpha-Adrenergic Blockers, Central Alpha-Adrenergic Agonists, and Direct Vasodilators (continued)	
Drug	**Some Available Oral Formulations**
Direct Vasodilators	
Hydralazine – generic	10, 25, 50, 100 mg tabs
Minoxidil – generic	2.5, 10 mg tabs

(coronary heart disease death, nonfatal myocardial infarction, stroke, angina, coronary revascularization, congestive heart failure, and peripheral arterial disease).[20] Alpha blockers provide symptomatic relief from benign prostatic hyperplasia in men, but may cause stress incontinence in women.

CENTRAL ALPHA-ADRENERGIC AGONISTS — **Clonidine**, **guanfacine**, and **methyldopa** decrease sympathetic outflow, but do not inhibit reflex responses as completely as sympatholytic drugs that act peripherally. They may, however, cause sedation, dry mouth, and erectile dysfunction. Once-daily guanfacine may be a reasonable add-on for treatment of refractory hypertension.

DIRECT VASODILATORS — Direct vasodilators frequently produce reflex tachycardia (especially early in treatment) and rarely cause orthostatic hypotension. They should generally be given with a beta blocker or a centrally acting drug to minimize the reflex increase in heart rate and cardiac output, and with a diuretic to avoid sodium and fluid retention. Direct vasodilators should generally be avoided in patients with coronary artery disease. The maintenance dosage of **hydralazine** should be limited to 200 mg per day to decrease the possibility of a lupus-like reaction. **Minoxidil**, a potent drug that rarely fails to lower blood

Usual Adult Dosage[1]	Frequent or Severe Adverse Effects[2]	Cost[3]
40-200 mg divided bid or qid	Tachycardia, aggravation of angina, headache, dizziness, fluid retention, nasal congestion, lupus-like syndrome, hepatitis	$11.50
5-40 mg once/d or divided bid	Tachycardia, aggravation of angina, marked fluid retention, pericardial effusion, hair growth on face and body	15.20

pressure, should be reserved for severe hypertension refractory to other drugs. It may cause hirsutism and tachycardia, and can also cause severe fluid retention.

SAFETY IN PREGNANCY — Drugs affecting the renin-angiotensin system (**ACE inhibitors**, **ARBs**, and **aliskiren**) are contraindicated for use during pregnancy; they have been associated with serious fetal toxicity, including renal and cardiac abnormalities and death.

Methyldopa has a long history of safe use in pregnancy, but the high doses often required to adequately lower blood pressure can cause significant sedation.

Calcium channel blockers are generally considered safe for use during pregnancy; **extended-release nifedipine** has been studied most extensively.[21] Immediate-release oral nifedipine is not recommended for chronic treatment of hypertension in pregnancy because it can cause an acute drop in blood pressure that may reduce uteroplacental perfusion.

Limited data suggest that the beta blocker **labetalol** is similar in efficacy and safety to methyldopa and nifedipine for use during pregnancy.[22,23] A

Table 7. Some Combination Products

Drug	Some Oral Formulations	Cost[1]
ACE Inhibitors and Diuretics		
Benazepril/HCTZ	5/6.25, 10/12.5, 20/12.5,	
generic	20/25 mg tabs	$38.20
Lotensin HCT[2] (Validus)		60.90
Captopril/HCTZ	25/15, 25/25, 50/15, 50/25 mg	
generic	tabs	29.20
Enalapril/HCTZ		
generic	5/12.5, 10/25 mg tabs	16.20
Vaseretic (Valeant)	10/25 mg tabs	391.10
Fosinopril/HCTZ	10/12.5, 20/12.5 mg tabs	
generic		43.20
Lisinopril/HCTZ	10/12.5, 20/12.5, 20/25 mg tabs	
generic		5.20
Zestoretic (Almatica)		381.60
Moexipril/HCTZ	7.5/12.5, 15/12.5, 15/25 mg tabs	
generic		27.10
Quinapril/HCTZ	10/12.5, 20/12.5, 20/25 mg tabs	
generic		27.10
Accuretic (Pfizer)		117.90
ARBs and Diuretics		
Azilsartan/chlorthalidone	40/12.5, 40/25 mg tabs	
Edarbyclor (Arbor)		170.90
Candesartan/HCTZ	16/12.5, 32/12.5, 32/25 mg tabs	
generic		105.80
Atacand HCT (AstraZeneca)		131.30
Irbesartan/HCTZ	150/12.5, 300/12.5 mg tabs	
generic		22.30
Avalide (Sanofi)		206.50
Losartan/HCTZ	50/12.5, 100/12.5, 100/25 mg	
generic	tabs	7.00
Hyzaar (Merck)		116.10

ACE = angiotension-converting enzyme; ARB = angiotensin receptor blocker; ER = extended-release; HCTZ = hydrochlorothiazide

1. Approximate wholesale acquisition cost (WAC) for 30 of the lowest strength tablets or capsules. WAC = wholesaler acquisition cost or manufacturer's published price to wholesalers; WAC represents a published catalogue or list price and may not represent an actual transactional price. Source: AnalySource® Monthly. February 5, 2017. Reprinted with permission by First Databank, Inc. All rights reserved. ©2017. www.fdbhealth.com/policies/drug-pricing-policy.
2. Not available in 5/6.25 mg tabs.

Continued on next page

Table 7. Some Combination Products (continued)		
Drug	**Some Oral Formulations**	**Cost[1]**
ACE Inhibitors and Diuretics (continued)		
Olmesartan/HCTZ	20/12.5, 40/12.5, 40/25 mg tabs	
generic		$158.30
Benicar HCT (Daiichi Sankyo)		192.00
Telmisartan/HCTZ	40/12.5, 80/12.5, 80/25 mg	
generic	tabs	115.00
Micardis HCT (Boehringer Ingelheim)		188.50
Valsartan/HCTZ	80/12.5, 160/12.5, 160/25,	
generic	320/12.5, 320/25 mg tabs	30.90
Diovan HCT (Novartis)		229.30
Direct Renin Inhibitor and Diuretic		
Aliskiren/HCTZ	150/12.5, 150/25, 300/12.5,	
Tekturna HCT (Novartis)	300/25 mg tabs	165.10
Beta-Adrenergic Blockers and Diuretics		
Atenolol/chlorthalidone	50/25, 100/25 mg tabs	
generic		16.40
Tenoretic (Almatica)		450.00[3]
Bisoprolol/HCTZ	2.5/6.25, 5/6.25, 10/6.25 mg	
generic	tabs	12.10
Ziac (Teva)		170.40
Metoprolol succinate/HCTZ	25/12.5, 50/12.5, 100/12.5 mg	
generic	ER tabs	1249.50
Dutoprol (Concordia)		184.00
Metoprolol tartrate/HCTZ	50/25, 100/25, 100/50 mg tabs	
generic		27.20
Lopressor HCT (Validus)	50/25 mg tabs	62.10
Nadolol/bendroflumethiazide	40/5, 80/5 mg tabs	
generic		111.80
Corzide (Pfizer)		149.40
Propranolol/HCTZ	40/25, 80/25 mg tabs	
generic		27.60

3. Cost for 100/25-mg tabs. The cost for thirty 50/25-mg tabs is $1080.00.

Continued on next page

Table 7. Some Combination Products (continued)		
Drug	**Some Oral Formulations**	**Cost[1]**
Beta-Adrenergic Blocker and ARB		
Nebivolol/valsartan	5/80 mg tabs	
Byvalson (Allergan)		$109.60
Calcium Channel Blockers and ACE Inhibitors		
Amlodipine/benazepril	2.5/10, 5/10, 5/20, 5/40 10/20,	
generic	10/40 mg caps	27.30
Lotrel[4] (Novartis)		246.50
Amlodipine/perindopril	2.5/3.5, 5/7, 10/14 mg tabs	
Prestalia (Symplmed)		156.20
Verapamil ER/trandolapril	180/2, 240/1, 240/2, 240/4 mg	
generic	tabs	127.00
Tarka (Abbvie)		167.90
Calcium Channel Blockers and ARBs		
Amlodipine/telmisartan	5/40, 5/80, 10/40, 10/80 mg	
generic	tabs	126.30
Twynsta (Boehringer Ingelheim)		202.80
Amlodipine/valsartan	5/160, 5/320, 10/160,	
generic	10/320 mg tabs	44.10
Exforge (Novartis)		230.20
Amlodipine/olmesartan	5/20, 5/40, 10/20, 10/40 mg	
generic	tabs	88.50
Azor (Daiichi Sankyo)		249.40
Calcium Channel Blocker and Direct Renin Inhibitor		
Amlodipine/aliskiren	5/150, 10/150, 5/300,	
Tekamlo (Novartis)	10/300 mg tabs	131.00
Diuretic Combinations		
HCTZ/spironolactone	25/25 mg tabs	
generic		36.00
Aldactazide (Pfizer)	25/25, 50/50 mg tabs	65.30
HCTZ/triamterene	25/37.5, 50/75 mg tabs,	
generic	25/37.5, 25/50 mg caps	9.00
Dyazide (GSK)	25/37.5 mg caps	62.60
Maxzide (Mylan)	25/37.5, 50/75 mg tabs	45.50

4. Not available in 2.5/10-mg caps.

Continued on next page

Table 7. Some Combination Products (continued)		
Drug	**Some Oral Formulations**	**Cost[1]**
Diuretic Combinations (continued)		
HCTZ/amiloride	50/5 mg tabs	
generic		$12.20
Central Alpha-Adrenergic Agonists and Diuretics		
Clonidine/chlorthalidone	0.1/15, 0.2/15, 0.3/15 mg tabs	
Clorpres (Mylan)		66.60
Methyldopa/HCTZ	250/15, 250/25 mg tabs	
generic		44.00
ARB/Calcium Channel Blocker/Diuretic Combinations		
Valsartan/amlodipine/HCTZ	160/5/12.5, 160/5/25,	
generic	160/10/12.5, 160/10/25,	111.70
Exforge HCT (Novartis)	320/10/25 mg tabs	230.20
Olmesartan/amlodipine/HCTZ	20/5/12.5, 40/5/12.5, 40/5/25,	
generic	40/10/12.5, 40/10/25 mg tabs	122.60
Tribenzor (Daiichi Sankyo)		239.40

review of 13 population-based studies found that use of **beta blockers** in the first trimester was not associated with an overall increase in congenital malformations, but in some studies, their use has been associated with increased rates of cleft lip/palate and cardiovascular and neural tube defects.[24] **Atenolol** has been associated with fetal growth retardation.[25]

Thiazide-like diuretics should not be initiated during pregnancy because the volume depletion caused by these drugs in their first weeks of use may reduce uretoplacental perfusion. Women already taking a thiazide-like diuretic who become pregnant can generally continue it.

1. PK Whelton et al. 2017 ACC/AHA/AAPA/ABC/ACPM/AGS/APhA/ASH/ASPC/NMA/PCNA guideline for the prevention, detection, evaluation, and management of high blood pressure in adults: executive summary: a report of the American College of Cardiology/American Heart Association Task Force on Clinical Practice Guidelines. J Am Coll Cardiol 2017 November 7 (epub).

2. American College of Cardiology. ASCVD risk estimator plus. Available at: http://tools.acc.org/ASCVD-Risk-Estimator-Plus. Accessed January 31, 2018.
3. A Qaseem et al. Pharmacologic treatment of hypertension in adults aged 60 years or older to higher versus lower blood pressure targets: a clinical practice guideline from the American College of Physicians and the American Academy of Family Physicians. Ann Intern Med 2017 Jan 17 (epub).
4. AAFP. AAFP decides to not endorse AHA/ACC hypertension guidelines. Available at: https://www.aafp.org/news/health-of-the-public/20171212notendorseaha-accgdlne.html. Accessed January 26, 2018.
6. JT Wright Jr et al. ALLHAT findings revisited in the context of subsequent analyses, other trials, and meta-analyses. Arch Intern Med 2009; 169:832.
7. GC Roush et al. Diuretics: a review and update. J Cardiovasc Pharmacol Ther 2014; 19:5.
8. VM Musini et al. Blood pressure-lowering efficacy of loop diuretics for primary hypertension. Cochrane Database Syst Rev 2015; 5:CD003825.
9. DA Calhoun et al. Refractory hypertension: determination of prevalence, risk factors, and comorbidities in a large, population-based cohort. Hypertension 2014; 63:451.
10. DA Calhoun and WB White. Effectiveness of the selective aldosterone blocker, eplerenone, in patients with resistant hypertension. J Am Soc Hypertens 2008; 2:462.
11. Drugs for chronic heart failure. Med Lett Drugs Ther 2015; 57:9.
12. Aliskiren (Tekturna) for hypertension. Med Lett Drugs Ther 2007; 49:29.
13. F Turnbull et al. Effects of different blood-pressure-lowering regimens on major cardiovascular events: results of prospectively-designed overviews of randomised trials. Lancet 2003; 362:1527.
14. K Jamerson et al. Benazepril plus amlodipine or hydrochlorothiazide for hypertension in high-risk patients. N Engl J Med 2008; 359:2417.
15. WH Frishman and E Saunders. ß-adrenergic blockers. J Clin Hypertens (Greenwich) 2011; 13:649.
16. CS Wiysonge et al. Beta-blockers for hypertension. Cochrane Database Syst Rev 2012; 11:CD002003.
17. GL Bakris et al. Metabolic effects of carvedilol vs metoprolol in patients with type 2 diabetes mellitus and hypertension: a randomized controlled trial. JAMA 2004; 292:2227.
18. Nebivolol (Bystolic) for hypertension. Med Lett Drugs Ther 2008; 50:17.
19. J Fongemie and E Felix-Getzik. A review of nebivolol pharmacology and clinical evidence. Drugs 2015; 75:1349.
20. The ALLHAT Officers and Coordinators for the ALLHAT Collaborative Research Group. Major cardiovascular events in hypertensive patients randomized to doxazosin vs chlorthalidone: the antihypertensive and lipid-lowering treatment to prevent heart attack trial (ALLHAT). JAMA 2000; 283:1967.
21. P Smith et al. Nifedipine in pregnancy. BJOG 2000; 107:299.
22. WF Peacock IV et al. A systematic review of nicardipine vs labetalol for the management of hypertensive crises. Am J Emerg Med 2012; 30:981.
23. SN Molvi et al. Role of antihypertensive therapy in mild to moderate pregnancy-induced hypertension: a prospective randomized study comparing labetalol with alpha methyldopa. Arch Gynecol Obstet 2012; 285:1553.

24. MY Yacoob et al. The risk of congenital malformations associated with exposure to β-blockers early in pregnancy: a meta-analysis. Hypertension 2013; 62:375.
25. C Lydakis et al. Atenolol and fetal growth in pregnancies complicated by hypertension. Am J Hypertens 1999; 12:541.

DRUGS FOR Migraine

Original publication date – February 2017 (revised March 2018)

TREATMENT OF MIGRAINE

An oral nonopioid analgesic may be sufficient for treatment of mild to moderate migraine without severe nausea or vomiting. A triptan is the drug of choice for treatment of moderate to severe migraine.[1,2] Use of a triptan early in an attack when pain is still mild to moderate in intensity improves headache response and reduces recurrence rates.

ANALGESICS — Aspirin and **acetaminophen,** used alone or together in combination with caffeine (*Excedrin Migraine*, and others), and **non-steroidal anti-inflammatory drugs (NSAIDs)** such as naproxen sodium (*Aleve*, and others) and ibuprofen (*Advil, Motrin*, and generics) are effective in relieving mild to moderate migraine pain.[3-5] The NSAID diclofenac is FDA-approved as a powder for oral solution *(Cambia)* for treatment of migraine; it has a rapid onset of action (about 15 minutes).[6] Some patients may respond better to one NSAID than to another.

Products that combine **butalbital** and caffeine with aspirin (*Fiorinal*, and others) or acetaminophen (*Fioricet*, and others) are used for treatment of migraine despite evidence that butalbital is not effective in relieving migraine pain. Their frequent use can lead to tolerance, addiction, and medication overuse headache. Oral combinations of aspirin or acetaminophen with an **opioid** can be effective for relief of migraine

Recommendations for Treatment and Prevention of Migraine
Treatment
▸ A nonopioid analgesic may be effective for mild to moderate migraine.
▸ A triptan is the drug of choice for moderate to severe migraine.
▸ The short-acting oral triptans sumatriptan, almotriptan, eletriptan, rizatriptan, and zolmitriptan are similar in efficacy and speed of onset.
▸ Intranasal triptan formulations have a faster onset of action than oral triptans.
▸ Subcutaneous sumatriptan is the fastest-acting and most effective triptan formulation.
▸ Patients who do not respond to one triptan may respond to another.
▸ Use of opioids and butalbital for migraine treatment is discouraged.
Prevention
▸ Topiramate, valproate, and the beta blockers propranolol, timolol, and metoprolol are effective for prevention of migraine.

pain, but they cause the usual opioid adverse effects (e.g., nausea, drowsiness, and constipation), and regular use can lead to dependence and addiction.

Pregnancy – Occasional use of acetaminophen for treatment of mild to moderate migraine during pregnancy is generally considered safe.

TRIPTANS — The short-acting oral serotonin (5-$HT_{1B/1D}$) receptor agonists (triptans) **sumatriptan** (*Imitrex*, and others), **almotriptan** (*Axert*, and generics), **eletriptan** *(Relpax)*, **rizatriptan** (*Maxalt*, and generics), and **zolmitriptan** (*Zomig*, and generics) are similar in efficacy.[7] Onset of pain relief generally occurs 30-60 minutes after administration. The longer-acting oral triptans **naratriptan** (*Amerge*, and generics) and **frovatriptan** (*Frova*, and generics) have a slower onset of action and lower initial response rate than other triptans, but they are better tolerated.[8] Patients with migraine who have nausea or vomiting may not be able to take an oral triptan.

An oral fixed-dose combination of sumatriptan and naproxen *(Treximet)* is more effective in relieving moderate or severe migraine pain than either of its components alone.[9]

Table 1. Triptans		
	Onset of action	**Elimination half-life**
Almotriptan	30-60 min	3-4 hrs
Eletriptan	30-60 min	~4 hrs
Frovatriptan	~2 hrs	~25 hrs
Naratriptan	1-3 hrs	~6 hrs
Rizatriptan	30-60 min	2-3 hrs
Sumatriptan		~2 hrs
tablets	30-60 min	
nasal spray and powder	10-15 min	
SC injection	~10 min	
Zolmitriptan		2-3 hrs
tablets	30-60 min	
nasal spray	10-15 min	

Intranasal triptan formulations have a more rapid onset of action than oral tablets, but their efficacy is partially dependent on GI absorption of the portion of the dose that is swallowed. Use of sumatriptan nasal powder *(Onzetra Xsail)* results in a faster rise in sumatriptan plasma concentrations and higher peak concentrations than use of a similar dose of sumatriptan nasal spray, suggesting that a larger portion of the dose is absorbed intranasally with the powder.[10]

Subcutaneously administered sumatriptan relieves pain faster (in about 10 minutes) and more effectively than other triptan formulations, but it causes more adverse effects.

Recurrence – In patients with moderate to severe migraine, the rate of recurrence within 24 hours after treatment with a triptan is generally 20-40%. Early treatment of an attack reduces recurrence rates. Recurrences may respond to a second dose of the triptan.

Adverse Effects – Tingling, flushing, dizziness, drowsiness, fatigue, and a feeling of heaviness, tightness, or pressure in the chest can occur

Table 2. Some Drugs for Treatment of Migraine	
Drug	**Formulations**
Triptans	
Almotriptan[3] – generic *Axert* (Janssen)	6.25, 12.5 mg tabs
Eletriptan – *Relpax* (Pfizer)	20, 40 mg tabs
Frovatriptan – generic *Frova* (Endo)	2.5 mg tabs
Naratriptan – generic *Amerge* (GSK)	1, 2.5 mg tabs
Rizatriptan[4] – generic	5, 10 mg tabs 5, 10 mg orally disintegrating tabs
Maxalt (Merck)	5, 10 mg tabs
Maxalt-MLT	5, 10 mg orally disintegrating tabs
Sumatriptan – generic *Imitrex* (GSK)	25, 50, 100 mg tabs 6 mg/0.5 mL, vials; 4, 6 mg/0.5 mL auto-injector pen and refill cartridge[7] 5, 20 mg/0.1 mL nasal spray
Onzetra Xsail (Avanir)	11 mg nasal powder capsules
Sumavel DosePro (Endo)	6 mg/0.5 mL needle-free delivery system
Zembrace SymTouch (Promius)	3 mg/0.5 mL auto-injector
Zolmitriptan – generic	2.5, 5 mg tabs 2.5, 5 mg orally disintegrating tabs
Zomig (Impax)	2.5, 5 mg tabs
Zomig-ZMT	2.5, 5 mg orally disintegrating tabs
Zomig nasal spray[3]	2.5, 5 mg/0.1 mL nasal spray
Triptan/NSAID Combination	
Sumatriptan/naproxen[3] – *Treximet* (Pernix)	10/60, 85/500 mg tabs

1. Dosage may need to be adjusted for renal or hepatic impairment or for drug interactions.
2. Approximate WAC for one dose at the lowest usual dosage. WAC = wholesaler acquisition cost or manufacturer's published price to wholesalers; WAC represents a published catalogue or list price and may not represent an actual transactional price. Source: AnalySource® Monthly. January 5, 2017. Reprinted with permission by First Databank, Inc. All rights reserved. ©2017. www.fdbhealth.com/policies/drug-pricing-policy.
3. Also approved for use in patients 12-17 years old.
4. Also approved for use in patients 6-17 years old.

Usual Adult Dosage[1]	Cost[2]
6.25 or 12.5 mg PO; can be repeated after 2 hrs (max 25 mg/d)	$33.00
	42.70
20 or 40 mg PO; can be repeated after 2 hrs (max 80 mg/d)	52.00
2.5 mg PO; can be repeated after 2 hrs (max 7.5 mg/d)	53.60
	73.60
2.5 mg PO; can be repeated after 4 hrs (max 5 mg/d)	11.00
	56.60
5 or 10 mg PO; can be repeated after 2 hrs (max 30 mg/d)[5,6]	1.60
	3.20
	36.60
	36.60
50 or 100 mg PO; can be repeated after 2 hrs (max 200 mg/d)	2.00
	60.40
6 mg SC; can be repeated after 1 hr (max 12 mg/d)	45.10
	176.10
5, 10, or 20 mg intranasally; can be repeated after 2 hrs (max 40 mg/d)	49.20
	75.40
22 mg intranasally; can be repeated after 2 hrs (max 44 mg/d)	65.00
6 mg SC; can be repeated after 1 hr (max 12 mg/d)	169.20[10]
3 mg SC; can be repeated after 1 hr (max 12 mg/d)	149.80
2.5 or 5 mg PO; can be repeated after 2 hrs (max 10 mg/d)[8]	26.20
	27.70
	89.40
	89.40
2.5 or 5 mg intranasally; can be repeated after 2 hrs (max 10 mg/d)	61.50
85/500 mg PO; can be repeated after 2 hrs (max 170/1000 mg/d)[9]	81.00

5. Dose for pediatric patients is 5 mg (<40 kg) or 10 mg (≥40 kg). In pediatric patients, the efficacy and safety of redosing within 24 hours have not been established.
6. Adults and children (≥40 kg) also taking propranolol should only use a 5-mg dose (max 15 mg/d for adults and 5 mg/d for children). Combined use not recommended for children weighing <40 kg.
7. Generic also available as a 6-mg syringe.
8. Patients also taking cimetidine should only use a 2.5-mg dose (max 5 mg/d).
9. Dosage for adolescents 12-17 years old is 10/60 mg (max 85/500 mg/d).
10. Product discontinued February 2018.

Continued on next page

Table 2. Some Drugs for Treatment of Migraine (continued)	
Drug	**Formulations**
Ergots	
Dihydroergotamine mesylate –	
generic	1 mg/mL ampules
D.H.E. 45 (Valeant)	
Migranal nasal spray (Valeant)	4 mg/mL nasal spray
Ergotamine/caffeine – generic	1/100 mg tabs
Cafergot (Sandoz)	
Migergot (Horizon)	2/100 mg rectal suppository

with all triptans, but most commonly with SC sumatriptan. A burning sensation at the injection site is also common with SC sumatriptan. Intranasal formulations of sumatriptan and zolmitriptan can have an unpleasant taste. CNS symptoms such as somnolence and asthenia following triptan therapy may be part of the migraine attack, unmasked by the successful treatment of pain, rather than adverse effects of the drugs. Sumatriptan is contraindicated for use in patients with severe hepatic impairment. Naratriptan is contraindicated in patients with severe renal or hepatic impairment.

Angina, myocardial infarction, cardiac arrhythmia, stroke, seizure, and death have occurred rarely with triptans.[11] All triptans are contraindicated for use in patients with ischemic or vasospastic coronary artery disease, Wolff-Parkinson-White syndrome, peripheral vascular disease, ischemic bowel disease, uncontrolled hypertension, or a history of stroke, transient ischemic attack, hemiplegic migraine, or migraine with brainstem aura. Triptans should be used with caution in patients with other significant risk factors for vascular disease, particularly diabetes.

Drug Interactions – The labels of all triptans state that a triptan should not be taken within 24 hours of another triptan or an ergot because vasoconstriction could be additive. MAO inhibitors increase serum con-

Usual Adult Dosage[1]	Cost[2]
1 mg IM or SC; can be repeated at 1 hr intervals (max 3 mg/d, 6 mg/wk)	$124.80 1176.80
1 spray (0.5 mg) into each nostril, repeated 15 min later (2 mg/dose; max 3 mg/d)	421.40
2 tabs PO at attack onset, then 1 tab q30 min PRN (max 6 tabs/attack)	11.10 12.40
1 supp at attack onset, repeat in 1 hr if needed (max 2 supp/attack)	63.90

centrations of rizatriptan, sumatriptan, and zolmitriptan; they should not be used within 2 weeks of each other. Propranolol increases serum concentrations of eletriptan, frovatriptan, rizatriptan, and zolmitriptan. Cimetidine increases serum concentrations of zolmitriptan. Inhibitors of CYP3A4 can increase serum concentrations of almotriptan and eletriptan.[12] Cases of serotonin syndrome have been reported with concurrent use of triptans and selective serotonin reuptake inhibitors (SSRIs) or serotonin-norepinephrine reuptake inhibitors (SNRIs), but data from large observational databases suggest that the risk is low.[13,14]

Pregnancy and Lactation – Based on available evidence, use of sumatriptan, or possibly rizatriptan, eletriptan, or zolmitriptan during pregnancy does not appear to be associated with an increased risk of birth defects.[15,16] Levels of sumatriptan and eletriptan in breast milk are low and these drugs would not be expected to cause adverse effects in most breastfed infants[17]; avoiding breastfeeding for 8-12 hours after taking a short-acting triptan would reduce the infant's risk of exposure to the drug.

ERGOTS — A fixed-dose combination of **ergotamine tartrate**, a nonspecific serotonin agonist and vasoconstrictor, and caffeine is available as tablets *(Cafergot)* and suppositories *(Migergot)* for treatment of moderate to severe migraine. The combination is less effective than a triptan for acute treatment of migraine.[18]

Dihydroergotamine, which can be administered subcutaneously, intramuscularly, intravenously (*D.H.E.*, and generics), or intranasally *(Migranal)*, is effective for acute treatment of migraine. Dihydroergotamine nasal spray relieves migraine after 2 hours in about 50% of patients, with a 15% incidence of recurrence within 24 hours. It can be effective in some patients who do not respond to triptans.

Adverse Effects – Dihydroergotamine is a weaker arterial vasoconstrictor than ergotamine and causes fewer serious adverse effects. Nausea and vomiting are fairly common with ergotamine, but pretreatment with or concurrent use of an antiemetic such as metoclopramide (*Reglan*, and generics) can reduce GI effects. Serious adverse effects, such as vascular (including coronary) occlusion and gangrene, are rare and are usually associated with overdosage (>6 mg in 24 hours or >10 mg per week). Hepatic impairment or fever can accelerate development of severe vasoconstriction. Ergots are contraindicated in patients with arterial disease or uncontrolled hypertension.

Drug Interactions – The effects of ergots can be potentiated by triptans, beta blockers, dopamine, nicotine, or CYP3A4 inhibitors. Use of ergots is contraindicated with strong CYP3A4 inhibitors such as clarithromycin (*Biaxin*, and generics) or itraconazole (*Sporanox*, and generics).[12] Ergots and triptans should not be taken within 24 hours of each other.

Pregnancy and Lactation – Ergots can reduce placental blood flow and are contraindicated for use during pregnancy. Ergotamine is excreted in human breast milk; women who take an ergot should avoid breastfeeding.

TRANSCRANIAL MAGNETIC STIMULATION — The FDA has approved the use of a transcranial magnetic stimulation device (*SpringTMS* – eNeura) for self-treatment of migraine with aura. In one trial, the pain-free response rate 2 hours after treatment of the first migraine attack was significantly higher with use of transcranial magnetic stimulation at the onset of aura than with sham stimulation (39% vs 22%).[19]

MEDICATION OVERUSE HEADACHE — Overuse of drugs for headache, particularly butalbital and opioids, can lead to chronic headache with structural and functional changes in the brain. Treatment of medication overuse headache involves withdrawing the overused drug(s); abrupt withdrawal may require hospitalization and bridge therapy with other drugs. Preventive treatment for migraine should be considered. Future use of acute migraine treatments should be limited to ≤2 days per week.[20,21]

PREVENTION OF MIGRAINE

Patients with frequent or severe migraine headaches and those who cannot take vasoconstrictors or are refractory to acute treatment should receive preventive treatment.[22,23] Menstrual migraine attacks may sometimes be prevented by a brief course of an NSAID or triptan, particularly frovatriptan or naratriptan, taken for several days before and after the onset of menstruation.[24,25] Preventive therapy is generally not recommended during pregnancy.

BETA BLOCKERS — Beta blockers are commonly used for prevention of migraine. Propranolol (*Inderal LA*, and others) and timolol are the only beta blockers approved by the FDA for this indication, but metoprolol (*Lopressor*, and others), nadolol (*Corgard*, and generics), and atenolol (*Tenormin*, and generics) are also effective in preventing migraine.[23] All beta blockers can cause fatigue, exercise intolerance, and orthostatic hypotension, and should not be used in patients with decompensated heart failure. All are relatively contraindicated in patients with asthma. Patients with migraine often have comorbid depression, which may be aggravated by beta blockers.

Pregnancy – Intrauterine growth retardation, small placentas, and congenital abnormalities have been reported with use of propranolol during pregnancy. Atenolol has been associated with the birth of small

Table 3. Some Drugs for Prevention of Migraine in Adults

Drug	Some Available Formulations
Beta Blockers	
Metoprolol[3] – generic	25, 50, 100 mg tabs
Lopressor (Validus)	50, 100 mg tabs
extended-release – generic	25, 50, 100, 200 mg ER tabs
Toprol-XL (AstraZeneca)	
Propranolol – generic	10, 20, 40, 60, 80 mg tabs
extended-release – generic	60, 80, 120, 160 mg ER caps
Inderal LA (Akrimax)	
Timolol – generic	5, 10, 20 mg tabs
Antiepileptic Drugs	
Valproate[4] – generic	125, 250, 500 mg delayed-release tabs;
Depakote (Abbvie)	125 mg sprinkle caps
extended-release – generic	250, 500 mg ER tabs
Depakote ER	
Topiramate[5] – generic	25, 50, 100, 200 mg tabs; 15, 25 mg
Topamax (Janssen)	sprinkle caps
Tricyclic Antidepressants[3]	
Amitriptyline – generic	10, 25, 50, 75, 100, 150 mg tabs
Nortriptyline – generic	10, 25, 50, 75 mg caps
SNRI[3]	
Venlafaxine – generic	25, 37.5, 50, 75, 100 mg tabs
extended-release – generic	37.5, 75, 150 mg caps;
	37.5, 75, 150, 225 mg tabs
Effexor XR (Pfizer)	37.5, 75, 150 mg caps
Botulinum Toxin Type A	
OnabotulinumtoxinA – *Botox* (Allergan)[7]	100, 200 unit vials

ER = extended-release

1. Dosage adjustments may be required for renal or hepatic impairment.
2. Approximate WAC for 30 days' treatment at the lowest usual dosage. WAC = wholesaler acquisition cost or manufacturer's published price to wholesalers; WAC represents a published catalogue or list price and may not represent an actual transactional price. Source: AnalySource® Monthly. January 5, 2017. Reprinted with permission by First Databank, Inc. All rights reserved. ©2017. www.fdbhealth.com/policies/drug-pricing-policy.
3. Not FDA-approved for this indication.
4. Oral formulations marketed as divalproex sodium (*Depakote*, and others) and valproic acid (*Depakene*, and others). Only divalproex sodium is FDA-approved for prevention of migraine.

Usual Adult Dosage[1]	Cost[2]
50-100 mg bid	$1.80
	57.60
100-200 mg once/d	36.30
	53.90
40-160 mg divided bid	20.40
60-160 mg once/d	50.10
	530.40
10-15 mg bid or 20 mg once/d	75.30
250-500 mg bid	17.80
	195.80
500-1000 mg once/d	87.60
	156.60
50 mg bid[6]	13.50
	574.60
25-150 mg once/d	9.50
25-150 mg once/d	8.00
25-50 mg tid	47.70
75-150 mg once/d	11.70
	352.50
155 units IM every 12 weeks[8]	1158.00[9]

5. Extended-release formulations of topiramate (*Trokendi XR*; *Qudexy XR*, and generic) are not FDA-approved for migraine prevention.
6. Dosage should be titrated to 100 mg/day over 4 wks: wk 1: 25 mg in the evening; wk 2: 25 mg morning and evening; wk 3: 25 mg morning and 50 mg evening; wk 4: 50 mg morning and evening.
7. *Botox* is FDA-approved for prevention of headaches in adult patients with chronic migraine. *Botox Cosmetic* is not FDA-approved for migraine prevention.
8. Total dosage of 155 units is divided over 7 specific head/neck muscle areas (detailed information provided in package insert).
9. Cost of one 200-unit vial.

for gestational age infants and, at high doses, with embryofetal resorptions in animals.

ANTIEPILEPTIC DRUGS — Valproate (*Depakote*, and others) and topiramate (*Topamax*, and generics) are similarly effective in decreasing migraine frequency and are FDA-approved for migraine prevention. About 50% of patients achieve a ≥50% reduction in headache frequency with these drugs.[26] In randomized, double-blind trials, topiramate was at least as effective as propranolol for migraine prevention.[27,28] Topiramate has reduced the number of migraine headache days per month and improved associated symptoms in patients with chronic migraine (≥15 headache days/month for ≥3 months) and medication overuse headache.[29,30] In a trial in pediatric patients, however, topiramate was no better than placebo in preventing migraine.[31]

Adverse Effects – Adverse effects of valproate include nausea, fatigue, tremor, weight gain, and hair loss. Acute hepatic failure, pancreatitis, and hyperammonemia (in patients with urea cycle disorders) occur rarely. Other adverse effects include polycystic ovary syndrome, hyperinsulinemia, lipid abnormalities, hirsutism, and menstrual disturbances. Topiramate commonly causes paresthesias; fatigue, language and cognitive impairment, taste perversion, weight loss, and nephrolithiasis can also occur. Topiramate can rarely cause secondary narrow-angle glaucoma, oligohydrosis, and symptomatic metabolic acidosis.

Pregnancy – Use of topiramate or valproate during pregnancy has been associated with congenital malformations[32,33]; neither drug should be used for migraine prevention in pregnant women.

ANTIDEPRESSANTS — Amitriptyline is the only **tricyclic** antidepressant shown to be effective for migraine prevention in clinical trials,[34] but it often causes sedation, dry mouth, and weight gain. Other tricyclics such as nortriptyline, which may have fewer adverse effects than amitriptyline, are frequently used for migraine prevention in adults. In a trial in pediatric patients, amitriptyline was no better than placebo in preventing migraine.[31]

The **SNRIs** venlafaxine (*Effexor*, and others) and duloxetine (*Cymbalta*, and generics) may also be effective in preventing migraine.[22,35,36] They can cause nausea, vomiting, sweating, tachycardia, urinary retention, and increased blood pressure.

Pregnancy – Tricyclic antidepressant use during pregnancy has been associated with jitteriness and seizures in newborns. Fetal malformations are uncommon with SNRIs, but increased risks of neonatal behavioral syndrome and perinatal complications have been reported with use of SNRIs during pregnancy.[37]

OTHER PREVENTIVE TREATMENTS — **NSAIDs**, such as naproxen and ibuprofen, have been used for prevention of migraine and for aborting acute attacks.[38]

The **angiotensin-converting enzyme (ACE) inhibitor** lisinopril (*Prinivil*, and others) and the **angiotensin receptor blocker (ARB)** candesartan (*Atacand*, and generics) have reduced migraine frequency by about 30-35% in small, double-blind trials.[39] In a randomized, placebo-controlled, crossover trial, candesartan was noninferior to propranolol for prevention of migraine.[40]

The **calcium channel blocker** verapamil (*Calan*, and others) was somewhat more effective than placebo in some small studies.[41]

The combination of **simvastatin** (*Zocor*, and others) and **vitamin D** was effective for migraine prevention in one small, randomized, placebo-controlled trial.[42]

The **dietary supplement** petasites (butterbur; *Petadolex*) 100-150 mg daily reduced migraine attack frequency by 36-60% in two randomized, placebo-controlled trials in about 300 patients,[38] but it has been associated with hepatic toxicity.[43] Melatonin, riboflavin, magnesium citrate, coenzyme Q10, and feverfew have also been effective in preventing migraine in small, randomized, placebo-controlled trials.[38,43,44]

Pericranial intramuscular injections of **onabotulinumtoxinA** *(Botox)* are FDA-approved for prevention of headaches in adults with chronic migraine (≥15 headaches/month).[45] Botulinum toxin is not recommended for prevention of episodic migraine.

A **transcutaneous electrical nerve stimulation device** *(Cefaly)* that is worn on the forehead has been approved by the FDA for prevention of episodic migraine in adults. In one small study, daily 20-minute treatments for 3 months were modestly effective in reducing the number of migraine days per month.[46]

1. EA MacGregor. In the clinic. Migraine. Ann Intern Med 2013; 159:ITC5-1.
2. MJ Marmura et al. The acute treatment of migraine in adults: the American Headache Society evidence assessment of migraine pharmacotherapies. Headache 2015; 55:3.
3. MJ Prior et al. A randomized, placebo-controlled trial of acetaminophen for treatment of migraine headache. Headache 2010; 50:819.
4. CC Suthisisang et al. Meta-analysis of the efficacy and safety of naproxen sodium in the acute treatment of migraine. Headache 2010; 50:808.
5. C Suthisisang et al. Efficacy of low-dose ibuprofen in acute migraine treatment: systematic review and meta-analysis. Ann Pharmacother 2007; 41:1782.
6. C Chen et al. Differential pharmacokinetics of diclofenac potassium for oral solution vs immediate-release tablets from a randomized trial: effect of fed and fasting conditions. Headache 2015; 55:265.
7. MM Johnston and AM Rapoport. Triptans for the management of migraine. Drugs 2010; 70:1505.
8. V Tullo et al. Frovatriptan versus zolmitriptan for the acute treatment of migraine: a double-blind, randomized, multicenter, Italian study. Neurol Sci 2010; 31 Suppl 1:S51.
9. S Law et al. Sumatriptan plus naproxen for the treatment of acute migraine attacks in adults. Cochrane Database Syst Rev 2016; 4:CD008541.
10. Onzetra Xsail - sumatriptan nasal powder. Med Lett Drugs Ther 2016; 58:92.
11. G Roberto et al. Triptans and serious adverse vascular events: data mining of the FDA Adverse Event Reporting System database. Cephalalgia 2014; 34:5.
12. Inhibitors and inducers of CYP enzymes and P-glycoprotein. Med Lett Drugs Ther 2016 Aug 2 (epub). Available at: http://secure.medicalletter.org/downloads/CYP_PGP_Tables.pdf. Accessed February 2, 2017.
13. FDA Public Health Advisory. Combined use of 5-hydroxytryptamine receptor agonists (triptans), selective serotonin reuptake inhibitors (SSRIs) or selective serotonin/norepinephrine reuptake inhibitors (SNRIs) may result in life-threatening serotonin syndrome. July 19, 2006. Last updated August 16, 2013. Available at: www.fda.gov/Drugs/DrugSafety/ucm124349.htm. Accessed February 2, 2017.
14. PE Rolan. Drug interactions with triptans: which are clinically significant? CNS Drugs 2012; 26:949.

15. ML Hilaire et al. Treatment of migraine headaches with sumatriptan in pregnancy. Ann Pharmacother 2004; 38:1726.
16. K Nezvalová-Henriksen et al. Triptan safety during pregnancy: a Norwegian population registry study. Eur J Epidemiol 2013; 28:759.
17. US National Library of Medicine. Drugs and Lactation Database (LactMed). Available at: https://toxnet.nlm.nih.gov/newtoxnet/lactmed.htm. Accessed February 2, 2017.
18. MJ Láinez et al. Crossover, double-blind clinical trial comparing almotriptan and ergotamine plus caffeine for acute migraine therapy. Eur J Neurol 2007; 14:269.
19. RB Lipton et al. Single-pulse transcranial magnetic stimulation for acute treatment of migraine with aura: a randomised, double-blind, parallel-group, sham-controlled trial. Lancet Neurol 2010; 9:373.
20. JR Saper and AN Da Silva. Medication overuse headache: history, features, prevention and management strategies. CNS Drugs 2013; 27:867.
21. SJ Tepper. Medication-overuse headache. Continuum (Minneap Minn) 2012; 18:807.
22. SD Silberstein et al. Evidence-based guideline update: pharmacologic treatment for episodic migraine prevention in adults: report of the Quality Standards Subcommittee of the American Academy of Neurology and the American Headache Society. Neurology 2012; 78:1337.
23. E Loder et al. The 2012 AHS/AAN guidelines for prevention of episodic migraine: a summary and comparison with other recent clinical practice guidelines. Headache 2012; 52:930.
24. T Pringsheim et al. Acute treatment and prevention of menstrually related migraine headache: evidence-based review. Neurology 2008; 70:1555.
25. EA MacGregor et al. Safety and tolerability of frovatriptan in the acute treatment of migraine and prevention of menstrual migraine: results of a new analysis of data from five previously published studies. Gend Med 2010; 7:88.
26. WM Mulleners et al. Antiepileptics in migraine prophylaxis: an updated Cochrane review. Cephalalgia 2015; 35:51.
27. HC Diener et al. Topiramate in migraine prophylaxis–results from a placebo-controlled trial with propranolol as an active control. J Neurol 2004; 251:943.
28. F Ashtari et al. A double-blind, randomized trial of low-dose topiramate vs propranolol in migraine prophylaxis. Acta Neurol Scand 2008; 118:301.
29. S Silberstein et al. Topiramate treatment of chronic migraine: a randomized, placebo-controlled trial of quality of life and other efficacy measures. Headache 2009; 49:1153.
30. HC Diener et al. Topiramate reduces headache days in chronic migraine: a randomized, double-blind, placebo-controlled study. Cephalalgia 2007; 27:814.
31. SW Powers et al. Trial of amitriptyline, topiramate, and placebo for pediatric migraine. N Engl J Med 2017; 376:115.
32. In brief: Warning against use of valproate for migraine prevention during pregnancy. Med Lett Drugs Ther 2013; 55:45.
33. J Weston et al. Monotherapy treatment of epilepsy in pregnancy: congenital malformation outcomes in the child. Cochrane Database Syst Rev 2016; 11:CD010224.
34. DW Dodick et al. Topiramate versus amitriptyline in migraine prevention: a 26-week, multicenter, randomized, double-blind, double-dummy, parallel-group noninferiority trial in adult migraineurs. Clin Ther 2009; 31:542.

35. S Tarlaci. Escitalopram and venlafaxine for the prophylaxis of migraine headache without mood disorders. Clin Neuropharmacol 2009; 32:254.
36. WB Young et al. Duloxetine prophylaxis for episodic migraine in persons without depression: a prospective study. Headache 2013; 53:1430.
37. C Bellantuono et al. The safety of serotonin-noradrenaline reuptake inhibitors (SNRIs) in pregnancy and breastfeeding: a comprehensive review. Hum Psychopharmacol 2015; 30:143.
38. S Holland et al. Evidence-based guideline update: NSAIDs and other complementary treatments for episodic migraine prevention in adults: report of the Quality Standards Subcommittee of the American Academy of Neurology and the American Headache Society. Neurology 2012; 78:1346.
39. BJ Gales et al. Angiotensin-converting enzyme inhibitors and angiotensin receptor blockers for the prevention of migraines. Ann Pharmacother 2010; 44:360.
40. LJ Stovner et al. A comparative study of candesartan versus propranolol for migraine prophylaxis: A randomised, triple-blind, placebo-controlled, double cross-over study. Cephalalgia 2014; 34:523.
41. JL Jackson et al. A comparative effectiveness meta-analysis of drugs for the prophylaxis of migraine headache. PLoS One 2015; 10:e0130733.
42. C Buettner et al. Simvastatin and vitamin D for migraine prevention: a randomized, controlled trial. Ann Neurol 2015; 78:970.
43. SJ Tepper. Nutraceutical and other modalities for the treatment of headache. Continuum (Minneap Minn) 2015; 21:1018.
44. AL GonÇalves et al. Randomised clinical trial comparing melatonin 3 mg, amitriptyline 25 mg and placebo for migraine prevention. J Neurol Neurosurg Psychiatry 2016; 87:1127.
45. Botulinum toxin for chronic migraine. Med Lett Drugs Ther 2011; 53:7.
46. A transcutaneous electrical nerve stimulation device (Cefaly) for migraine prevention. Med Lett Drugs Ther 2014; 56:78.

DRUGS FOR Opioid Use Disorder

Original publication date – March 2017 (revised March 2018)

Opioid use disorder is a chronic, relapsing disease with both physical and psychiatric components. It is associated with economic hardship, social isolation, incarceration, increased rates of blood-borne infections such as HIV and viral hepatitis, adverse pregnancy outcomes, and increased mortality. According to the CDC, there were 33,091 deaths related to opioid overdose in the US in 2015, more than in any previous year.[1] Diagnostic criteria for opioid use disorder were updated in the DSM-5.[1a] Several guidelines on the management of opioid use disorder have recently been published.[2-5]

MAINTENANCE TREATMENT

METHADONE — Methadone was the first successful treatment for opioid addiction; it is a synthetic mu-opioid receptor agonist with a slow onset of action and a long, variable elimination half-life. At high doses, methadone induces cross-tolerance with other opioid agonists. Patients tolerant to other opioid agonists, however, may have only an incomplete cross-tolerance to methadone.[6]

Availability – Methadone is classified as a schedule II controlled substance (highest potential for abuse; recognized medical use). In the US, methadone maintenance treatment is only available through government-licensed opioid treatment programs which offer supervised

Recommendations for Treatment of Opioid Use Disorder
▸ Maintenance pharmacotherapy is more effective than only treating withdrawal symptoms. ▸ Maintenance treatment with methadone has been shown to reduce mortality, but the drug's adverse effects and potential drug interactions are a concern. Methadone should be used in patients who do not have access to buprenorphine, those whose disorder does not respond to buprenorphine, and those who would benefit from daily supervised dosing. ▸ Buprenorphine with or without naloxone is the maintenance treatment of choice for most patients. It is safer than methadone, can be prescribed in an outpatient setting, and at higher doses appears to be similarly effective. ▸ Extended-release naltrexone is an alternative for highly motivated patients who do not have access to buprenorphine or methadone or do not want to take an opioid, and for those who also have alcohol use disorder. Naltrexone has not been shown to lower mortality. ▸ In pregnant or breastfeeding women, maintenance treatment with methadone or buprenorphine (without naloxone) is recommended. ▸ Naloxone is the drug of choice for emergency treatment of opioid overdose. New laws have increased its availability to relatives and friends of opioid users and to first responders.

administration of the drug. The drug is available in oral tablets, tablets for oral suspension, an oral solution, and an oral concentrate. To reduce the risk of drug diversion, treatment programs usually do not dispense the tablet formulation.[7]

Efficacy – Methadone maintenance therapy can improve treatment retention, productivity, and social engagement, and decrease crime rates, heroin use, injection risk behaviors, mortality rates, and the spread of blood-borne infections such as hepatitis C and HIV.[8-11] Use of higher doses of methadone (≥100 mg/day) in patients with opioid use disorder and HIV infection has been associated with increased adherence to antiretroviral therapy, lower viral loads, and higher CD4 cell counts.[12]

Safety – The risk of methadone-associated mortality is highest in the first weeks after starting or stopping treatment.[13] The drug accumulates during induction; it takes 4-7 days to achieve a stable dose. In overdosage, or if the dose is increased too rapidly during initiation of therapy, methadone can cause sedation and respiratory depression. The respiratory depressant effect of methadone peaks later and lasts longer than that of buprenorphine and other opioid agonists, and it persists longer than the analgesic effect of the drug.

Methadone can prolong the QT interval and cause arrhythmias such as torsades de pointes, particularly in patients taking other QT interval-prolonging drugs[14] and in those with congenital long QT syndrome or a history of QT-interval prolongation.[15]

Drug Interactions – Methadone is a substrate of CYP3A4 and CYP2B6; inhibitors of these isozymes can increase serum concentrations of methadone, and inducers can reduce them.[16] Concurrent use of methadone and other QT interval-prolonging drugs should be avoided if possible.[14] As with any opioid, concomitant use of methadone with selective serotonin reuptake inhibitors (SSRIs), serotonin and norepinephrine reuptake inhibitors (SNRIs), tricyclic antidepressants, or other serotonergic drugs could result in serotonin syndrome. Concurrent use of methadone and benzodiazepines or other sedating drugs can result in additive CNS effects.

Dosage and Administration – Because methadone has a long half-life, initial titration of the drug should be performed slowly. Federal law prohibits administration of an initial methadone dose >30 mg or a total first daily dose >40 mg.[17] For most patients, a maintenance dose of 60-120 mg/day can suppress cravings and block the euphoric effects of other opioid agonists.[18]

BUPRENORPHINE — Buprenorphine is a mu-opioid receptor partial agonist and kappa-opioid receptor antagonist. It is available alone and in combination with the opioid antagonist naloxone.[19-22] Taken orally, naloxone is poorly absorbed and generally has no clinical effects; combining it with buprenorphine in sublingual or buccal formulations is intended to counteract intravenous or intranasal abuse.

Table 1. Some Drugs for Maintenance Treatment of Opioid Use Disorder	
Drug	**Some Available Formulations**
Buprenorphine	
generic	2, 8 mg sublingual tabs
Probuphine (Braeburn)[2]	74.2 mg subdermal implant
Sublocade (Indivior)[4]	100 mg/0.5 mL, 300 mg/1.5 mL prefilled syringes for subcutaneous injection[5]
Buprenorphine/Naloxone	
generic	2/0.5, 8/2 mg sublingual tabs
Bunavail (BioDelivery Sciences)	2.1/0.3, 4.2/0.7, 6.3/1 mg buccal films
Suboxone (Indivior)	2/0.5, 4/1, 8/2, 12/3 mg sublingual films
Zubsolv (Orexo)	0.7/0.18, 1.4/0.36, 2.9/0.71, 5.7/1.4, 8.6/2.1, 11.4/2.9 mg sublingual tabs
Methadone	
generic	5, 10 mg tabs; 5, 10 mg/5 mL oral solution; 10 mg/mL oral concentrate; 40 mg tabs for oral suspension[7]
Dolophine (Roxane)	5, 10 mg tabs[7]
Naltrexone	
generic *Revia* (Duramed)	50 mg tabs
extended-release microspheres – *Vivitrol* (Alkermes)	380 mg ER suspension for injection

1. Approximate WAC for 6 months' treatment at the lowest target maintenance dosage. WAC = wholesaler acquisition cost or manufacturer's published price to wholesalers; WAC represents a published catalogue or list price and may not represent an actual transactional price. Source: AnalySource® Monthly. February 5, 2018. Reprinted with permission by First Databank, Inc. All rights reserved. ©2018. www.fdbhealth.com/policies/drug-pricing-policy.
2. Approved for 6 or 12 months' treatment of patients with opioid use disorder in whom prolonged clinical stability has been achieved and sustained with transmucosal doses of buprenorphine ≤8 mg/day. Not approved for initial treatment or for more than 12 months of use.
3. Buprenorphine levels after insertion of 4 *Probuphine* implants are comparable to those achieved with 8 mg/day of sublingual buprenorphine.
4. Approved for treatment of moderate to severe opioid use disorder in patients who have received treatment with a transmucosal buprenorphine-containing product for ≥7 days with dose adjustment to 8-24 mg/day of buprenorphine sublingual tablets or equivalent. Not approved for initial treatment.

Target Maintenance Dosage	Cost[1]
16 mg once/d	$1083.60
4 implants for 6 months[3]	4950.00
100 mg once/month[6]	9480.00
16/4 mg once/d	2339.10
8.4/1.4 mg once/d	2793.60
16/4 mg once/d	2933.30
11.4/2.9 mg once/d	2989.40
80-120 mg once/d[8]	73.50[9]
	850.80
50 mg once/day	371.00 1648.90
380 mg IM q4 wks or once/month	7854.00

5. Syringes should be refrigerated during storage; they should be discarded if left at room temperature for >7 days.
6. 300 mg/month for the first two doses. The monthly maintenance dose can be increased to 300 mg if patients do not have a satisfactory clinical response to the 100-mg dose. Steady-state buprenorphine levels with the target maintenance dosage are about 10% higher than those achieved with 24 mg/day of sublingual buprenorphine tablets.
7. To reduce the risk of drug diversion, the liquid formulation, diluted in colored water or juice, is generally used in treatment programs.
8. Some rapid metabolizers may require more frequent dosing.
9. Cost of oral concentrate.

Availability – Buprenorphine is classified as a schedule III controlled substance (less potential for abuse than schedule II; recognized medical use). In the US, prescribers who complete a training course and obtain a special DEA number can treat a limited number of patients for opioid use disorder with buprenorphine in an outpatient setting; current laws relating to outpatient prescription of buprenorphine are available at the website for the Substance Abuse and Mental Health Services Administration.[23]

Efficacy – Buprenorphine significantly improves treatment retention and reduces illicit opioid use compared to placebo.[24] It appears to be at least as effective as methadone in reducing mortality.[13] Office-based buprenorphine/naloxone maintenance therapy has been shown to improve abstinence rates, occupational stability, and psychosocial outcomes.[25]

Administering buprenorphine via subdermal implant *(Probuphine)*[22] or once-monthly extended-release subcutaneous injection *(Sublocade)*[25a] should reduce the risks of treatment nonadherence and drug diversion, but these formulations are more expensive than transmucosal buprenorphine. *Sublocade* has not been studied in active-controlled clinical trials.

Safety – Even without naloxone, buprenorphine is safer than methadone because it has a ceiling on its respiratory depressant effect. As a partial agonist, it also has a lower abuse potential than methadone; the presence of naloxone may further reduce the abuse potential of buprenorphine products.

In a retrospective analysis of about 5 million adverse drug events reported to the FDA over 42 years, events mentioning methadone, but not those mentioning buprenorphine, were disproportionately likely to involve QT-interval prolongaton, ventricular arrhythmia, or cardiac arrest.[26]

In a retrospective study in the United Kingdom of about 20 million prescriptions for methadone or buprenorphine over a 6-year period, prescriptions for methadone were 6.23 times more likely to be associated with a subsequent overdose death than prescriptions for buprenorphine with or without naloxone.[27]

Hepatic impairment reduces naloxone clearance to a greater extent than it does buprenorphine clearance. Use of fixed-dose buprenorphine/naloxone combinations in patients with severe hepatic impairment can lead to withdrawal symptoms when treatment is started and may decrease the efficacy of buprenorphine maintenance treatment.

Buprenorphine subdermal implants, like other drug-eluting implants, can cause adverse effects such as pain, pruritus, and erythema at the insertion site, and insertion and removal of implants have been associated with nerve injury and implant migration and extrusion. Healthcare providers must complete a live training session and become certified through a Risk Evaluation and Mitigation Strategy (REMS) program before they can prescribe, insert, or remove buprenorphine implants.[22]

Injection-site reactions can occur with subcutaneous administration of buprenorphine. Healthcare facilities must become certified through a REMS program before they can order and dispense *Sublocade*.[27a]

Drug Interactions – Concurrent use of benzodiazepines or other sedating drugs with opioids such as buprenorphine can result in additive effects. Buprenorphine is metabolized primarily by CYP3A4; concomitant use with a 3A4 inducer can decrease buprenorphine serum concentrations and use with a 3A4 inhibitor can increase them.[16] Buprenorphine is a substrate of P-glycoprotein (P-gp); concomitant use with inhibitors of P-gp could increase buprenorphine serum concentrations. Use of an opioid with serotonergic drugs such as selective serotonin reuptake inhibitors (SSRIs) may result in serotonin syndrome, though the risk is lower with buprenorphine than it is with directly serotonergic opioids such as methadone.

Buprenorphine may interfere with the analgesic efficacy of full opioid agonists. It should generally be discontinued 24-36 hours before elective surgery (except Cesarean section; stopping buprenorphine could cause fetal withdrawal).

Dosage and Administration – Buprenorphine has a greater affinity for opioid receptors than full opioid agonists such as heroin and can displace them, causing opioid withdrawal. The risk of withdrawal can be reduced by not starting treatment until the patient is already experiencing mild-to-moderate opioid withdrawal (Clinical Opiate Withdrawal Scale score ~11-12)[28] and by using a low initial dose of buprenorphine (2-4 mg of *Suboxone*, or equivalent). The daily dose should then be uptitrated, usually to at least 8 mg; most patients can readily achieve their target dose within 2-3 days. Higher doses (12-16 mg/day) should be considered if opioid misuse or abuse persists. Data supporting increased efficacy with doses >16 mg/day up to the maximum recommended dose of 24 mg/day are limited.

NALTREXONE — The mu-opioid receptor antagonist naltrexone is available as a once-daily oral tablet (*Revia*, and generics) and as a once-monthly extended-release (ER) microsphere suspension given by intramuscular (IM) injection *(Vivitrol)*. It is not addictive or readily abused, and tolerance to its effects does not develop with long-term use. Both oral and extended-release IM naltrexone are also approved for treatment of alcohol use disorder.[29]

Availability – Naltrexone is not a controlled substance, and there are no special restrictions on its prescription.

Efficacy – Adherence and outcomes have been better with extended-release IM naltrexone than with the oral formulation, though neither formulation has been conclusively shown to have a mortality benefit. In a randomized, double-blind, placebo-controlled, 24-week trial in 250 patients with opioid dependence, addition of injectable naltrexone to biweekly counseling was found to significantly increase the likelihood of abstinence from opioid use, improve retention in the treatment program, and reduce cravings and relapse to physiological opioid dependence, compared to addition of placebo.[30] In an open-label, randomized,

Table 2. Recommendations for Switching Treatments for Opioid Use Disorder[1]
Methadone to Buprenorphine
▸ Use buprenorphine without naloxone when initially switching therapies
▸ Tapering to 30-40 mg/day of methadone before transition can reduce patient discomfort
▸ Administer first dose (2-4 mg of *Suboxone*, or equivalent) ≥24 hours after last dose of methadone
▸ Observe patient for 1 hour after first dose
▸ If withdrawal symptoms improve, dispense 2 additional doses (2-4 mg) to be taken as needed later in the day
Methadone or Buprenorphine to Naltrexone
▸ Patient must be completely withdrawn from methadone or buprenorphine before starting naltrexone (may take up to 14 days)
▸ Consider naloxone challenge (0.4-0.8 mg) to confirm absence of physiological dependence, except in pregnant women
Buprenorphine to Methadone
▸ No special time delay or precautions required
Naltrexone to Buprenorphine or Methadone
▸ Use of naltrexone can reduce tolerance to opioids
▸ Administer first dose of methadone or buprenorphine about 1 day after last dose of oral naltrexone or 30 days after last dose of IM naltrexone

1. Adapted from: American Society of Addiction Medicine. National practice guideline for the use of medications in the treatment of addiction involving opioid use. 2015. Available at: www.asam.org/docs/default-source/practice-support/guidelines-and-consensus-docs/asam-national-practice-guideline-supplement.pdf. Accessed May 25, 2017.

24-week trial in 308 patients with a history of opioid dependence who were abstinent from opioids at the time of randomization, those who received extended-release IM naltrexone had a significantly longer median time to relapse (10.5 vs 5.0 weeks) and significantly lower rates of relapse (43% vs 64%) than those who received usual care, which consisted of brief counseling and referral to community treatment programs.[31] In an open-label study, treatment failure during induction occurred significantly more often with once-monthly IM naltrexone than with sublingual buprenorphine/naloxone, but among those successfully inducted, the two treatments were similar in efficacy and safety.[31a]

In a meta-analysis of 13 studies, oral naltrexone was no more effective than placebo, nonpharmacologic treatment, or benzodiazepines or buprenorphine in reducing opioid use, and treatment retention was poor.[32] Oral naltrexone was more effective than placebo in sustaining abstinence in studies where patients were legally mandated to take the drug.[31-33]

Safety – Naltrexone is generally well tolerated. Adverse effects reported in opioid-dependent patients given IM naltrexone have included injection-site reactions, nasopharyngitis, insomnia, headache, nausea, and toothache. Depressed mood and suicidality have occurred rarely; a cause-and-effect relationship has not been established. Hepatic enzyme elevations and toxicity have been reported with use of naltrexone, but these findings occur frequently in opioid- and alcohol-dependent patients. Use of naltrexone can reduce tolerance to opioids; patients who relapse after receiving naltrexone may be at greater risk of a serious, potentially fatal opioid overdose.

Drug Interactions – Naltrexone blocks the effects of usual doses of opioids, including opioid-derivative antidiarrheals and antitussives.[34] It should not be used in patients taking an opioid for treatment of pain. Oral naltrexone should be discontinued 72 hours before and IM naltrexone 30 days before elective surgery.

Dosage and Administration – Administration of naltrexone to a patient with physiological opioid dependence can precipitate a severe opioid withdrawal syndrome; patients should be free of dependence for at least 7 days before naltrexone is initiated. A naloxone challenge can be used to confirm the absence of physiological opioid dependence, but it is contraindicated in pregnant women because it can induce preterm labor or fetal distress.

Vivitrol is supplied in single-use cartons containing a vial of microspheres, a diluent for suspension, needles, and a syringe. It should be given as a 380-mg IM gluteal injection in alternating buttocks every 4 weeks or once monthly. The dose pack should be stored in the refrigerator; if left unrefrigerated, it may be used for up to 7 days as long as it is not exposed to temperatures >77°F (25°C).

Patients starting treatment with oral naltrexone should receive an initial dose of 25 mg. If withdrawal symptoms do not occur, they can then be given a maintenance dosage of 50 mg once daily.

ALTERNATIVES — Limited data suggest that **24-hour extended-release oral morphine** may be effective for maintenance treatment of opioid use disorder. Morphine may be better tolerated and more effective than methadone in some patients; it has less of an effect on the QT interval, but it may have a greater risk of opioid-related adverse effects.[35] In a 22-week, randomized, open-label, crossover study in 157 patients being treated in methadone maintenance clinics, 24-hour oral morphine was noninferior to methadone in preventing positive urine tests for heroin. Adverse effects were similar in the two groups.[36]

Addition of supervised **heroin** injections to flexible-dose methadone therapy has been shown to improve treatment retention and may also reduce criminal activity, incarceration rates, and social functioning, but it also increases the risk of adverse events.[37]

In a 12-week, randomized, double-blind trial in 196 opioid-dependent patients, addition of the antitussive **dextromethorphan** 60 mg/day to methadone maintenance therapy significantly improved treatment retention and decreased plasma morphine levels compared to placebo, but addition of dextromethorphan 120 mg/day did not.[38]

In a 24-week randomized trial in 141 opioid-dependent patients, addition of **cognitive behavioral therapy** to primary care-based maintenance treatment with buprenorphine did not improve self-reported opioid use or opioid abstinence.[39]

PREGNANCY — Opioid use during pregnancy is associated with an increased risk of complications such as preeclampsia, miscarriage, reduced fetal growth, fetal death, and premature delivery.[40] Pregnant women who are physically dependent on opioids or are likely to resume opioid misuse should receive opioid agonist maintenance therapy; it is safer than detoxification alone.[41]

Methadone has a long history of use in pregnancy and is generally considered the standard of care for maintenance treatment of pregnant women with opioid use disorder. More recently, **buprenorphine** (without naloxone) has been used as an effective and safe alternative. In a randomized, double-blind, double-dummy trial in 175 opioid-dependent pregnant women, neonates whose mothers were treated with buprenorphine during pregnancy required less morphine and had shorter durations of treatment for neonatal abstinence syndrome and hospital stays than those whose mothers received methadone, but treatment retention was significantly greater among women taking methadone.[42]

Combination **buprenorphine/naloxone** products are considered safe for use during pregnancy, but data on their efficacy in pregnant women are limited.[43] Buprenorphine without naloxone is preferred.

Data on the safety and efficacy of **naltrexone** use in pregnancy are limited. In general, women taking naltrexone who become pregnant and are at high risk for relapse can continue treatment.

LACTATION — Use of **methadone** or **buprenorphine** monotherapy by breastfeeding women is generally considered safe. Women taking **naltrexone** should not breastfeed because the drug and its major metabolite can pass into breast milk to a clinically significant extent.

TREATMENT OF OPIOID OVERDOSE

NALOXONE — Naloxone is the drug of choice for emergency treatment of opioid overdose. It is available in various dosage forms for intravenous (IV), intramuscular (IM), subcutaneous (SC), or intranasal administration (see Table 3).[44,45]

Table 3. Some Naloxone Formulations

Drug	Formulations	Usual Dosage	Cost[1]
Parenteral			
generic	0.4 mg/mL vials and syringes; 1 mg/mL syringes	0.4-2 mg IV, IM, or SC[2]	$13.70[3]
Evzio (Kaleo)	0.4, 2 mg/0.4 mL prefilled auto-injectors	0.4 or 2 mg IM or SC[4]	1875.00[5]
Intranasal			
Narcan nasal spray (Adapt)	4 mg/0.1 mL nasal spray[6]	4 mg intranasally[4]	62.50[7,8]

1. Approximate WAC for a single dose at the lowest usual dosage. WAC = wholesaler acquisition cost or manufacturer's published price to wholesalers; WAC represents a published catalogue or list price and may not represent an actual transactional price. Source: AnalySource® Monthly. May 5, 2017. Reprinted with permission by First Databank, Inc. All rights reserved. ©2017. www.fdbhealth.com/policies/drug-pricing-policy.
2. Dose can be repeated every 2-3 minutes up to a total of 10 mg.
3. Cost for a 1-mL vial.
4. Dose can be repeated every 2-3 minutes until the patient responds or emergency medical personnel arrive.
5. Manufacturer's list price for insurers for one 0.4-mg auto-injector, but it is supplied in packages containing 2 auto-injectors. The list price for one 2-mg auto-injector is $2050. Insurers and pharmacy benefit managers may negotiate with the manufacturer for a lower price or decide not to pay for *Evzio* at all. According to the manufacturer, the out-of-pocket cost is $0 for all commercially insured patients, whether or not their insurer covers the device. The cash price for patients without government or commercial insurance is $360 for those with a household income ≥$100,000/year and $0 for those with a household income <$100,000/year.
6. A 2 mg/0.1 mL formulation of *Narcan* nasal spray has been approved by the FDA, but is not yet available.
7. Cost for one nasal spray device, but supplied in cartons containing two nasal spray devices.
8. Available from the manufacturer at a discounted price of $37.50 per 4-mg nasal spray device to law enforcement, firefighters, first responders, departments of health, local school districts, colleges and universities, and community-based organizations.

Availability – A number of jurisdictions now have naloxone access laws that make the drug available to first responders and to relatives and close friends of persons using heroin or taking prescription opioids. These laws may also grant civil and criminal immunity to laypeople who carry or administer naloxone, to healthcare professionals who prescribe or dispense the drug to laypeople, and to persons who call emergency medical services in good faith to reverse an overdose. A regularly updated database of state naloxone access laws is available (http://lawatlas.org/datasets/laws-regulating-administration-of-naloxone).

Pharmacology – Naloxone is a competitive mu-opioid receptor antagonist and has no opioid agonist effects. In opioid overdose, naloxone begins to reverse sedation, respiratory depression, and hypotension within 1-2 minutes after IV administration, 2-5 minutes after IM or SC administration, and 8-13 minutes after intranasal administration.

The half-life of naloxone is much shorter than that of most opioids and repeated administration may be necessary, especially for overdose with a long-acting opioid agonist such as methadone or a sustained-release formulation of a short-acting agonist such as oxycodone. Pure heroin has a shorter half-life than naloxone (2-6 minutes), but heroin is a prodrug that is rapidly metabolized to 6-acetylmorphine and morphine. The risk of respiratory depression is related to those active metabolites, and it may persist well beyond the clearance of heroin from the blood. Other drugs used to "cut" heroin may have longer half-lives.[46] If not already present, emergency medical services should always be called immediately after administration of naloxone.

Adverse Effects – Whether naloxone itself has any toxicity is unclear, but it can precipitate acute withdrawal symptoms in opioid-dependent patients. Acute opioid withdrawal is associated with anxiety, piloerection, yawning, sneezing, rhinorrhea, nausea, vomiting, diarrhea, and abdominal or muscle cramps, which are uncomfortable but generally not life-threatening, except in neonates. In a pharmacokinetic study of intranasal naloxone *(Narcan)*, the most common adverse effects were increased blood pressure, constipation, toothache, muscle spasms, musculoskeletal pain, headache, rhinalgia, xeroderma, and intranasal effects including dryness, edema, congestion, and inflammation.

Pregnancy – No embryotoxic or teratogenic effects were observed in pregnant mice and rats treated with large doses of naloxone. Naloxone does cross the placenta, however, and may cause fetal opioid withdrawal or induce preterm labor.

1. Centers for Disease Control and Prevention. Drug overdose death data. Available at: www.cdc.gov/drugoverdose/data/statedeaths.html. Accessed May 25, 2017.
1a. American Psychiatric Association. Opioid use disorder: diagnostic criteria. Available at: https://pcssmat.org/wp-content/uploads/2014/02/5B-DSM-5-Opioid-Use-Disorder-Diagnostic-Criteria.pdf. Accessed February 15, 2018.
2. American Society of Addiction Medicine. National practice guideline for the use of medications in the treatment of addiction involving opioid use. 2015. Available at: www.asam.org/docs/default-source/practice-support/guidelines-and-consensus-docs/asam-national-practice-guideline-supplement.pdf. Accessed May 25, 2017.
3. Department of Veterans Affairs and Department of Defense. VA/DoD clinical practice guideline for the management of substance use disorders. 2015. Available at: www.healthquality.va.gov/guidelines/MH/sud/VADoDSUDCPGRevised22216.pdf. Accessed May 25, 2017.
4. MA Schuckit. Treatment of opioid-use disorders. N Engl J Med 2016; 375:357.
5. British Columbia Ministry of Health. A guideline for the clinical management of opioid use disorder. Available at: www2.gov.bc.ca/assets/gov/health/practitioner-pro/bc-guidelines/bc_oud_guidelines.pdf. Accessed May 25, 2017.
6. Institute for Safe Medication Practices. Keeping patients safe from iatrogenic methadone overdoses. February 14, 2008. Available at: www.ismp.org/newsletters/acutecare/articles/ 20080214.asp. Accessed May 25, 2017.
7. Substance Abuse and Mental Health Services Administration. Substance abuse treatment advisory. News for the treatment field. Emerging issues in the use of methadone. 2009. Available at: https://store.samhsa.gov/shin/content/SMA09-4368/SMA09-4368.pdf. Accessed May 25, 2017.
8. RP Mattick et al. Methadone maintenance therapy versus no opioid replacement therapy for opioid dependence. Cochrane Database Syst Rev 2009; 3:CD002209.
9. F Faggiano et al. Methadone maintenance at different dosages for opioid dependence. Cochrane Database Syst Rev 2003; 3:CD002208.
10. L Gowing et al. Oral substitution treatment of injecting opioid users for prevention of HIV infection. Cochrane Database Syst Rev 2011; 8:CD004145.
11. S Nolan et al. The impact of methadone maintenance therapy on hepatitis C incidence among illicit drug users. Addiction 2014; 109:2053.
12. L Lappalainen et al. Dose-response relationship between methadone dose and adherence to antiretroviral therapy among HIV-positive people who use illicit opioids. Addiction 2015; 110:1330.
13. L Sordo et al. Mortality risk during and after opioid substitution treatment: systematic review and meta-analysis of cohort studies. BMJ 2017; 357:j1550.
14. RL Woosley and KA Romero. QT drugs list. Available at: www.crediblemeds.org. Accessed May 25, 2017.
15. FDA. Information for healthcare professionals methadone hydrochloride text version. Available at: www.fda.gov/Drugs/DrugSafety/PostmarketDrugSafetyInformationforPatientsandProviders/ucm142841.htm. Accessed May 25, 2017.

16. Inhibitors and inducers of CYP enzymes and p-glycoprotein. Med Lett Drugs Ther 2017. May 18 (epub). Available at: medicalletter.org/downloads/CYP_PGP_Tables.pdf. Accessed May 25, 2017.
17. U.S. Government Publishing Office. 42 CFR 8.12 – Federal opioid treatment standards. Available at: www.gpo.gov/fdsys/pkg/CFR-2002-title42-vol1/pdf/CFR-2002-title42-vol1-sec8-12.pdf. Accessed May 25, 2017.
18. LE Baxter Sr et al. Safe methadone induction and stabilization: report of an expert panel. J Addict Med 2013; 7:377.
19. Buprenorphine: an alternative to methadone. Med Lett Drugs Ther 2003; 45:13.
20. In brief: Buprenorphine/naloxone (Zubsolv) for opioid dependence. Med Lett Drugs Ther 2013; 55:83.
21. Bunavail: another buprenorphine/naloxone formulation for opioid dependence. Med Lett Drugs Ther 2015; 57:19.
22. Buprenorphine implants (Probuphine) for opioid dependence. Med Lett Drugs Ther 2016; 58:94.
23. Substance Abuse and Mental Health Services Administration. Buprenorphine waiver management. 2017. Available at: www.samhsa.gov/medication-assisted-treatment/buprenorphine-waiver-management. Accessed May 25, 2017.
24. RP Mattick et al. Buprenorphine maintenance versus placebo or methadone maintenance for opioid dependence. Cochrane Database Syst Rev 2014; 2:CD002207.
25. TV Parran et al. Long-term outcomes of office-based buprenorphine/naloxone maintenance therapy. Drug Alcohol Depend 2010; 106:56.
26. DP Kao et al. Arrhythmia associated with buprenorphine and methadone reported to the Food and Drug Administration. Addiction 2015; 110:1468.
27. D Marteau et al. The relative risk of fatal poisoning by methadone or buprenorphine within the wider population of England and Wales. BMJ Open 2015; 5:e007629.
27a. Once-monthly subcutaneous buprenorphine (Sublocade) for opioid use disorder. Med Lett Drugs Ther 2018; 60:35.
28. DR Wesson and W Ling. The Clinical Opiate Withdrawal Scale (COWS). J Psychoactive Drugs 2003; 35:253.
29. Naltrexone (Vivitrol) – a once-monthly injection for alcoholism. Med Lett Drugs Ther 2006; 48:62.
30. E Krupitsky et al. Injectable extended-release naltrexone for opioid dependence: a double-blind, placebo-controlled, multicentre randomised trial. Lancet 2011; 377:1506.
31. JD Lee et al. Extended-release naltrexone to prevent opioid relapse in criminal justice offenders. N Engl J Med 2016; 374:1232.
31a. JD Lee et al. Comparative effectiveness of extended-release naltrexone versus buprenorphine-naloxone for opioid relapse prevention (X:BOT): a multicentre, open-label, randomised controlled trial. Lancet 2018; 391:309.
32. S Minozzi et al. Oral naltrexone maintenance treatment for opioid dependence. Cochrane Database Syst Rev 2011; 4:CD001333.
33. Y Adi et al. Oral naltrexone as a treatment for relapse prevention in formerly opioid-dependent drug users: a systematic review and economic evaluation. Health Technol Assess 2007; 11:iii.

34. SD Comer et al. Depot naltrexone: long-lasting antagonism of the effects of heroin in humans. Psychopharmacology 2002; 159:351.
35. M Ferri et al. Slow-release oral morphine as maintenance therapy for opioid dependence. Cochrane Database Syst Rev 2013; 6:CD009879.
36. T Beck et al. Maintenance treatment for opioid dependence with slow-release oral morphine: a randomized cross-over, non-inferiority study versus methadone. Addiction 2014; 109:617.
37. M Ferri et al. Heroin maintenance for chronic heroin-dependent individuals. Cochrane Database Syst Rev 2011; 12:CD003410.
38. SY Lee et al. A placebo-controlled trial of dextromethorphan as an adjunct in opioid-dependent patients undergoing methadone maintenance treatment. Int J Neuropsychopharmacol 2015 February 25 (epub).
39. DA Fiellin et al. A randomized trial of cognitive behavioral therapy in primary care-based buprenorphine. Am J Med 2013; 126:74.
40. ACOG Committee on Health Care for Underserved Women and American Society of Addiction Medicine. ACOG committee opinion No. 524: opioid abuse, dependence, and addiction in pregnancy. Obstet Gynecol 2012; 119:1070.
41. KA Saia et al. Caring for pregnant women with opioid use disorder in the USA: expanding and improving treatment. Curr Obstet Gynecol Rep 2016; 5:257.
42. HE Jones et al. Neonatal abstinence syndrome after methadone or buprenorphine exposure. N Engl J Med 2010; 363:2320.
43. SL Wiegand et al. Buprenorphine and naloxone compared with methadone treatment in pregnancy. Obstet Gynecol 2015; 125:363.
44. In brief: A naloxone auto-injector (Evzio). Med Lett Drugs Ther 2014; 56:45.
45. Naloxone (Narcan) nasal spray for opioid overdose. Med Lett Drugs Ther 2016; 58:1.
46. EW Boyer. Management of opioid analgesic overdose. N Engl J Med 2012; 367:146.

DRUGS FOR Postmenopausal Osteoporosis

Original publication date – December 2017

Diagnosis of osteoporosis is based on the results of bone mineral density (BMD) testing or by the occurrence of a fragility fracture. Bone densitometry results are generally reported in terms of standard deviations (SD) from the mean value for young adults (T-score).[1] The World Health Organization (WHO) defines osteoporosis in women as a T-score of -2.5 or below in the spine, femoral neck, or total hip. A computerized model (FRAX) is available that estimates the 10-year probability of a hip fracture or other major osteoporotic fracture based on clinical risk factors and BMD at the femoral neck.[2]

CALCIUM AND VITAMIN D

DIETARY REQUIREMENTS — The Institute of Medicine (IOM) recommends a total daily elemental **calcium** intake of 1000 mg for all women (including pregnant or lactating women) 19-50 years old and men 19-70 years old, and 1200 mg for women >50 years old and men >70 years old.[3]

The IOM recommends a total daily **vitamin D** intake of 600 IU for men and women ≤70 years old (including pregnant or lactating women) and 800 IU for those >70 years old.[3] Intake of ≥600 IU of vitamin D is difficult to achieve by diet and sunlight exposure alone. For postmenopausal women, many experts recommend a daily intake of 800-2000 IU of vitamin D and 25-hydroxyvitamin D serum levels between 30 and 60 ng/mL.

Table 1. Diagnosis of Osteoporosis in Postmenopausal Women[1]

- Hip or spine fragility fracture
- T-score of-2.5 or below in the lumbar spine, femoral neck, total hip, and/or distal one-third radius
- T-score between -1.0 and -2.5 and a FRAX 10-year probability of ≥3% for hip fracture or ≥20% for major osteoporotic fracture (hip, spine, proximal humerus, or forearm)
- T-score between -1.0 and -2.5 and a proximal humerus, pelvic, or distal forearm fracture

1. Adapted from PM Camacho et al. Endo Pract 2016; 22(suppl 4).

SUPPLEMENTATION — Although evidence for the efficacy of calcium and vitamin D supplementation in preventing osteoporotic fractures is conflicting,[4] calcium and vitamin D supplements are generally recommended for postmenopausal women with osteoporosis who have an inadequate dietary intake of calcium (<1200 mg/day) and vitamin D (<800 mg/day).[5-8] Postmenopausal women receiving a bisphosphonate or another antiresorptive drug for osteoporosis should maintain an adequate intake of both calcium and vitamin D through diet and supplementation.

Efficacy – A meta-analysis of 11 randomized, placebo-controlled trials conducted mostly in postmenopausal women ≥65 years old, including the Women's Health Initiative, found that a combination of calcium (500-1200 mg/day) and vitamin D (300-1000 IU/day) decreased fracture risk by 12%. The benefit was greatest in institutionalized patients, who often have a low calcium intake and may be deficient in vitamin D; the risk reduction was smaller among community-dwelling elderly persons and postmenopausal women and there was no risk reduction among community-dwelling women with a history of fracture.[9] Another review found that postmenopausal women and older men taking calcium and vitamin D had fewer hip fractures (1 fewer per 1000 community-dwelling patients per year; 9 fewer per 1000 institutionalized patients per year) and other nonvertebral fractures.[10]

Recommendations for Treatment of Postmenopausal Osteoporosis

- Postmenopausal women with osteoporosis who have an inadequate dietary intake of calcium (<1200 mg) and vitamin D (<800 IU) should take calcium and vitamin D supplements to reduce their risk of fractures.
- The oral bisphosphonates alendronate (*Fosamax*, and others) and risedronate (*Actonel*, and others) can reduce the risk of vertebral and hip and other nonvertebral fractures in postmenopausal women with osteoporosis. Weekly or monthly doses are as effective as daily doses in increasing bone mineral density and may be preferred by patients. IV administration of ibandronate (*Boniva*, and generics) once every 3 months or zoledronic acid (*Reclast*, and generics) once a year is an alternative to oral therapy. Ibandronate has not been shown to reduce the risk of hip and other nonvertebral fractures.
- Denosumab *(Prolia)* injected subcutaneously once every 6 months can reduce the risk of vertebral and hip and other nonvertebral fractures in women with postmenopausal osteoporosis. It is an alternative for patients at high risk for fracture or who have not responded to or cannot tolerate bisphosphonates.
- Teriparatide *(Forteo)* and abaloparatide *(Tymlos)* can increase bone mineral density and reduce the risk of vertebral and nonvertebral fractures, but they are expensive, must be injected daily, and can only be used for a maximum of 2 years in the patient's lifetime.
- Selective estrogen receptor modulators can increase bone mineral density. They have been shown to reduce the risk of vertebral fractures, but not nonvertebral fractures.

A recent systematic review that included 2 randomized, controlled trials and 44 cohort studies in patients ≥50 years old found no association between dietary calcium intake and fracture risk. The authors concluded that there was no evidence that increasing calcium intake from dietary sources prevents fractures and that evidence that calcium supplementation prevents fractures is weak.[11]

A pooled analysis of 11 randomized, double-blind trials of oral vitamin D supplementation, with or without calcium, in patients ≥65 years old (91% women) found that high-dose vitamin D supplementation (median ≥800 IU) reduced the risk of hip fracture by 30% and the risk of any nonvertebral fracture by 14%, compared to controls.[12]

Table 2. Calcium Content of Some Foods[1]

Food[2]	Serving size	Calcium content (mg)[3]
Breakfast cereals, *Cheerios*[4]	1 cup	112
Broccoli, raw	1 cup	43
Cheddar cheese, reduced fat	1 slice	160
Collards, boiled	1 cup	268
Cottage cheese, creamed	4 oz	94
Kale, cooked	1 cup	94
Milk, soy (calcium fortified)	8 oz	299
Milk, skim	1 cup	299
Mozzarella cheese, part-skim	1 cup	945
Oatmeal, instant (regular)	1 packet	21
Parmesan cheese, shredded	1 tbsp	63
Provolone cheese	1 cup	998
Spinach, boiled	1 cup	245
Swiss cheese	1 slice	269
Tofu, raw, firm	½ cup	861
Yogurt, fruit, lowfat	6 oz	258

1. US Department of Agriculture. USDA national nutrient database for standard reference, release 28. Available at http://www.ars.usda.gov/ba/bhnrc/ndl. Accessed December 8, 2017.
2. Some foods, such as spinach, contain oxalic acid, which may limit the absorption of calcium.
3. Content per serving.
4. Calcium content of cereal varies; *Total Whole Grain* cereal (General Mills) contains 1000 mg of calcium per ¾ cup serving.

Products – Calcium supplements are available in a variety of salts. Calcium carbonate should be taken with food to enhance calcium absorption. Calcium citrate does not require acid for absorption and can be taken with or without food; it is preferred for patients taking a proton pump inhibitor (PPI) or an H2-receptor antagonist. Absorption of calcium is reduced at higher doses; patients who require doses >600 mg/day should take divided doses. Vitamin D supplements are available as ergocalciferol (vitamin D2) or cholecalciferol (vitamin D3), often in combination with calcium.

Adverse Effects – Calcium supplements are generally well tolerated; they can cause constipation, intestinal bloating, and excess gas. Their use has been associated with an increased risk of nephrolithiasis.[13]

Table 3. Vitamin D Content of Some Foods[1]

Food[2]	Serving size	Vitamin D content (IU)[3]
Egg, whole large	1 egg	41
Halibut, cooked (Atlantic and Pacific)	3 oz	196
Herring, pickled (Atlantic)	1 cup	158
Milk, skim (fortified)	1 cup	115
Milk, soy (fortified)	8 oz	105
Milk, whole (fortified)	1 cup	124
Salmon, sockeye, cooked	3 oz	447
Sardines, canned	1 cup	288
Tuna, light, canned	1 cup	393

1. US Department of Agriculture. USDA national nutrient database for standard reference, release 28. Available at http://www.ars.usda.gov/ba/bhnrc/ndl. Accessed December 8, 2017.
2. Many other products, including breakfast cereal and margarine, are often fortified with vitamin D.
3. Content per serving.

Some reports have suggested that calcium supplementation could increase the risk of myocardial infarction,[14,15] but in the Women's Health Initiative, among 36,282 postmenopausal women randomized to receive either calcium (1000 mg/day) plus vitamin D (400 IU/day) or placebo, 7 years of calcium plus vitamin D supplementation did not increase the incidence of coronary heart disease, myocardial infarction, or stroke.[16] A recent systematic review found that a daily calcium intake of 2000-2500 mg was not associated with an increased risk of cardiovascular disease in generally healthy adults.[17]

Hypercalciuria and hypercalcemia can occur with high doses of vitamin D.

BISPHOSPHONATES

These nonhormonal drugs decrease bone resorption by binding to active sites of bone remodeling and inhibiting osteoclasts. Alendronate, risedronate, and zoledronic acid have been shown to reduce the risk of vertebral and hip and other nonvertebral fractures in postmenopausal women; ibandronate has only been shown to reduce the risk of vertebral frac-

Table 4. Some Calcium and Vitamin D Supplements		
Drug	**Ca (mg)**[1]	**D_3 (IU)**[1]
Calcium Carbonate[2]		
Caltrate 600+D_3 (Pfizer)	600	800
Os-Cal Calcium + D_3 (GSK)	500	200
Tums Extra Strength 750 (GSK)	300	–
Viactiv Calcium plus D (Viactiv Lifestyle)[3]	500	500
Calcium Citrate[2]		
Citracal Maximum (Bayer)	315	250
Citracal Petites (Bayer)	200	250
Calcium Complex (carbonate, lactate)		
Calcet Petites (Mission)	200	250
Calcium Phosphate[2]		
Citracal Calcium Gummies (Bayer)[4]	250	500
Posture-D (International Vitamins Corp)[5]	600	500

1. Elemental calcium and vitamin D content per tablet.
2. Also available generically.
3. Content of milk chocolate and caramel soft chews; also contains 40 mcg vitamin K.
4. Also contains 107 mg phosphorous.
5. Also contains 280 mg phosphorus and 50 mg magnesium.

tures.[5] In clinical trials of these drugs, patients were also taking calcium and vitamin D supplements.

ALENDRONATE — Oral alendronate (*Fosamax*, and others) is FDA-approved for prevention and treatment of osteoporosis in postmenopausal women. Once-weekly dosing appears to be as effective as daily dosing in increasing BMD and may be better tolerated.

RISEDRONATE — Oral risedronate (*Actonel*, and others) is FDA-approved for prevention and treatment of osteoporosis in postmenopausal women. Once-weekly and once-monthly regimens appear to have similar effects on BMD.

IBANDRONATE — Oral ibandronate (*Boniva*, and generics) is FDA-approved for prevention and treatment of postmenopausal osteoporosis.

IV administration of ibandronate once every three months is only approved for treatment of postmenopausal osteoporosis. It appears to be more effective than the oral formulation in increasing BMD.[18] Ibandronate has not been shown to reduce the risk of hip and other nonvertebral fractures.

ZOLEDRONIC ACID — IV zoledronic acid (*Reclast*, and generics) is FDA-approved for treatment (once-yearly) or prevention (once every two years) of osteoporosis in postmenopausal women.[19] Studies in postmenopausal women with osteoporosis have found that IV administration of a 5-mg dose once-yearly for 3 years reduces bone turnover, increases BMD, and reduces the risk of vertebral, hip, and other fractures.[20,21] In patients at high risk for fracture, treatment for an additional 3 years has been shown to continue to decrease the incidence of vertebral fractures.[21]

ORAL ADMINISTRATION — Food, calcium supplements, antacids, and other medications containing polyvalent cations, such as iron, interfere with the absorption of bisphosphonates from the GI tract. To ensure adequate absorption and prevent esophageal injury, oral bisphosphonates must be taken after an overnight fast, while in an upright position, along with 6-8 ounces of plain (not mineral) water. After taking the drug, the patient must take nothing by mouth except plain water for at least 30 minutes (60 minutes for ibandronate) and avoid lying down. The enteric-coated, delayed-release, once-weekly formulation of risedronate *(Atelvia)* can be taken immediately after breakfast with at least 4 ounces of plain water, but the patient must remain upright for at least 30 minutes.

ADVERSE EFFECTS — Oral bisphosphonates can cause heartburn, esophageal irritation, esophagitis, abdominal pain, diarrhea, and other GI adverse effects. Severe bone, joint, and muscle pain have occurred infrequently with bisphosphonates.[22] Ocular inflammation has also been reported.[23] Hypocalcemia can occur, typically in patients with vitamin D deficiency. An increased risk of atrial fibrillation has been reported with use of bisphosphonates in some studies.

IV bisphosphonates have been associated with acute phase reactions (low-grade fevers, myalgias, and arthralgias) within 1-3 days of the infusion, most frequently after the first infusion; NSAIDs or acetaminophen can decrease these symptoms. Acute phase reactions have also been reported with use of the monthly formulations of oral bisphosphonates. Renal failure and death have occurred in patients with renal impairment (creatinine clearance <35 mL/min) treated with *Reclast*; the drug is contraindicated for use is such patients.[24]

Osteonecrosis of the jaw (ONJ) has occurred rarely with chronic use of oral bisphosphonates.[25] The incidence of ONJ has been higher in patients with cancer or immunosuppression treated with high-dose IV bisphosphonates. Risk factors for ONJ in patients with osteoporosis include bisphosphonate or denosumab use, dental extractions, and supparation.[26]

Numerous cases of atypical femoral fractures have been reported in patients on bisphosphonate therapy.[27] The absolute risk of these fractures is low, ranging from 3.2 to 50 cases per 100,000 person-years; the risk increases with long-term use (~100 cases per 100,000 person-years).[28] Among >52,000 women taking a bisphosphonate for at least 5 years, a subtrochanteric or femoral shaft fracture occurred during the subsequent year in 0.13% of women and within 2 years in 0.22%.[29]

Some reports have suggested an association between use of bisphosphonates and esophageal cancer, but the data are conflicting.[30,31] The FDA has not concluded that bisphosphonates increase the risk of esophageal cancer, but has recommended that they not be used in patients with Barrett's esophagus.

DURATION OF TREATMENT — The optimal duration of treatment with bisphosphonates is unclear. Among 1099 postmenopausal women who had received alendronate for 5 years and were randomized to receive an additional 5 years of alendronate or placebo, those who were treated for 5 or more years had a significantly lower risk of developing clinically recognized vertebral fractures (2.4% vs 5.3%), but not nonvertebral fractures; women considered to be at high risk for fracture were excluded from the trial.[32] Because of the association between long-term bisphosphonate use and atypical femoral fractures, some experts discontinue bisphosphonates temporarily after 5 years of oral use (or 3 years of IV administration) in patients at low risk for fracture (stable bone density, femoral neck T-score >-2.5, no history of hip or spine fracture). How long to wait before restarting these drugs is unclear.

DENOSUMAB

Denosumab *(Prolia)* is a fully human anti-RANK ligand monoclonal antibody that inhibits osteoclast formation and reduces bone resorption. It is FDA-approved for treatment of osteoporosis in postmenopausal women at high risk for fracture.[33] Injected subcutaneously once every 6 months, denosumab has been shown to increase BMD and reduce the incidence of new vertebral and hip and other nonvertebral fractures in postmenopausal women.[34] It has been shown to increase BMD more than alendronate, but no studies directly comparing the efficacy of denosumab and bisphosphonates for prevention of fractures are available.

The optimal duration of treatment with denosumab is not known. Data are available supporting its continued efficacy for 10 years.[35] Denosumab's effects on BMD and bone turnover are reversible with discontinuation of the drug. Stopping the drug after 24 months of treatment resulted in increased bone turnover markers within 3 months and a decline in BMD to pretreatment values within 2 years.[36] Vertebral fractures have been reported 8-16 months after stopping denosumab.[37] Drug holidays are not recommended. If denosumab is stopped, administering another drug, typically a bisphosphonate, is recommended to prevent a rapid decline in BMD. Switching from denosumab to teriparatide has resulted in progressive or transient bone loss.[38]

ADVERSE EFFECTS — Denosumab can cause hypocalcemia, especially in patients with renal impairment. In clinical trials, rash, eczema, and dermatitis occurred more commonly with denosumab than with placebo. Denosumab is a potent antiresorptive agent; osteonecrosis of the

Table 5. Some Drugs for Postmenopausal Osteoporosis

Drug	Some Formulations
Bisphosphonates	
Alendronate – generic	5, 10, 35, 70 mg tabs[3]
Fosamax (Merck)	70 mg tabs
Fosamax Plus D	70 mg/2800 IU D_3, 70 mg/5600 IU D_3 tabs
Binosto (Mission Pharma)	70 mg effervescent tabs
Ibandronate – generic *Boniva* (Genentech)	150 mg tabs; 3 mg/3 mL prefilled syringe
Risedronate – generic *Actonel* (Allergan)	5, 35, 75, 150 mg tabs[7]
delayed-release – *Atelvia* (Allergan)	35 mg delayed-release tabs
Zoledronic acid[8] – generic *Reclast* (Novartis)	5 mg/100 mL soln
Anti-RANK Ligand Antibody	
Denosumab – *Prolia* (Amgen)[10]	60 mg/mL prefilled syringe
Parathyroid Hormone[12]	
Abaloparatide – *Tymlos* (Radius)	3120 mcg/1.56 mL prefilled pen
Teriparatide – *Forteo* (Lilly)	600 mcg/2.4 mL prefilled pen
Selective Estrogen Receptor Modulator	
Raloxifene – generic	60 mg tabs
Conjugated Estrogens and Selective Estrogen Receptor Modulator[13]	
Conjugated estrogens and bazedoxifene – *Duavee* (Pfizer)	0.45 mg/20 mg tabs

1. Dosage adjustment may be needed for renal or hepatic impairment.
2. Cost based on lowest dosage or frequency used for treatment. Cost of *Duavee* is based on dosage used for prevention. Approximate WAC for 28 days. WAC = wholesaler acquisition cost or manufacturer's published price to wholesalers; WAC represents a published catalogue or list price and may not represent an actual transactional price. Source: AnalySource® Monthly. December 5, 2017. Reprinted with permission by First Databank, Inc. All rights reserved. ©2017. www.fdbhealth.com/policies/drug-pricing-policy.
3. Alendronate is available in a 40-mg tablet for treatment of Paget's disease of bone.
4. Cost for 70-mg tablets.
5. Effervescent tablet should be dissolved in 4 oz of room-temperature plain water.
6. Cost of one 3 mg/3 mL *Boniva* syringe. Cost of one generic 3 mg/mL syringe is $245.00.

Usual Adult Dosage[1]	Cost[2]
Prevention: 5 mg once/d or 35 mg once/wk PO	$9.20
Treatment: 10 mg once/d or 70 mg once/wk PO	127.80[4]
Treatment: 70 mg/2800 IU D_3 or 70 mg/5600 IU D_3 once/wk PO	173.30
Treatment: 70 mg once/wk[5]	192.00
Prevention: 150 mg PO once/mo	32.60
Treatment: 150 mg PO once/mo or	190.90
3 mg IV once every 3 mo	527.40[6]
Prevention: 5 mg once/d, 35 mg once/wk,	149.40
or 150 mg once/mo PO	321.50
Treatment: 5 mg once/d, 35 mg once/wk, 75 mg 2 consecutive days/mo, or 150 mg once/mo PO	
Treatment: 35 mg PO once/wk	232.10
Prevention: 5 mg IV once every 2 years	262.50[9]
Treatment: 5 mg IV once/yr	1083.80[9]
Treatment: 60 mg SC once every 6 mo	1128.20[11]
Treatment: 80 mcg SC once/d	1166.70
Treatment: 20 mcg SC once/d	2798.00
Prevention: 60 mg PO once/d	99.10
Treatment: 60 mg PO once/d	
Prevention: 0.45 mg/20 mg PO once/d	148.10

7. *Actonel* is also available in a 30-mg tablet for treatment of Paget's disease.
8. Zoledronic acid is also available in a 4-mg formulation (*Zometa*, and generics) for treatment of hypercalcemia of malignancy, multiple myeloma, and bone metastases from solid tumors.
9. Cost of one 5 mg/100 mL infusion bottle.
10. Denosumab is also available in a 120 mg/1.7 mL formulation (*Xgeva*) for prevention of skeletal-related events in patients with bone metastases from solid tumors.
11. Cost of one 60 mg/mL syringe.
12. Cumulative use for $\geq$2 years during a patient's lifetime is not recommended.
13. Conjugated estrogens are no longer recommended for first-line treatment of postmenopausal osteoporosis because of an increased risk of breast cancer, stroke, and venous thromboembolism.

Continued on next page

Table 5. Some Drugs for Postmenopausal Osteoporosis (continued)	
Drug	**Some Formulations**
Calcitonin[14]	
Miacalcin Injection (Mylan)	400 IU/2 mL vial

14. Due to limited evidence of efficacy and safety concerns, many experts no longer recommend use of salmon calcitonin. Calcitonin is also available in an intranasal formulation, but availability is limited.

jaw and atypical femoral fractures, which can occur with bisphosphonates, have also been reported with denosumab.[39,40]

PARATHYROID HORMONE

Unlike other drugs available for osteoporosis, which inhibit bone resorption and decrease bone turnover, low-dose daily subcutaneous injection of parathyroid hormone (PTH) or parathyroid hormone-related protein (PTHrP) analogs increase BMD by stimulating bone formation. **Teriparatide** *(Forteo)*, the recombinant 1-34 sequence of human PTH, and **abaloparatide** *(Tymlos),* a synthetic analog of human parathyroid hormone-related peptide, are FDA-approved for treatment of osteoporosis for up to 2 years (in the patient's lifetime) in postmenopausal women at high risk for fracture. Experts usually start a bisphosphonate or another antiresorptive drug after stopping these drugs.

Once-daily injections of **teriparatide** have been shown to increase BMD at the lumbar spine, femoral neck, and hip and decrease the incidence of vertebral and nonvertebral fractures by 50% or more, but the effect of the drug on hip fractures is unknown. BMD decreases after the drug is stopped, but retreatment after a drug-free period has been shown to produce further small gains in BMD.[41] Switching from teriparatide or a combination of teriparatide and denosumab to denosumab monotherapy results in further increases in BMD.[38]

In a double-blind trial in 1360 postmenopausal women with ≥2 moderate or one severe vertebral fracture and a T-score ≤-1.5, teriparatide was

Usual Adult Dosage[1]	Cost[2]
Treatment: 100 IU SC or IM once/d	$17,391.10

significantly more effective than risedronate in preventing new vertebral fractures (5.4% vs 12%).[42]

In a double-blind trial in 2463 postmenopausal women with osteoporosis, 63% of whom had a history of fracture, once-daily injections of **abaloparatide** significantly increased BMD at the hip, femoral neck, and lumbar spine at 18 months and reduced the rate of new vertebral fractures (0.6% vs 4.2% with placebo). The estimated rate of nonvertebral fractures was also significantly lower with abaloparatide than with placebo (2.7% vs 4.7%).[43,44]

ADVERSE EFFECTS — Teriparatide can cause nausea, arthralgia, and pain. Hypotension and tachycardia may occur with the first few doses. Transient hypercalcemia and hypercalciuria can occur; they can generally be corrected by reducing calcium intake. A boxed warning is included in the labeling of teriparatide regarding a risk of osteosarcoma (based on animal data), but a postmarketing surveillance study found that among 1448 cases of osteosarcoma identified in the US in a 7-year period, none of those that were investigated were associated with prior use of the drug.[45]

Abaloparatide can cause injection-site reactions, dizziness, nausea, headache, palpitations, tachycardia, orthostatic hypotension, hypercalcemia, hypercalciuria, and increased serum uric acid concentrations. The incidence of adverse events leading to study discontinuation in one trial was higher with abaloparatide (9.9%) than with either teriparatide (6.8%) or placebo (6.1%). The incidence of hypercalcemia was significantly lower with abaloparatide (3.4%) than with teriparatide (6.1%) at 4 hours post-dose, but not at 16-24 hours.[43] As with teriparatide, the labeling of abaloparatide includes a boxed warning regarding a risk of osteosarcoma based on animal data.

SELECTIVE ESTROGEN RECEPTOR MODULATORS

RALOXIFENE — Raloxifene (*Evista*, and generics), a selective estrogen receptor modulator (SERM) with estrogen-like effects on bone and anti-estrogen effects on the uterus and breast, is FDA-approved for prevention and treatment of postmenopausal osteoporosis. It has reduced the risk of vertebral fractures, but not nonvertebral fractures.[46] Raloxifene can reduce the risk of invasive breast cancer and may be a reasonable alternative to bisphosphonate therapy in younger postmenopausal women at high risk for invasive breast cancer. Bisphosphonates are generally preferred over raloxifene for treatment of osteoporosis in postmenopausal women because they are more effective in preventing nonvertebral and hip fractures.[47]

Adverse Effects – Hot flashes, leg cramps, and peripheral edema can occur with raloxifene. Like estrogens, raloxifene increases the risk of venous thromboembolic events and stroke.

CONJUGATED ESTROGENS/BAZEDOXIFENE — A fixed-dose combination *(Duavee)* of conjugated estrogens and the SERM bazedoxifene is FDA-approved for prevention of osteoporosis in postmenopausal women with an intact uterus. Like raloxifene, bazedoxifene inhibits the stimulating effect of estrogen on the endometrium and breast. The combination has been shown to increase BMD in postmenopausal women, and bazedoxifene alone (not available commercially) has been shown to decrease the risk of vertebral fractures.[48,49]

Adverse Effects – In short-term clinical trials of conjugated estrogens/bazedoxifene, the combination did not increase the incidence of breast cancer, endometrial cancer, ovarian cancer, venous thromboembolism, stroke, myocardial infarction, or death from any cause. In a randomized, double-blind trial in postmenopausal women with osteoporosis, venous thromboembolic events, primarily DVT, occurred more frequently in women taking bazedoxifene for 5 years than in those taking placebo.[50] Use of the combination for up to two years did not increase the risk of breast cancer.[51]

CALCITONIN

Salmon calcitonin, a peptide hormone given intranasally, subcutaneously, or intramuscularly, is approved by the FDA for treatment of osteoporosis in women >5 years after menopause when alternative treatments are not suitable. It decreases bone resorption by inhibiting osteoclast function. A 5-year trial in women with osteoporosis found new vertebral fractures in 51 of 287 (18%) receiving a 200-IU dose of calcitonin nasal spray once daily and in 70 of 270 (26%) receiving a placebo, a statistically significant difference.[52]

ADVERSE EFFECTS — Serious allergic reactions, including anaphylaxis, have occurred with use of calcitonin. An increased risk of malignancy has been reported with use of calcitonin nasal spray.[53]

Given the limited evidence of its efficacy, concerns about its safety, and the availability of other options, many experts no longer recommend calcitonin. It has been removed from the market in Canada and Europe.

ROMOSOZUMAB

Romosozumab (*Evenity* – Amgen/UCB Pharma) is an investigational monoclonal antibody that binds to and inhibits sclerostin, increasing bone formation and decreasing bone resorption. Romosozumab, which was originally being investigated for accelerated fracture healing, is undergoing an extended FDA review for treatment of postmenopausal osteoporosis; the FDA required additional data from an active-comparator trial.[54] In one trial, 7180 postmenopausal women with osteoporosis and a T-score of -2.5 to -3.5 in the total hip or femoral neck were randomized to receive subcutaneous romosozumab or placebo for 12 months; new vertebral fractures occurred in 0.5% of women receiving romosozumab and in 1.8% of those receiving placebo, a statistically significant difference. There was no significant difference between the groups in the occurrence of nonvertebral fractures.[55] In the active-comparator trial in 4093 postmenopausal women with osteoporosis and a fragility fracture, patients randomized to receive romosozumab for 12 months followed by alendronate for an additional 12 months had a 48% lower risk of new vertebral fractures, a 19% lower risk of nonvertebral fractures, and a 38% lower risk of hip fracture at 24 months compared to those who received alendronate for 12 months followed by open-label alendronate. In this trial, serious cardiovascular adverse events were reported more often in the romosozumab group (2.5% vs 1.9% with alendronate).[54]

1. DM Black and CJ Rosen. Clinical practice. Postmenopausal osteoporosis. N Engl J Med 2016; 374:254.
2. FRAX. Fracture risk assessment tool. Available at www.sheffield.ac.uk/FRAX/tool.jsp. Accessed December 7, 2017.
3. Institute of Medicine (US) Committee to Review Dietary Reference Intakes for Vitamin D and Calcium. Dietary reference intakes for calcium and vitamin D. Available at http://www.iom.edu/Reports/2010/Dietary-Reference-Intakes-for-Calcium-and-Vitamin-D.aspx. Accessed December 7, 2017.
4. DC Bauer. Clinical practice. Calcium supplements and fracture prevention. N Engl J Med 2013; 369:1537.
5. PM Camacho et al. American Association of Clinical Endocrinologists and American College of Endocrinology Clinical practice guidelines for the diagnosis and treatment of postmenopausal osteoporosis – 2016 – executive summary. Endocr Pract 2016; 22:1111.
6. A Qaseem et al. Treatment of low bone density or osteoporosis to prevent fractures in men and women: a clinical practice guideline update from the American College of Physicians. Ann Intern Med 2017; 166:818.
7. NB Watts and JE Manson. Osteoporosis and fracture risk evaluation and management: shared decision making in clinical practice. JAMA 2017; 317:253.
8. US Preventive Services Task Force. Draft recommendation statement. Vitamin D, calicum, or combined supplementation for the primary prevention of fractures in community-dwelling adults: preventive medication. Available at: www.uspreventiveservicestaskforce.org/Page/Document/draft-recommendation-statement/vitamin-d-calcium-or-combined-supplementation-for-the-primary-prevention-of-fractures-in-adults-preventive-medication. Accessed December 8, 2017.
9. M Chung et al. Vitamin D with or without calcium supplementation for prevention of cancer and fractures: an updated meta-analysis for the U.S. Preventive Services Task Force. Ann Intern Med 2011; 155:827.

10. A Avenell et al. Vitamin D and vitamin D analogues for preventing fractures in postmenopausal women and older men. Cochrane Database Syst Rev 2014; 4:CD000227.
11. MJ Bolland et al. Calcium intake and risk of fracture: systematic review. BMJ 2015; 351:h4580.
12. HA Bischoff-Ferrari et al. A pooled analysis of vitamin D dose requirements for fracture prevention. N Engl J Med 2012; 367:40.
13. RB Wallace et al. Urinary tract stone occurrence in the Women's Health Initiative (WHI) randomized clinical trial of calcium and vitamin D supplements. Am J Clin Nutr 2011; 94:270.
14. K Li et al. Associations of dietary calcium intake and calcium supplementation with myocardial infarction and stroke risk and overall cardiovascular mortality in the Heidelberg cohort of the European Prospective Investigation into Cancer and Nutrition study (EPIC-Heidelberg). Heart 2012; 98:920.
15. IR Reid. Cardiovascular effects of calcium supplements. Nutrients 2013; 5:2522.
16. RL Prentice et al. Health risks and benefits from calcium and vitamin D supplementation: Women's Health Initiative clinical trial and cohort study. Osteoporo Int 2013; 24:567.
17. M Chung et al. Calcium intake and cardiovascular disease risk: an updated systematic review and meta-analysis. Ann Intern Med 2016; 165:856.
18. JA Eisman et al. Efficacy and tolerability of intravenous ibandronate injections in postmenopausal osteoporosis: 2-year results from the DIVA study. J Rheumatol 2008; 35:488.
19. A once-yearly IV bisphosphonate for osteoporosis. Med Lett Drugs Ther 2007; 49:89.
20. DM Black et al. Once-yearly zoledronic acid for treatment of postmenopausal osteoporosis. N Engl J Med 2007; 356:1809.
21. DM Black et al. The effect of 3 versus 6 years of zoledronic acid treatment of osteoporosis: a randomized extension to the HORIZON-Pivotal Fracture Trial (PFT). J Bone Miner Res 2012; 27:243.
22. DK Wysowski and JT Chang. Alendronate and risedronate: reports of severe bone, joint, and muscle pain. Arch Intern Med 2005; 165:346.
23. M Pazianas et al. Inflammatory eye reactions in patients treated with bisphosphonates and other osteoporosis medications: cohort analysis using a national prescription database. J Bone Miner Res 2013; 28:455.
24. FDA drug safety communication: new contraindication and updated warning on kidney impairment for Reclast (zoledronic acid). Available at www.fda.gov/Drugs/DrugSafety/ucm270199.htm. Accessed December 7, 2017.
25. S Fedele et al. Nonexposed variant of bisphosphonate-associated osteonecrosis of the jaw: a case series. Am J Med 2010; 123:1060.
26. AA Khan et al. Case-based review of osteonecrosis of the jaw (ONJ) and application of the International Recommendations for Management from the International Task Force on ONJ. J Clin Densitom 2017; 20:8.
27. J Schilcher et al. Bisphosphonate use and atypical fractures of the femoral shaft. N Engl J Med 2011; 364:1728.
28. E Shane et al. Atypical subtrochanteric and diaphyseal femoral fractures: second report of a task force of the American Society for Bone and Mineral Research. J Bone Miner Res 2014; 29:1.

29. LY Park-Wyllie et al. Bisphosphonate use and the risk of subtrochanteric or femoral shaft fractures in older women. JAMA 2011; 305:783.
30. Y Vinogradova et al. Exposure to bisphosphonates and risk of gastrointestinal cancers: series of nested case-control studies with QResearch and CPRD data. BMJ 2013; 346:f114.
31. NE Morden et al. Oral bisphosphonates and upper gastrointestinal toxicity: a study of cancer and early signals of esophageal injury. Osteoporos Int 2015; 26:663.
32. DM Black et al. Effects of continuing or stopping alendronate after 5 years of treatment: the Fracture Intervention Trial Long-term Extension (FLEX): a randomized trial. JAMA 2006; 296:2927.
33. Denosumab (Prolia) for postmenopausal osteoporosis. Med Lett Drugs Ther 2010; 52:81.
34. SR Cummings et al. Denosumab for prevention of fractures in postmenopausal women with osteoporosis. N Engl J Med 2009; 361:756.
35. HG Bone et al. 10 years of denosumab treatment in postmenopausal women with osteoporosis: results from the phase 3 randomised FREEDOM trial and open-label extension. Lancet Diabetes Endocrinol 2017; 5:513.
36. HG Bone et al. Effects of denosumab treatment and discontinuation on bone mineral density and bone turnover markers in postmenopausal women with low bone mass. J Clin Endocrinol Metab 2011; 96:972.
37. AD Anastasilakis et al. Clinical features of 24 patients with rebound-associated vertebral fractures after denosumab discontinuation: systematic review and additional cases. J Bone Miner Res 2017; 32:1291.
38. BZ Leder et al. Denosumab and teriparatide transitions in postmenopausal osteoporosis (the DATA-Switch study): extension of a randomised controlled trial. Lancet 2015; 386:1147.
39. TD Rachner et al. Osteonecrosis of the jaw after osteoporosis therapy with denosumab following long-term bisphosphonate therapy. Mayo Clin Proc 2013; 88:418.
40. S Papapoulos et al. The effect of 8 or 5 years of denosumab treatment in postmenopausal women with osteoporosis: results from the FREEDOM Extension study. Osteoporos Int 2015; 26:2773.
41. JS Finkelstein et al. Effects of teriparatide retreatment in osteoporotic men and women. J Clin Endocrinol Metab 2009; 94:2495.
42. DL Kendler et al. Effects of teriparatide and risedronate on new fractures in postmenopausal women with severe osteoporosis (VERO): a multicentre, double-blind, double-dummy, randomised controlled trial. Lancet 2017 November 9 (epub).
43. PD Miller et al. Effect of abaloparatide vs placebo on new vertebral fractures in postmenopausal women with osteoporosis: a randomized clinical trial. JAMA 2016; 316:722.
44. Abaloparatide (Tymlos) for postmenopausal osteoporosis. Med Lett Drugs Ther 2017; 59:97.
45. EB Andrews et al. The US postmarketing surveillance study of adult osteosarcoma and teriparatide: study design and findings from the first 7 years. J Bone Miner Res 2012; 27:2429.
46. KE Ensrud et al. Effects of raloxifene on fracture risk in postmenopausal women: the raloxifene use for the heart trial. J Bone Miner Res 2008; 23:112.
47. CJ Crandall et al. Comparative effectiveness of pharmacologic treatments to prevent fractures: an updated systematic review. Ann Intern Med 2014; 161:711.

48. Conjugated estrogens/bazedoxifene (Duavee) for menopausal symptoms and prevention of osteoporosis. Med Lett Drugs Ther 2014; 56:33.
49. JV Pinkerton et al. Effects of bazedoxifene/conjugated estrogens on the endometrium and bone: a randomized trial. J Clin Endocrinol Metab 2014; 99:e189.
50. TJ de Villiers et al. Safety and tolerability of bazedoxifene in postmenopausal women with osteoporosis: results of a 5-year, randomized, placebo-controlled phase 3 trial. Osteoporos Int 2011; 22:567.
51. JH Pickar and BS Komm. Selective estrogen receptor modulators and the combination therapy conjugated estrogens/bazedoxifene: a review of effects on the breast. Post Reprod Health 2015; 21:112.
52. JA Knopp-Sihota et al. Calcitonin for treating acute and chronic pain of recent and remote osteoporotic vertebral compression fractures: a systematic review and meta-analysis. Osteoporos Int 2012; 23:17.
53. In brief: Cancer risk with salmon calcitonin. Med Lett Drugs Ther 2013; 55:29.
54. KG Saag et al. Romosozumab or alendronate for fracture prevention in women with osteoporosis. N Engl J Med 2017; 377:1417.
55. F Cosman et al. Romosozumab treatment in postmenopausal women with osteoporosis. N Engl J Med 2016; 375:1532.

DRUGS FOR Parkinson's Disease

Original publication date – November 2017 (revised March 2018)

The motor symptoms of Parkinson's disease (PD) are caused primarily by degeneration of dopaminergic neurons in the substantia nigra. The nonmotor symptoms of the disease are thought to be caused by degeneration of other neurotransmitter systems.

LEVODOPA — Dopamine itself cannot be used to treat PD because it does not cross the blood-brain barrier. Levodopa, the immediate precursor of dopamine, is decarboxylated to dopamine in both the brain and peripheral tissues. Combining levodopa with carbidopa, a peripheral decarboxylase inhibitor, makes more levodopa available for transport to the brain and prevents peripheral adverse effects such as nausea, vomiting, and orthostatic hypotension. The combination is the most effective treatment available for the motor symptoms of PD.

Limitations – For the first 2-5 years of treatment, levodopa produces a sustained response, but over time the duration of benefit from each dose becomes shorter ("wearing-off" effect), and some patients develop sudden, unpredictable fluctuations between mobility and immobility ("on-off" effect). After 5-8 years, the majority of patients have motor fluctuations and dyskinesia. As the disease progresses, levodopa-resistant motor problems such as difficulties with balance, gait, speech, and swallowing and nonmotor symptoms such as autonomic, cognitive, sleep, and psychiatric difficulties become more prominent. Sudden discontinuation of levodopa or an abrupt reduction in dosage can cause a severe, potentially fatal return of parkinsonian symptoms.

Dosage – When levodopa is given with carbidopa, its pharmacological half-life is only 60-90 minutes, but its clinical benefits ("on" time) usually last 5-6 hours. The daily dosage of levodopa usually ranges from 300-1500 mg divided into 3 to 6 doses; some patients, such as those who develop "wearing-off" phenomena, may require more frequent or higher doses. High-protein foods may decrease the effectiveness of levodopa by competing with the drug for absorption from the intestine and transport across the blood-brain barrier.

Relatively complete inhibition of peripheral decarboxylation of levodopa requires 75-100 mg of carbidopa daily; some patients require up to 200 mg daily.

Carbidopa/levodopa is available as immediate- and sustained-release tablets (*Sinemet, Sinemet CR,* and generics) and as orally disintegrating tablets that can be taken without liquid.[1] Although not FDA-approved, some clinicians have used "liquid" levodopa (crushed immediate-release tablets dissolved in a carbonated beverage for rapid absorption) as rescue treatment for hypomobility ("off" episodes).

An oral capsule formulation that contains carbidopa and levodopa in a 1:4 ratio *(Rytary)* was approved in 2015 for treatment of PD.[2,3] The capsules contain both immediate-release and extended-release beads. Doses of *Rytary* are not interchangeable with those of other carbidopa/levodopa products; the drug's labeling includes dosage conversion tables.

In patients with advanced PD, stomach emptying may be delayed and unpredictable, which can affect the rate and amount of absorption of carbidopa/levodopa and its efficacy. A carbidopa/levodopa enteral suspension (intestinal gel; *Duopa*) can be used as an alternative to oral formulations in patients with advanced disease and motor fluctuations.

Recommendations for Treatment of Parkinson's Disease

- The combination of levodopa and carbidopa is the most effective treatment for the motor symptoms of Parkinson's disease, but its long-term use leads to motor fluctuations and dyskinesia.
- Dopamine agonists are less effective than levodopa; they can be used as monotherapy before the introduction of levodopa or as an adjunct to levodopa in patients with motor fluctuations.
- Addition of a peripherally-acting COMT inhibitor or an MAO-B inhibitor to levodopa can reduce motor fluctuations in patients with advanced disease.
- Amantadine can be used as monotherapy in early PD and as an adjunct in later stages; it may modestly improve PD symptoms and can decrease levodopa-induced dyskinesia.
- Anticholinergics can help control tremor and drooling, but are rarely used because of their adverse effects.
- Subcutaneous apomorphine can be used for rescue treatment of "off" episodes.
- Deep brain stimulation is an option for patients with levodopa-induced motor complications and relatively intact cognition.
- Other drugs are available to treat the nonmotor complications of PD such as depression, psychosis, and cognitive impairment.
- Combining pharmacologic therapy with exercise therapy can improve physical function and quality of life.

In a randomized, double-blind, 12-week trial, the intestinal gel reduced daily mean "off" time from baseline significantly more than oral immediate-release carbidopa/levodopa (by 4.04 hours vs 2.14 hours).[4,5]

The gel is administered via a percutaneous gastrojejunostomy tube connected to a portable infusion pump. It is delivered to the proximal jejunum as a continuous 16-hour infusion during the day. After the infusion period, the delivery pump is disconnected from the jejunal tube and the patient can take a nighttime dose of oral immediate-release carbidopa/levodopa if needed. The infusion rate and total dose administered can be customized to control symptoms and minimize dyskinesia, and patients can self-administer extra doses to manage acute "off" symptoms. *Duopa* is available in single-use cassettes containing 2000 mg of levodopa. The maximum dose is one cassette daily.

Carbidopa is available alone as 25-mg tablets (*Lodosyn*, and generics) that can be added to fixed-dose carbidopa/levodopa formulations if patients continue to have nausea.

Adverse Effects – Peripheral adverse effects of levodopa, including anorexia, nausea, vomiting, and orthostatic hypotension, may be prominent during initiation of therapy. With chronic therapy, somnolence, vivid dreams, hallucinations, delusions, confusion, and agitation can occur, especially in older patients with dementia. Impulsive and hypersexual behaviors have also been associated with levodopa therapy.

Drug Interactions – Concurrent administration of carbidopa/levodopa and a nonselective monoamine oxidase (MAO) inhibitor such as phenelzine or tranylcypromine could result in severe hypertension and is contraindicated. Use of carbidopa/levodopa with an antipsychotic drug should be avoided because it could result in reduced effectiveness of levodopa due to antagonism of its dopaminergic effects. Coadministration of an antihypertensive drug could increase the risk of orthostatic hypotension.

Strategy – Some expert clinicians prefer to start treatment with low doses of levodopa or with another drug because of concerns about inducing early dyskinesias and "wearing-off" effects. This strategy is used particularly in younger patients, who have a higher risk of developing motor fluctuations and dyskinesia and a longer life expectancy.

DOPAMINE AGONISTS — Dopamine agonists are less effective than levodopa in treating the motor symptoms of PD, but they are less likely to cause motor fluctuations or dyskinesia. They are effective as monotherapy in early, mild disease, but within a few years most patients require addition of levodopa. Used as adjuncts to levodopa in advanced disease, dopamine agonists can reduce motor fluctuations and permit use of lower doses of levodopa.

Two oral nonergot dopamine agonists, **pramipexole** (*Mirapex*, and generics) and **ropinirole** (*Requip*, and generics), are widely used in both early and advanced disease. **Rotigotine** *(Neupro)*, another nonergot dopamine agonist, is available as a transdermal patch. Older ergot-derivative dopamine agonists, such as bromocriptine (*Parlodel*, and generics), can cause serious adverse effects and are no longer recommended for treatment of PD.

Dosage – Pramipexole should be started at a dosage of 0.125 mg tid, which can be gradually increased to 0.25 mg tid and then to 0.5 mg tid over 3 weeks. Further dose increases should be made in smaller increments and no more frequently than every 5-7 days. The FDA-approved maximum daily dosage is 4.5 mg, but some studies have found no significant benefit and an increase in adverse effects at doses higher than 1.5 mg daily. Ropinirole should be started at 0.25 mg tid and slowly titrated upward in 0.25-mg increments over 4 weeks to 1 mg tid. After week 4, the dose can continue to be increased gradually to a maximum of 8 mg tid.

Both pramipexole and ropinirole are also available in extended-release formulations that can be taken once daily. The usual starting dosage of extended-release pramipexole (*Mirapex ER*, and generics) is 0.375 mg once daily. The daily dose is slowly titrated upward at weekly (or even longer) intervals first to 0.75 mg and then, in increments of 0.75 mg, to a maximum of 4.5 mg. The recommended initial dosage of extended-release ropinirole (*Requip XL*, and generics) is 2 mg once daily for 1-2 weeks. The daily dose can be increased in increments of 2 mg at weekly intervals to a maximum of 24 mg.

The rotigotine transdermal patch should be applied to intact hairless skin and changed every 24 hours; the usual starting dosage is 2 mg/24 hours for early-stage disease and 4 mg/24 hours for advanced disease. The dose can be increased weekly by 2 mg/24 hours to a target of 4-6 mg/24 hours for early-stage and 6-8 mg/24 hours for advanced-stage PD.

As the dosage of the dopamine agonist increases, the dosage of levodopa may have to be decreased.

Table 1. Some Drugs for Parkinson's Disease

Drug	Some Available Formulations
Carbidopa/Levodopa	
immediate-release – generic	10/100, 25/100, 25/250 mg tabs
Sinemet (Merck)	
orally disintegrating – generic	10/100, 25/100, 25/250 mg ODTs
sustained-release – generic	25/100, 50/200 mg tabs
Sinemet CR (Merck)	
extended-release – *Rytary* (Impax)	23.75/95, 36.25/145, 48.75/195, 61.25/245 mg ER caps[3]
intrajejunal infusion – *Duopa* (Abbvie)	100 mL single-use cassettes (4.63 mg/20 mg/mL)
Dopamine Agonists	
Oral	
Pramipexole – generic	0.125, 0.25, 0.5, 0.75, 1, 1.5 mg tabs
Mirapex (Boehringer Ingelheim)	
extended-release – generic	0.375, 0.75, 1.5, 2.25, 3, 3.75, 4.5 mg ER tabs
Mirapex ER	
Ropinirole – generic	0.25, 0.5, 1, 2, 3, 4, 5 mg tabs
Requip (GSK)	
extended-release – generic	2, 4, 6, 8, 12 mg ER tabs
Requip XL	
Transdermal	
Rotigotine – *Neupro* (UCB)	1, 2, 3, 4, 6, 8 mg/24 hr patches[6]
Subcutaneous	
Apomorphine – *Apokyn* (US Worldmeds)	30 mg/3 mL cartridges
COMT Inhibitors	
Entacapone – generic	200 mg tabs
Comtan (Novartis)	

ER = extended-release; levo = levodopa; ODTs = orally disintegrating tabs; N.A. = cost not available

1. Dosage adjustment may be needed for renal or hepatic impairment.
2. Approximate WAC for 30 days' treatment with the lowest to highest dose of levodopa or the lowest usual dosage. WAC = wholesaler acquisition cost or manufacturer's published price to wholesalers; WAC represents a published catalogue or list price and may not represent an actual transactional price. Source: AnalySource® Monthly. November 5, 2017. Reprinted with permission by First Databank, Inc. All rights reserved. ©2017. www.fdbhealth.com/policies/drug-pricing-policy.
3. Capsules may be opened, and the contents sprinkled on 1-2 tablespoons of applesauce and taken immediately.
4. Dosages of *Rytary* are not interchangeable with those of other carbidopa/levodopa products.

Usual Dosage[1]	Cost[2]
300-1500 mg levo/d, divided	$6.70-18.30
	117.90-298.00
300-1500 mg levo/d, divided	79.00-201.30
400-1600 mg levo/d, divided	75.90-303.60
	168.00-672.00
285-1170 mg levo/d, divided[4]	232.60-465.10
2000 mg levo/d (1 cassette)[5]	6055.20
0.5-1.5 mg tid	13.30
	552.00
1.5-4.5 mg once/d	295.00
	522.20
3-8 mg tid	31.50
	499.60
8-24 mg once/d	132.00
	422.00
4-8 mg/24 hrs[7]	621.80
2-6 mg SC 3-5x/d prn[8]	1008.00[9]
200 mg tid or qid[10]	450.00
	661.60

5. Daily dosage is individualized based on clinical response and tolerability. Maximum recommended daily dose is 2000 mg of levodopa. Administered as a 16-hour infusion through a nasojejunal (NJ) or percutaneous endoscopic gastrostomy with jejunal (PEG-J) tube with the *CADD-Legacy 1400* portable infusion pump.
6. The 1 mg/24 hour formulation is not FDA-approved for Parkinson's disease.
7. Usual dose is 4-6 mg/day for early-stage disease and 6-8 mg/day for advanced-stage disease.
8. Should be administered with the antiemetic trimethobenzamide.
9. Cost of one 3-mL cartridge.
10. With each dose of carbidopa/levodopa (max 8 tabs/day).

Continued on next page

Table 1. Some Drugs for Parkinson's Disease (continued)

Drug	Some Available Formulations
COMT Inhibitors (continued)	
Tolcapone – generic *Tasmar* (Valeant)	100 mg tabs
Carbidopa/Levodopa/Entacapone	
generic *Stalevo* (Orion)	12.5/50/200, 18.75/75/200, 25/100/200, 31.25/125/200, 37.5/150/200, 50/200/200 mg tabs
MAO-B Inhibitors	
Rasagiline – generic *Azilect* (Teva)	0.5, 1 mg tabs
Safinamide – *Xadago* (US Worldmeds)	50, 100 mg tabs
Selegiline – generic	5 mg tabs, caps
Eldepryl (Somerset)	5 mg caps
orally disintegrating – *Zelapar* (Valeant)	1.25 mg ODTs
Other Drugs	
Amantadine – generic	100 mg caps, tabs; 50 mg/5 mL syrup
extended-release – *Gocovri* (Adamas)	68.5, 137 mg ER caps
Osmolex ER (Osmotica)	129, 193, 258 mg ER tabs
Carbidopa – generic *Lodosyn* (Aton)	25 mg tabs[14]

ER = extended-release; levo = levodopa; ODTs = orally disintegrating tabs; N.A. = cost not available
11. Tolcapone does not need to be taken at the same time as carbidopa/levodopa. Discontinue within 3 weeks if no clinical benefit.
12. Dose is 1 mg as monotherapy and 0.5-1 mg when given with carbidopa/levodopa.
13. Equivalent to 340 mg of amantadine HCl. Capsules may be opened and the contents sprinkled over soft food such as applesauce and taken immediately.

Adverse Effects – Compulsive behaviors such as pathologic gambling, hypersexuality and obsessive viewing of pornography, uncontrollable spending, and excessive computer use are now recognized as common complications of dopaminergic drugs, especially dopamine agonists, and are defined as impulse control disorders (ICDs).[6] The patient often denies and minimizes ICD symptoms, but the abnormal behavior can be severe and lead to serious personal and financial problems. When ICD symp-

Usual Dosage[1]	Cost[2]
100 mg tid[11]	$8319.20
	10,668.50
300-1500 mg levo/d, divided	180.00-900.20
	437.40-2186.80
0.5-1 mg once/d[12]	428.80
	694.40
50-100 mg once/d	669.90
5 mg once/d with breakfast	54.00
	99.90
1.25-2.5 mg once/d in the morning	2034.90
200-400 mg/d, divided	130.10
	38.80
274 mg once/d at bedtime[13]	2375.00
129-322 mg once/d in the morning[16]	N.A.
25 mg tid or qid[15]	1117.80
	2369.70

14. Tablets are scored.
15. Starting dosage for patients who require individual titration of levodopa and carbidopa. Dosage for patients who need additional carbidopa is 25 mg given with the first dose of carbidopa/levodopa each day; additional doses of 12.5 or 25 mg may be needed.
16. A 129-mg tablet and a 193-mg tablet are taken together for a 322-mg dose.

toms are recognized, dopamine agonists should be tapered and stopped, and levodopa used as dopaminergic treatment.

Dopamine agonists can cause peripheral dopaminergic adverse effects such as nausea and orthostatic hypotension; nausea can be blocked by trimethobenzamide (*Tigan*, and generics) or possibly ondansetron (*Zofran*, and generics). Somnolence, lower-extremity edema, and hallucinations can also occur. In a controlled trial comparing pramipexole with levodopa for initial treatment, pramipexole was associated with a higher incidence of somnolence, edema, and hallucinations than levodopa.[7] Sudden sleep attacks (falling asleep without preceding drowsiness) can occur with use of dopamine agonists alone or in combination with levodopa. Rather than sacrifice motor performance by reducing the dose or eliminating the dopamine agonist, some expert clinicians treat excessive daytime sleepiness (off-label) with once-daily modafinil (*Provigil*, and generics) or armodafinil *(Nuvigil)*, the R-enantiomer of modafinil.

Dopamine agonists, used alone or in low doses, can cause confusion and psychosis, particularly in elderly patients. They should generally not be used in patients with dementia. Application-site reactions and nail dyschromia have occurred with the rotigotine patch.[8]

Withdrawal of dopamine agonists can lead to development of physical and psychological symptoms in some patients, particularly those with ICDs; these can include anxiety, dysphoria, irritability, suicidal ideation, fatigue, generalized pain, and drug cravings.[9]

Drug Interactions – All antipsychotic drugs antagonize dopamine to some extent and may reduce the efficacy of dopamine agonists. Concomitant use of any drug that causes CNS depression could increase the risk of somnolence and confusion in patients taking a dopamine agonist.

An Injectable Dopamine Agonist – Apomorphine *(Apokyn)*, a potent nonergot dopamine agonist, can be used as rescue treatment for "off" episodes in patients with advanced PD.[10] Administered subcutaneously, it can cause emesis and must be taken with an antiemetic. Trimethobenzamide 300 mg tid should be started 3 days before starting apomorphine and continued for the first 2 months or until tolerance develops. Serotonin receptor antagonists such as ondansetron are contraindicated for use with apomorphine because the combination can cause severe hypotension with loss of consciousness.

Injection-site reactions can occur. Like oral dopamine agonists, apomorphine can cause nausea, orthostatic hypotension, confusion, hallucinations, and psychosis. Yawning and drowsiness are common. Hypersexuality and frequent erections can occur and have been associated with abuse of the drug.

COMT INHIBITORS — Levodopa is metabolized in the periphery by dopa decarboxylase and catechol-O-methyltransferase (COMT). **Entacapone** (*Comtan*, and generics) and **tolcapone** (*Tasmar*, and generics) inhibit the activity of COMT. Used in combination with levodopa, they prolong the half-life of levodopa (without affecting peak serum concentrations) and decrease parkinsonian disability, but they can increase dyskinesia.

Entacapone acts peripherally and has been effective in decreasing daily "off" time by about 1 hour, improving motor scores and reducing levodopa requirements in patients with motor fluctuations. It is available both alone and in a fixed-dose combination with carbidopa and levodopa (*Stalevo*, and generics). Tolcapone inhibits both peripheral and central COMT. It is more effective than entacapone, but it has been associated with fatal hepatotoxicity and was taken off the market in Canada and other countries. It is available in the US for patients with normal liver function who have not responded to entacapone.[11]

Dosage – Entacapone has a short half-life; the recommended dosage is 200 mg taken with each dose of carbidopa/levodopa (maximum 8 times/day). The initial dosage of tolcapone is 100 mg tid, which can be increased to a maximum of 200 mg tid; it does not need to be taken at the same time as carbidopa/levodopa. Tolcapone should be stopped if no benefit is observed within 3 weeks of starting therapy.

Adverse Effects – Dyskinesia, nausea, diarrhea (worse with tolcapone), and urine discoloration can occur with both COMT inhibitors. Use of tolcapone requires written informed consent and monitoring of liver function every 2-4 weeks for the first 6 months of treatment and periodically thereafter. Serious hepatotoxicity has not been reported with entacapone.

The levodopa dose may have to be reduced in patients who develop dyskinesia, nausea, or hallucinations. Increased daytime sleepiness and sleep attacks have been reported with both entacapone and tolcapone.

Drug Interactions – COMT inhibitors may decrease the metabolism of COMT substrates such as methyldopa and isoproterenol, possibly resulting in tachycardia, arrhythmias, and hypertension. MAO and COMT are both involved in the metabolism of catecholamines; coadministration of a COMT inhibitor and a nonselective MAO inhibitor could result in decreased metabolism of catecholamines and catecholamine toxicity. Additive CNS depressant effects could occur if entacapone or tolcapone is used concurrently with any drug that causes CNS depression or sedation.

MAO-B INHIBITORS — **Selegiline** (*Eldepryl*, and others), an irreversible inhibitor of monoamine oxidase type B (MAO-B), inhibits catabolism of dopamine in the brain. Its effect on PD symptoms is modest, but used as monotherapy in early disease (not an FDA-approved indication) selegiline can delay initiation of levodopa treatment. Added to levodopa in advanced disease, it can permit use of lower doses of levodopa. Selegiline is available as a conventional tablet or capsule and as a lower-dose orally disintegrating tablet *(Zelapar)*. Absorption of the orally disintegrating tablet through the oral mucosa minimizes first-pass metabolism, increases bioavailability, and reduces serum concentrations of amphetamine metabolites.

Rasagiline (*Azilect*, and generics), another irreversible MAO-B inhibitor, is FDA-approved for use as monotherapy or adjunctive therapy in the treatment of PD; it appears to be modestly effective when taken alone for early disease or in addition to carbidopa/levodopa for advanced disease.[12,13] In a double-blind trial, patients with untreated PD received rasagiline 1 or 2 mg daily for 72 weeks (early-start) or placebo for 36 weeks followed by rasagiline for 36 weeks (delayed-start). After 72 weeks, the 1-mg early-start group had significantly less disability than the 1-mg delayed-start group, but early-start treatment with 2-mg doses did not differ significantly from delayed-start treatment for the change in disability scores from baseline.[14] In levodopa-treated patients with advanced disease, the decrease in "off" time with addition of rasagiline is similar to that with entacapone.[15]

In 2017, the FDA approved the reversible MAO-B inhibitor **safinamide** *(Xadago)* as an adjunct to carbidopa/levodopa in patients experiencing motor fluctuations; it has not been approved for use as monotherapy. Safinamide can modestly increase "on" time without troublesome dyskinesia in patients with mid- to late-stage PD.[16] Whether safinamide is more effective or has a more favorable safety profile than the older irreversible MAO-B inhibitors is unknown.[17]

Dosage – The initial/usual dosage of the conventional formulation of selegiline is 5 mg once daily with breakfast; the dosage can be increased to 5 mg with breakfast and with lunch, but the higher dosage may not provide an additional benefit. The starting dosage of selegiline orally disintegrating tablets is 1.25 mg once daily in the morning. Patients should not eat or drink for 5 minutes before or after taking the drug. After 6 weeks, the dosage can be increased to a maximum of 2.5 mg once daily. The recommended dosage of rasagiline as monotherapy is 1 mg once daily and as an adjunct to levodopa is 0.5-1 mg once daily. The starting dosage of safinamide is 50 mg once daily; after two weeks, it can be increased to 100 mg once daily if needed.

Adverse Effects – Nausea and orthostatic hypotension can occur with use of MAO-B inhibitors. At higher-than-recommended doses, safinamide loses its selectivity for MAO-B and could cause severe hypertension. MAO-B inhibitors can increase levodopa adverse effects, particularly dyskinesia and psychosis in elderly patients.

Drug Interactions – Use of other MAO inhibitors (including the antibacterial linezolid), serotonin-norepinephrine reuptake inhibitors (SNRIs), selective serotonin reuptake inhibitors (SSRIs), tricyclic or triazolopyridine antidepressants, cyclobenzaprine, St. John's wort, or opioids such as methadone, tramadol, or meperidine during or within

14 days after use of an MAO-B inhibitor could result in hypertensive crisis and/or serotonin syndrome and is contraindicated. Concomitant use of methylphenidate, amphetamines, or sympathomimetic amines such as pseudoephedrine with an MAO-B inhibitor can also result in severe hypertension.

Unlike MAO-A inhibitors used for treatment of depression, MAO-B inhibitors at recommended doses generally do not cause hypertension after ingestion of tyramine-rich foods or when used concomitantly with levodopa. Nevertheless, some manufacturers recommend dietary restrictions. The cough suppressant dextromethorphan can cause episodes of psychosis in patients taking an MAO-B inhibitor.

In vitro data suggest that safinamide may inhibit breast cancer resistance protein (BCRP) at a dose of 100 mg/day, possibly resulting in increased serum concentrations of BCRP substrates, such as rosuvastatin (*Crestor*, and generics), taken concurrently.

AMANTADINE — Amantadine, an antiviral drug, has been used as monotherapy in early PD and as an adjunct in later stages, usually in patients with levodopa-induced dyskinesia. It is a weak noncompetitive antagonist of glutamatergic *N*-methyl-D-aspartate (NMDA) receptors; glutamate is thought to play a role in dyskinesia. Amantadine may also be effective in controlling tremor, which is often resistant to dopaminergic treatment. In some patients, however, the symptomatic benefit only lasts a few weeks. A new extended-release formulation of amantadine *(Gocovri)* is FDA-approved for once-daily treatment of levodopa-induced dyskinesia; it has not been compared with immediate-release amantadine and it is very expensive.[18]

Dosage – Amantadine is usually started at a dose of 100 mg once daily, which can be increased to 100 mg twice daily; some patients may benefit from higher doses (300 or 400 mg daily in divided doses). The starting dosage of extended-release amantadine is 137 mg once daily at bedtime; after 1 week, the nightly dose should be increased to 274 mg.

Adverse Effects – Amantadine has anticholinergic-like adverse effects; it commonly causes dry mouth, constipation, and urinary retention. Nausea, dizziness, insomnia, confusion, hallucinations, peripheral edema, and livedo reticularis can occur. High serum concentrations of amantadine can cause severe psychosis, particularly in the elderly. QT interval prolongation and torsades de pointes have been associated with amantadine overdose.[19] Sudden withdrawal of amantadine may cause severe exacerbation of parkinsonian symptoms, confusion, neuroleptic malignant syndrome, and acute delirium.

Drug Interactions – Coadministration of drugs with anticholinergic properties may exacerbate adverse effects of amantadine such as dry mouth and constipation, and could cause additive CNS adverse effects. Torsades de pointes has been associated with concurrent use of amantadine and other QT interval-prolonging drugs.[19]

Elimination of amantadine is dependent on urine acidity; drugs that alkalinize the urine, such as carbonic anhydrase inhibitors, can increase amantadine concentrations and the risk of adverse effects.

Because amantadine has antiviral properties, it may reduce the efficacy of live vaccines.

Consumption of alcohol may increase the risk of CNS adverse effects in patients taking amantadine, and could cause dose dumping with the extended-release formulation; patients taking amantadine should be advised not to consume alcohol.

ANTICHOLINERGICS — Anticholinergics such as trihexyphenidyl and benztropine (*Cogentin*, and generics) can be useful in some patients with PD, especially for treatment of tremor and drooling.

Adverse Effects – Adverse effects include dry mouth, constipation, urinary retention, and aggravation of narrow-angle glaucoma. CNS adverse effects, including impaired memory, confusion, and hallucinations, may be particularly severe in elderly patients; anticholinergics are generally contraindicated in this age group. Abrupt discontinuation of any of these drugs can cause a severe exacerbation of symptoms.

OTHER DRUGS — The glucagon-like peptide-1 (GLP-1) receptor agonist **exenatide** *(Byetta; Bydureon),* which is FDA-approved only for treatment of type 2 diabetes, has been shown to have neuroprotective effects in animal models of PD. In one single-center, randomized, double-blind, 48-week trial in patients with moderate PD receiving dopaminergic treatment, addition of extended-release exenatide 2 mg SC once weekly significantly improved off-medication motor scores, compared to addition of placebo.[20]

The tyrosine kinase inhibitor **nilotinib** *(Tasigna),* which is FDA-approved for treatment of chronic myelogenous leukemia, targets a molecular pathway that might interfere with pathogenic mechanisms relevant to PD. In one small, open-label, uncontrolled trial in patients with advanced PD, use of nilotinib in a low dose of 150 or 300 mg daily for 24 weeks improved motor and cognitive outcomes.[21]

SURGICAL TREATMENT — Surgical ablation or deep brain stimulation (DBS) have generally been recommended for patients with advanced PD and intolerable dyskinesia or motor fluctuations on levodopa, although DBS is now also being used in some patients with early motor complications.[22,23] Appropriate candidates for surgery are those who have relatively intact cognition, are not depressed, and have no medical contraindications.

Deep Brain Stimulation (DBS) – High-frequency electrical stimulation of the subthalamic nucleus or globus pallidus from implanted electrodes has largely replaced ablative surgical procedures and is now the surgical treatment of choice for PD.[24]

In a randomized trial in 255 patients with advanced PD and motor complications, those who underwent bilateral DBS of the subthalamic nucleus or globus pallidus had improved motor function compared to patients treated with medical therapy.[25] A trial comparing bilateral subthalamic to bilateral pallidal DBS in 299 patients with advanced PD found that both procedures resulted in similar improvements in motor function at 24 months.[26]

In a randomized, 2-year trial (EARLYSTIM) in 251 patients 18-60 years old with PD (duration ≥4 years) and early motor complications (fluctuations or dyskinesia for ≤3 years), bilateral subthalamic neurostimulation plus medical therapy was significantly superior to medical therapy alone in improving quality of life (the primary endpoint) and motor function.[27]

After DBS, reductions in levodopa dosage may be maintained for several years. In general, treated patients have marked improvement in off-medication motor function and improvement in dyskinesia when taking medication. Some symptoms, such as speech disturbances, postural instability, freezing of gait, and cognitive problems, do not improve with DBS and may become worse.

Adverse Effects – Adverse effects of DBS have included intracranial hemorrhage, hemiparesis, infection, confusion, attention/cognition deficits, dysarthria, depression, and death. Even with successful surgery, decreased verbal fluency and a variety of psychosocial problems have occurred. Hardware problems, including lead migration, fracture, or malfunction, can also occur. Cognitive decline is common after DBS in patients with pre-existing intellectual impairment and in those ≥70 years old.

EXERCISE THERAPY — Combining pharmacologic therapy with physical activity, such as an exercise or dance program, can improve physical function, particularly gait, mobility, posture, and balance, and quality of life in patients with PD.[28]

TREATMENT OF DEPRESSION — Depression commonly accompanies PD and must be treated if the patient is to benefit adequately from antiparkinson drugs. In one small study, the tricyclic antidepressant nortriptyline was more effective than an SSRI, but tricyclics can cause cognitive impairment and increase the risk of falls. A systematic review and meta-analysis of randomized, controlled trials found that use of SSRIs or cognitive behavioral therapy significantly improved depression in patients with PD.[29] Antidepressants may also help the sleep abnormalities commonly associated with PD. Electroconvulsive therapy (ECT) may alleviate refractory major depression and transiently improve the underlying parkinsonian symptoms.

TREATMENT OF PSYCHOSIS — **Pimavanserin** *(Nuplazid)*, a 5-HT_{2A} selective serotonin inverse agonist with no dopamine blocking activity, was approved by the FDA in 2016 specifically for treatment of hallucinations and delusions associated with PD psychosis.[30] It appears to be effective in the short term for treatment of psychotic symptoms, without exacerbating motor symptoms.[31] The recommended dosage is 34 mg (two 17-mg tablets) once daily, with no need for titration. Peripheral edema has been reported in patients taking pimavanserin. It is metabolized primarily by CYP3A; the dose should be adjusted when it is used concomitantly with CYP3A4 inhibitors or inducers.[32] Pimavanserin can prolong the QT interval, and should not be used in patients with risk factors for QT interval prolongation or in combination with other QT interval-prolonging drugs.[19] Like other antipsychotics, it may increase the risk of mortality in elderly patients with psychosis.

Clozapine (*Clozaril*, and generics), a potent antipsychotic agent, has been used to control psychosis associated with use of levodopa or dopamine agonists. Drowsiness is a common adverse effect. Clozapine has caused agranulocytosis in 0.6% of patients; blood counts should be obtained weekly for the first six months of treatment and biweekly thereafter. **Quetiapine** (*Seroquel*, and generics), another antipsychotic drug often used in patients with PD psychosis, does not cause agranulocytosis and does not have anticholinergic effects. Like clozapine, quetiapine can cause drowsiness. Both clozapine and quetiapine block dopamine receptors and could reduce the effectiveness of levodopa. Atypical antipsychotics have a warning in their labeling about an increased risk of mortality in elderly patients with dementia-related psychosis.

TREATMENT OF DEMENTIA — The oral acetylcholinesterase inhibitors **donepezil** (*Aricept*, and generics), **rivastigmine** (*Exelon*, and generics), and **galantamine** (*Razadyne*, and generics) that are used to treat Alzheimer's disease may improve the cognitive and behaviorial symptoms associated with PD dementia, but they may worsen tremor in some patients.[33] Only rivastigmine is FDA-approved for treatment of dementia in PD. **Memantine** *(Namenda)*, an NMDA-receptor antagonist, is also used to treat dementia; it may be helpful for cognitive impairment and potentially has an antiparkinson effect, but it may also aggravate parkinsonian symptoms.

1. Parcopa: a rapidly dissolving formulation of carbidopa/levodopa. Med Lett Drugs Ther 2005; 47:12.
2. R Pahwa et al. Randomized trial of IPX066, carbidopa/levodopa extended release, in early Parkinson's disease. Parkinsonism Relat Disord 2014; 20:142.
3. Carbidopa/levodopa extended-release capsules (Rytary). Med Lett Drugs Ther 2015; 57:59.
4. CW Olanow et al. Continuous intrajejunal infusion of levodopa-carbidopa intestinal gel for patients with advanced Parkinson's disease: a randomised, controlled, double-blind, double-dummy study. Lancet Neurol 2014; 13:141.
5. In brief: Duopa – a carbidopa/levodopa enteral suspension for Parkinson's disease. Med Lett Drugs Ther 2015; 57:112.
6. HD Weiss and L Marsh. Impulse control disorders and compulsive behaviors associated with dopaminergic therapies in Parkinson disease. Neurol Clin Pract 2012; 2:267.
7. KM Biglan et al. Risk factors for somnolence, edema, and hallucinations in early Parkinson disease. Neurology 2007; 69:187.
8. HA Teive and RP Munhoz. Rotigotine-induced nail dyschromia in a patient with Parkinson's disease. Neurology 2011; 76:1605.
9. MJ Nirenberg. Dopamine agonist withdrawal syndrome: implications for patient care. Drugs Aging 2013; 30:587.
10. Apomorphine (Apokyn) for Parkinson's disease. Med Lett Drugs Ther 2005; 47:7.
11. SZ Marsala et al. A systematic review of catechol-O-methyltransferase inhibitors: efficacy and safety in clinical practice. Clin Neuropharmacol 2012; 35:185.
12. Rasagiline (Azilect) for Parkinson's disease. Med Lett Drugs Ther 2006; 48:97.
13. LW Elmer. Rasagiline adjunct therapy in patients with Parkinson's disease: post hoc analyses of the PRESTO and LARGO trials. Parkinsonism Relat Disord 2013;19:930.
14. CW Olanow et al. A double-blind, delayed-start trial of rasagiline in Parkinson's disease. N Engl J Med 2009; 361:1268.

15. O Rascol et al. Rasagiline as an adjunct to levodopa in patients with Parkinson's disease and motor fluctuations (LARGO, Lasting effect in Adjunct therapy with Rasagiline Given Once daily, study): a randomised, double-blind, parallel-group trial. Lancet 2005; 365:947.
16. AH Schapira et al. Assessment of safety and efficacy of safinamide as a levodopa adjunct in patients with Parkinson disease and motor fluctuations: a randomized clinical trial. JAMA Neurol 2017; 74:216.
17. Safinamide (Xadago) for Parkinson's Disease. Med Lett Drugs Ther 2017; 59:151.
18. Extended-release amantadine (Gocovri) for dyskinesia in Parkinson's disease. Med Lett Drugs Ther 2017 Nov 8 (epub).
19. RL Woosley and KA Romero. QT drugs list. Available at: www.crediblemeds.org. Accessed November 9, 2017.
20. D Athauda et al. Exenatide once weekly versus placebo in Parkinson's disease: a randomised, double-blind, placebo-controlled trial. Lancet 2017; 390:1664.
21. F Pagan et al. Nilotinib effects in Parkinson's disease and dementia with Lewy bodies. J Parkinsons Dis 2016; 6:503.
22. Deep brain stimulation for Parkinson's disease with early motor complications. Med Lett Drugs Ther 2013; 55:81.
23. G Suarez-Cedeno et al. Earlier intervention with deep brain stimulation for Parkinson's disease. Parkinsons Dis 2017 Aug 16 (epub).
24. MS Okun. Deep-brain stimulation for Parkinson's disease. N Engl J Med 2012; 367:1529.
25. FM Weaver et al. Bilateral deep brain stimulation vs best medical therapy for patients with advanced Parkinson disease: a randomized controlled trial. JAMA 2009; 301:63.
26. KA Follett et al. Pallidal versus subthalamic deep-brain stimulation for Parkinson's disease. N Engl J Med 2010; 362:2077.
27. WM Schuepbach et al. Neurostimulation for Parkinson's disease with early motor complications. N Engl J Med 2013; 368:610.
28. M Lauzé et al. The effects of physical activity in Parkinson's disease: a review. J Parkinsons Dis 2016; 6:685.
29. E Bomasang-Layno et al. Antidepressive treatments for Parkinson's disease: a systematic review and meta-analysis. Parkinsonism Relat Disord 2015; 21: 833.
30. Pimavanserin (Nuplazid) for Parkinson's disease psychosis. Med Lett Drugs Ther 2016; 58:74.
31. J Cummings et al. Pimavanserin for patients with Parkinson's disease psychosis: a randomised, placebo-controlled phase 3 trial. Lancet 2014; 383:533.
32. Inhibitors and inducers of CYP enzymes and p-glycoprotein. Med Lett Drugs Ther 2017 September 18 (epub). Available at: medicalletter.org/downloads/CYP_PGP_Tables.pdf. Accessed November 9, 2017.
33. Drugs for cognitive loss and dementia. Med Lett Drugs Ther 2017; 59:155.

DRUGS FOR
Sexually Transmitted Infections

Original publication date – July 2017 (revised March 2018)

The text and tables that follow include recommendations for management of sexually transmitted infections (STIs) other than HIV and viral hepatitis. Some of the indications and dosages recommended here have not been approved by the FDA.

PARTNER TREATMENT — Management of STIs should include evaluation and treatment of sex partners of infected persons. If possible, partners should be examined and tested for STIs, but in most cases treatment should be initiated regardless of symptoms and without waiting for laboratory test results.

An alternative approach, particularly for heterosexual patients infected with gonorrhea or chlamydia, is to treat sex partners without direct examination or testing, either by prescription or by giving the medication for the partner to the index patient, a practice called expedited partner therapy (EPT).[1]

CHLAMYDIA — A single dose of azithromycin (*Zithromax*, and generics) or 7 days' treatment with doxycycline (*Vibramycin*, and generics) is effective for treatment of uncomplicated urogenital infection caused by *Chlamydia trachomatis*.[2] Levofloxacin (*Levaquin*, and generics) or ofloxacin for 7 days is an effective alternative. Erythromycin may also be effective, but gastrointestinal adverse effects are common and can lead

Table 1. Drugs of Choice for Some Sexually Transmitted Infections

Type or Stage	Regimen(s) of Choice
Chlamydial Infection and Related Clinical Syndromes[1]	
Urogenital or rectal (except LGV)	Azithromycin 1 g PO once[2] Doxycycline 100 mg PO bid x 7d[2-5]
Infection in pregnancy	Azithromycin 1 g PO once
Neonatal ophthalmia or pneumonia	Erythromycin 12.5 mg/kg PO qid x 14d[10-12]
LGV	Doxycycline 100 mg PO bid x 21d[3,14]
Gonorrhea[15]	
Urogenital or rectal	Ceftriaxone 250 mg IM once plus azithromycin 1 g PO once[16]
Pharyngeal	Ceftriaxone 250 mg IM once plus azithromycin 1 g PO once
Infection in pregnancy	Ceftriaxone 250 mg IM once plus azithromycin 1 g PO once[21]
Neonatal ophthalmia	Ceftriaxone 25-50 mg/kg IV or IM once (max 125 mg)

LGV = lymphogranuloma venereum

1. Related clinical syndromes include nongonococcal urethritis (NGU) and cervicitis.
2. For cases of persistent or recurrent NGU, azithromycin should be used if initial treatment was with doxycycline and vice versa. Some experts add a single 2-g dose of tinidazole or metronidazole to also treat trichomoniasis. Moxifloxacin can be used for persistent or recurrent NGU due to *Mycoplasma genitalium*.
3. Not recommended for use during pregnancy or in breastfeeding women.
4. Less effective than azithromycin against NGU associated with *Mycoplasma genitalium*.
5. Delayed-release doxycycline *(Doryx)* 200 mg once daily x 7d is as effective as twice-daily doxycycline, with less gastrointestinal toxicity, but it costs more (WM Geisler et al. Clin Infect Dis 2012; 55:82).
6. Should be used only if *Neisseria gonorrhoeae* has been excluded.
7. Fluoroquinolones are generally not recommended for patients <18 years old or in pregnant or breastfeeding women.
8. Erythromycin ethylsuccinate 800 mg may be substituted for erythromycin base 500 mg. Erythromycin estolate is contraindicated during pregnancy.
9. Erythromycin base 250 mg PO qid x 14d can be used if gastrointestinal adverse effects are bothersome.
10. Effectiveness of erythromycin for chlamydial pneumonia and neonatal ophthalmia is about 80%; some experts would use a second course.

Some Alternatives
Levofloxacin 500 mg PO once/d x 7d[4,6,7] Ofloxacin 300 mg PO bid x 7d[4,6,7] Erythromycin base 500 mg PO qid x 7d
Amoxicillin 500 mg PO tid x 7d Erythromycin base 500 mg PO qid x 7d[8,9]
Azithromycin 20 mg/kg PO once/d x 3d[11,13]
Erythromycin base 500 mg PO qid x 21d
Cefixime 400 mg PO once plus azithromycin 1 g PO once[17]
Gentamicin 240 mg IM once[3] plus azithromycin 2 g PO once[18] Gemifloxacin 320 mg PO once[7,19] plus azithromycin 2 g PO once[18]
Gemifloxacin 320 mg PO once[7,19] plus azithromycin 2 g PO once[18,20] Gentamicin 240 mg IM once[3] plus azithromycin 2 g PO once[18,20]

11. Hypertrophic pyloric stenosis has been reported in infants <6 weeks old.
12. Erythromycin base or ethylsuccinate.
13. No data available for efficacy in pneumonia.
14. Azithromycin 1 g PO once/wk for 3 weeks is probably effective, but data are lacking.
15. Dual antibiotic therapy is recommended for gonorrhea regardless of the presence of chlamydial infection.
16. Azithromycin is the preferred dual agent along with ceftriaxone (preferred) or cefixime (alternative); doxycycline 100 mg PO bid x 7d can be used as dual agent if patient is allergic to azithromycin.
17. Only when treatment with IM ceftriaxone is not possible. Cefixime is not effective for pharyngeal gonorrhea.
18. If severe allergy to penicillin or cephalosporins. Whether these regimens are effective for treatment of rectal or pharyngeal infection is unclear. Monotherapy with azithromycin is no longer recommended due to resistance concerns and reports of treatment failure.
19. Gemifloxacin is currently unavailable in the US due to patent issue.
20. Consider ID consult regarding treatment. If an alternative treatment regimen is used, test-of-cure 14 days post-treatment is recommended.
21. Consultation with an ID specialist is recommended for patients with a cephalosporin allergy.

Continued on next page

Table 1. Drugs of Choice for Some Sexually Transmitted Infections (continued)	
Type or Stage	**Regimen(s) of Choice**
Epididymitis (acute)	
	Ceftriaxone 250 mg IM once plus doxycycline 100 mg PO bid x 10d[22]
Proctitis (acute)[23]	
	Ceftriaxone 250 mg IM once plus doxycycline 100 mg PO bid x 7d[3]
Pelvic Inflammatory Disease	
Parenteral	Cefotetan 2 g IV q12h or cefoxitin 2 g IV q6h[24] plus doxycycline 100 mg IV or PO bid to complete 14d[3,25] Clindamycin 900 mg IV q8h plus gentamicin 2 mg/kg IV or IM once, then 1.5 mg/kg IV q8h[24,26,27]
IM/Oral	Ceftriaxone 250 mg IM once[29] plus doxycycline 100 mg PO bid x 14d[3] +/- metronidazole 500 mg PO bid x 14d Cefoxitin 2 g IM once plus probenecid 1 g PO once plus doxycycline 100 mg PO bid x 14d[3] +/- metronidazole 500 mg PO bid x 14d
Syphilis[31]	
Primary, secondary, or early latent (<1 year)	Benzathine penicillin G 2.4 MU IM once
Late latent, latent of unknown duration, or tertiary	Benzathine penicillin G 2.4 MU IM wkly x 3wks

MU = million units

22. For treatment of epididymitis likely caused by sexually transmitted chlamydia or gonorrhea. Men at risk for chlamydia or gonorrhea and infection with enteric organisms (history of insertive anal intercourse) should receive a single 250-mg dose of ceftriaxone IM and a 10-day course of levofloxacin 500 mg PO once/d or ofloxacin 300 mg PO bid. Older men and those who have had urinary tract instrumentation, surgery, or obstruction, or are immunosuppressed may have epididymitis due to enteric gram-negative bacilli; they should be treated with levofloxacin or ofloxacin alone (if not at risk for sexually transmitted chlamydia or gonorrhea).
23. Men who have sex with men who have bloody discharge, perianal ulcers, or mucosal ulcers, and a positive rectal chlamydia NAAT or HIV infection should be offered presumptive treatment for LGV with doxycycline 100 mg bid for 3 weeks.
24. Parenteral therapy can be stopped 24-48 hours after clinical improvement occurs, and oral doxycycline should be given to complete 14 days' treatment.
25. For tubo-ovarian abscess, also add clindamycin 450 mg PO qid or metronidazole 500 mg PO bid.

Some Alternatives
Ampicillin/sulbactam 3 g IV q6h[24] plus doxycycline 100 mg PO bid to complete 14d[3,28]
Levofloxacin 500 mg PO once/d x 14d[7,30] or ofloxacin 400 mg PO bid x 14d[7,30] or moxifloxacin 400 mg PO once/d x 14d[7,30] plus metronidazole 500 mg PO bid x 14d
Doxycycline 100 mg PO bid x 14d[3,32] Ceftriaxone 1-2 g IV or IM once/d x 10-14d[32]
Doxycycline 100 mg PO bid x 4wks[3,32]

26. Gentamicin 3-5 mg/kg once/d is probably effective, but has not been studied in pelvic inflammatory disease.
27. Doxycycline 100 mg PO bid or clindamycin 450 mg PO qid should be used to complete 14 days' treatment.
28. Azithromycin monotherapy (500 mg IV once/d x 1-2d, then 250 mg PO x 5-6d) for 7d or with a 12-day course of metronidazole may also be effective.
29. Or other third-generation cephalosporin.
30. Only if IV cephalosporins cannot be administered, *N. gonorrhoeae* infection is unlikely, and the patient can be followed.
31. Syphilis in pregnant women should be treated with penicillin in doses appropriate to the stage of the disease. If allergic to penicillin, hospitalization, desensitization, and treatment with penicillin is recommended.
32. Efficacy not established; for use only when patient is allergic to penicillin. Adherence must be ensured.

Continued on next page

Table 1. Drugs of Choice for Some Sexually Transmitted Infections (continued)

Type or Stage	Regimen(s) of Choice
Syphilis[31] (continued)	
Neurosyphilis, including ocular syphilis	Aqueous crystalline penicillin G 3-4 MU IV q4h or 18-24 MU continuous IV infusion x 10-14d
Trichomoniasis	
	Metronidazole 2 g PO once[33] Tinidazole 2 g PO once[3,33]
Bacterial Vaginosis	
	Metronidazole 500 mg PO bid x 7d Metronidazole gel 0.75% 5 g intravaginally once/d x 5d Clindamycin 2% cream 5 g intravaginally at bedtime x 7d[35]
Vulvovaginal Candidiasis[36]	
Uncomplicated	Intravaginal azole (butoconazole, clotrimazole, miconazole, tioconazole, terconazole) once/d x 1-14d[35,37] Fluconazole 150 mg PO once[38]
Recurrent	Intravaginal azole once/d x 7-14d or fluconazole 100-200 mg PO 3x/wk, then fluconazole 150 mg once/wk x 6 mos
Chancroid	
	Azithromycin 1 g PO once Ceftriaxone 250 mg IM once

MU = million units

33. HIV-positive women with trichomoniasis should be treated with metronidazole 500 mg PO bid x 7d.
34. A meta-analysis found a lower rate of treatment failure with the multidose regimen compared with the single-dose regimen in HIV-negative women (K Howe and PJ Kissinger. Sex Transm Dis 2017; 44:29).
35. May weaken latex condoms and diaphragms.
35a. Approved by the FDA in September 2017. Secnidazole oral granules should be sprinkled onto applesauce, yogurt, or pudding and be consumed within 30 minutes. The granules should not be chewed or crushed.

Some Alternatives
Procaine penicillin G 2.4 MU IM once/d x 10-14d plus probenecid 500 mg PO qid x 10-14d
Metronidazole 500 mg PO bid x 7d[33,34]
Tinidazole 1 g PO once/d x 5d[3] Tinidazole 2 g PO once/d x 2d[3] Clindamycin 300 mg PO bid x 7d Clindamycin ovules 100 mg intravaginally at bedtime x 3d[35] Secnidazole 2g PO once[35a]
Itraconazole 200 mg PO bid x 1d
Clotrimazole 200 mg 2x/wk or 500 mg once/wk intravaginally
Ciprofloxacin 500 mg PO bid x 3d[7] Erythromycin base 500 mg PO tid x 7d

36. Due to *Candida albicans*. Other *Candida* spp., such as *Candida glabrata* and *Candida krusei*, may respond to an azole other than fluconazole for 7-14 days, boric acid 600 mg intravaginally once/d x 14d, or topical 17% flucytosine cream (P Nyirjesy. Obstet Gynecol 2014; 124:1135).
37. Duration of treatment varies with drug and formulation.
38. May be repeated every 72 hours x 3 doses if patient remains symptomatic.

Continued on next page

Table 1. Drugs of Choice for Some Sexually Transmitted Infections (continued)

Type or Stage	Regimen(s) of Choice
Genital Herpes	
First episode	Acyclovir 400 mg PO tid x 7-10d Famciclovir 250 mg PO tid x 7-10d Valacyclovir 1 g PO bid x 7-10d
Episodic treatment[39,40]	Acyclovir 800 mg PO bid x 5d or 800 mg tid x 2d or 400 mg PO tid x 5d Famciclovir 1 g PO bid x 1d or 125 mg PO bid x 5d or 500 mg once, then 250 mg bid x 2d Valacyclovir 500 mg PO bid x 3d or 1 g PO once/d x 5d
Suppression[41,42]	Acyclovir 400 mg PO bid Valacyclovir 500 mg-1 g PO once/d[43] Famciclovir 250 mg PO bid
Genital Warts[44]	
Provider-administered	Trichloroacetic acid once/wk until resolved Bichloroacetic acid 80-90% once/wk until resolved Cryotherapy with liquid nitrogen or cryoprobe
Patient-applied	Imiquimod 5% once/d 3x/wk up to 16 weeks[3,35,45] Imiquimod 3.75% once/d up to 8 weeks[3,35,45] Podofilox 0.5% bid x 3d, then 4 days rest, repeat up to 4x[3] Sinecatechins 15% ointment tid up to 16 weeks[3,35]

39. Antiviral therapy is variably effective for episodic treatment of recurrences; it is only effective if started early.
40. For recurrent HSV in HIV-positive patients, treat with valacyclovir 1 g bid, famciclovir 500 mg bid, or acyclovir 400 mg tid for 5-10 days.
41. Some expert clinicians recommend discontinuing preventive treatment for 1 to 2 months once/year to reassess the frequency of recurrence.
42. Suppressive therapy with acyclovir 400 mg tid or valacyclovir 500 mg bid should be offered to pregnant women with recurrent genital herpes beginning at 36 weeks to reduce the risk of recurrence at delivery and possibly the need for cesarean section.

Some Alternatives
Acyclovir 200 mg PO 5x/d x 7-10d
Surgical removal Laser surgery

43. Use 500 mg once daily in immunocompetent patients with <10 recurrences per year and 500 mg bid or 1 g daily in patients with ≥10 recurrences per year. For HIV-infected patients, the dosage is 500 mg bid.
44. Recommendations for external genital warts. Cryotherapy with liquid nitrogen can also be used for vaginal, urethral meatus, and anal warts. Cryoprobe should not be used in the vagina due to the risk of vaginal perforation. Trichloroacetic or bichloroacetic acid can be used for vaginal and anal warts.
45. Imiquimod should be washed off 6-10 hours after application.

Continued on next page

Table 1. Drugs of Choice for Some Sexually Transmitted Infections (continued)

Type or Stage	Regimen(s) of Choice
Pediculosis[46]	
	Permethrin 1% 2 applications ≥7d apart[47] Pyrethrins with piperonyl butoxide 2 applications ≥7d apart[47]
Scabies	
	Permethrin 5% 2 applications ≥7d apart

46. Pediculocides should not be used for infestations of the eyelashes. Such infestations are treated with petrolatum ointment applied 2-4x/d x 8-10d.
47. Permethrin and pyrethrin are pediculocidal; retreatment in 7-10 days is needed to eradicate the infestation. Some lice are resistant to pyrethrins and permethrin.
48. Ivermectin is pediculocidal, but not ovicidal; more than one dose is generally necessary to eradicate the infestation. Safety of ivermectin in pregnant women remains to be established; animal studies have shown adverse effects on the fetus. Taking ivermectin with a meal increases its bioavailability.

to poor adherence and treatment failure. Rectal chlamydia can be treated with the same drugs as those used for urogenital infection, but some data suggest that doxycycline might be more effective than azithromycin for this indication.[3]

Pregnancy – Azithromycin is the drug of choice for treatment of chlamydial infection in pregnant women.[4] Erythromycin (base or ethylsuccinate) and amoxicillin are effective alternatives. Tetracyclines and fluoroquinolones should not be used during pregnancy.

Neonatal Ophthalmia and Pneumonia – Neonates born to women with untreated cervical *C. trachomatis* infection are at risk for conjunctivitis and pneumonia. Prenatal screening and treatment of pregnant women can prevent perinatal chlamydial infection. Ophthalmic antibiotics used for prophylaxis of neonatal gonococcal ophthalmia do not prevent ocular chlamydial infection in the newborn. For newborns with conjunctivitis or pneumonia caused by *C. trachomatis*, treatment with oral erythromycin is recommended; azithromycin may be an effective

Some Alternatives
Ivermectin 250 mcg/kg PO 2x ≥7d apart[48] Malathion 0.5% 1 application for 8-10 hrs, then wash off[49]
Ivermectin 200 mcg/kg PO 2x ≥7d apart[48]

49. Can be used when treatment failure due to resistance is thought to have occurred. Odor and long duration of application may be difficult to tolerate.

alternative. Use of oral erythromycin or azithromycin in infants <6 weeks old (especially those <2 weeks old) has been associated with hypertrophic pyloric stenosis.[5]

Lymphogranuloma Venereum – In the US, infections with *C. trachomatis* serovars L1-L3 that cause lymphogranuloma venereum (LGV) present primarily as proctocolitis, typically in patients with rectal exposure.[6] The classic presentation, a self-limited genital ulcer or papule with lymphadenopathy, is now rare. Patients who present with symptoms consistent with LGV (proctocolitis or genital ulcer with lymphadenopathy) should be offered presumptive treatment.[4,7] A 3-week course of doxycycline is recommended for treatment of LGV.

Follow-Up – Test-of-cure is generally not needed for nonpregnant patients who are treated for chlamydia with a recommended or alternative regimen. Pregnant women should be tested 3-4 weeks after treatment is completed. Retesting is recommended 3 months after treatment for all patients.[4]

Partner Treatment – Sex partners should be offered standard treatment for chlamydia. EPT should not be offered to men who have sex with men (MSM).

NONGONOCOCCAL URETHRITIS AND CERVICITIS — Up to 40% of **nongonococcal urethritis (NGU)** cases are caused by *C. trachomatis*. *Mycoplasma genitalium* is now responsible for up to 30% of NGU cases in the US. Other possible pathogens include *Trichomonas vaginalis*, herpes simplex virus (HSV), and adenovirus. Data on the role of *Ureaplasma urealyticum* in NGU are inconsistent.[8] Enteric organisms can cause NGU in patients with a history of insertive anal intercourse.

Most cases of NGU respond to treatment with azithromycin or doxycycline.[9] Persistent or recurrent NGU (in an adherent patient who has not been re-exposed to an untreated sex partner) is most commonly caused by *M. genitalium*. Azithromycin can be used if doxycycline was used initially, but up to 50% of *M. genitalium* are now resistant to azithromycin.[10-12] Men who have persistent or recurrent NGU after treatment with azithromycin can be treated with moxifloxacin (*Avelox*, and generics) 400 mg once daily for 7 days. A single 2-g dose of metronidazole (*Flagyl*, and generics) or tinidazole (*Tindamax*, and generics) should be added for possible trichomoniasis in men who have sex with women.

As with NGU, azithromycin or doxycycline is recommended for presumptive treatment of **non-gonococcal cervicitis**. Women at increased risk of gonorrhea, such as those <25 years old and those with a new sex partner, a sex partner with concurrent partners, or a sex partner who has an STI, should also be treated empirically for gonorrhea.[4]

GONORRHEA — The treatment of choice for uncomplicated urogenital, rectal, or pharyngeal gonorrhea, regardless of the presence of chlamydial infection, is an IM injection of ceftriaxone (*Rocephin*, and generics) plus a single dose of oral azithromycin. Doxycycline is no longer recommended as part of the standard dual regimen because of a high prevalence of gonococcal resistance to tetracyclines in the US, but it can be used with ceftriaxone as dual therapy in patients who are allergic to azithromycin.[4]

When treatment with ceftriaxone is not possible, cefixime (*Suprax*, and generics) plus azithromycin can be used to treat urogenital or rectal gonorrhea. In patients with severe penicillin allergy or allergy to cephalosporins, gentamicin plus azithromycin or gemifloxacin *(Factive)* plus azithromycin are effective in treating urogenital gonorrhea, but whether either regimen is effective for treatment of rectal or pharyngeal infection is unclear, and resistance of *Neisseria gonorrhoeae* to azithromycin in MSM is increasing. These regimens have a high incidence of gastrointestinal adverse effects, and gemifloxacin is currently unavailable in the US due to a patent issue.[13]

Resistance – Over the past several decades, *N. gonorrhoeae* has developed resistance to penicillin, sulfonamides, tetracyclines, and fluoroquinolones.[14] Gonococci have also recently demonstrated decreased susceptibility to azithromycin and third-generation cephalosporins (cefixime and ceftriaxone), and treatment failures have been reported in other countries.[15-18] A possible case of pharyngeal gonorrhea resistant to azithromycin and ceftriaxone has been reported in the US,[19] and a cluster of gonococcal isolates with high-level resistance to azithromycin and decreased susceptibility to ceftriaxone was recently reported in Hawaii.[20]

Pregnancy – Pregnant women with gonorrhea should be treated with the recommended regimen of ceftriaxone plus azithromycin. Doxycycline is contraindicated for use during pregnancy.

Neonatal Ocular Prophylaxis – Prenatal screening and treatment of pregnant women can prevent gonococcal infection in neonates. Neonatal ocular prophylaxis can prevent gonococcal ophthalmia and is required by law in most states in the US; it is no longer standard practice in Canada. Erythromycin 0.5% ophthalmic ointment is the only formulation approved for this indication in the US; a one-time instillation in both eyes is recommended for all newborn infants. An infant born to a mother with untreated gonorrhea should receive a single dose of ceftriaxone.

Follow-Up – Test-of-cure is generally not needed for patients who are treated for uncomplicated urogenital or rectal gonorrhea with a recommended or alternative regimen. It is recommended 14 days after treatment in patients with pharyngeal gonorrhea treated with an alternative regimen. Rescreening is recommended 3 months after treatment for all patients with gonococcal infection.[4]

Partner Treatment – Sex partners of patients with gonorrhea should ideally be treated with ceftriaxone plus azithromycin. Cefixime plus azithromycin is an EPT option for heterosexual partners not willing to be examined or treated with ceftriaxone.[21]

EPIDIDYMITIS — Acute epididymitis in men <35 years old is frequently caused by *C. trachomatis* or *N. gonorrhoeae*; empiric treatment with ceftriaxone plus doxycycline is recommended. Acute epididymitis with urethritis caused by sexually transmitted enteric organisms can occur in men who practice insertive anal intercourse; ceftriaxone plus either levofloxacin or ofloxacin is recommended for such patients. Older men and those who have had urinary tract instrumentation, surgery or obstruction, or are immunosuppressed may also have epididymitis due to enteric gram-negative bacilli; they should be treated with levofloxacin or ofloxacin.

PROCTITIS — Proctitis occurs predominantly in men who are the receptive partner during anal intercourse. It is commonly caused by *N. gonorrhoeae*, *C. trachomatis* (including LGV serovars), *Treponema pallidum*, or HSV. Empiric treatment with a single dose of ceftriaxone plus 7 days of doxycycline is recommended. If LGV is suspected, doxycycline treatment should be continued for a total of 3 weeks.

PELVIC INFLAMMATORY DISEASE — *C. trachomatis* or *N. gonorrhoeae* can cause acute, nonrecurrent pelvic inflammatory disease

(PID), but *M. genitalium*, *Mycoplasma hominis,* and various facultative and anaerobic bacteria may also be involved. Treatment regimens should include broad-spectrum antimicrobial coverage of likely pathogens, including *C. trachomatis* and *N. gonorrhoeae*. Parenteral regimens include cefotetan (*Cefotan*, and generics) plus doxycycline, cefoxitin (*Mefoxin*, and generics) plus doxycycline, or clindamycin (*Cleocin*, and generics) plus an aminoglycoside. Parenteral therapy is continued until 24-48 hours after clinical improvement occurs, and then oral doxycycline is used to complete 14 days' therapy (oral clindamycin can be used for the clindamycin/gentamicin regimen).[22] When tubo-ovarian abscess is present, clindamycin or metronidazole should be added to doxycycline for anaerobic coverage to complete 14 days of treatment.[23] An oral alternative regimen for mild-to-moderate acute PID is doxycycline, with or without metronidazole, after a single IM dose of a third-generation cephalosporin such as ceftriaxone. Levofloxacin, ofloxacin, or moxifloxacin plus metronidazole can be considered in patients with a cephalosporin allergy if infection with *N. gonorrhoeae* is unlikely and the patient can be followed.[4]

SYPHILIS — Parenteral penicillin G remains the drug of choice for treating all stages of syphilis.[24] Primary, secondary, or early latent syphilis (less than one year's duration) should be treated with a single IM injection of benzathine penicillin G. In patients with severe penicillin allergy, doxycycline or tetracycline is usually effective if adherence is ensured. The emergence of azithromycin-resistant *T. pallidum* precludes the use of azithromycin for treatment of syphilis in the US.[4] For late latent syphilis (more than one year's duration or when the duration is unknown) or tertiary syphilis (gumma or cardiovascular), treatment with 3 once-weekly doses of IM benzathine penicillin G is recommended. All persons with tertiary syphilis should have a lumbar puncture prior to treatment; those with neurosyphilis require treatment with an appropriate regimen (see Table 1, p. 274).

Syphilis and HIV – The majority of syphilis cases in HIV-infected patients respond to standard benzathine penicillin G regimens appropriate to the stage of infection.[25-27]

Pregnancy – Pregnant women with syphilis should be treated with parenteral penicillin G. In pregnant women with syphilis who are allergic to penicillin, hospitalization, desensitization, and treatment with penicillin is recommended.

TRICHOMONIASIS — A single dose of oral tinidazole or metronidazole is generally used for treatment of trichomoniasis.[28] Tinidazole may be less likely than metronidazole to cause gastrointestinal adverse effects, but it costs more. Tinidazole is often effective against metronidazole-resistant *T. vaginalis*.[29,30] Treatment with intravaginal metronidazole gel is not recommended. Reinfection is common; retesting within 3 months after treatment is recommended for all sexually active women. Sex partners of patients with trichomoniasis should be treated.

Pregnancy – Trichomoniasis has been associated with adverse pregnancy outcomes. Metronidazole appears to be safe during all stages of pregnancy and should be used to treat symptomatic trichomoniasis in pregnant women. The safety of tinidazole in pregnancy has not been established.

BACTERIAL VAGINOSIS — In bacterial vaginosis (BV), normal hydrogen peroxide-producing lactobacilli are replaced by overgrowth of various species of bacteria such as *Prevotella* spp., *Gardnerella vaginalis, U. urealyticum, M. hominis, Atopobium vaginae,* and BV-associated bacterium 1 and 2.[31] BV has been associated with an increased risk of STIs, including HIV.

Oral or intravaginal metronidazole or intravaginal clindamycin cream are usually effective for treatment of BV. Oral tinidazole or oral or intravaginal clindamycin ovules are alternatives.[32] A single 2-gm dose of secnidazole *(Solosec)*, a nitroimidazole similar to metronidazole with a longer half-life, was noninferior to seven days of oral metronidazole 500 mg twice daily in the rate of therapeutic cure in women with BV.[47] It is more expensive than other drugs for treatment of BV. Recurrent BV is common; retreatment with the same drug or an alternative is usually effective in the short term, but symptomatic recurrences are frequent.

Maintenance suppressive therapy with twice-weekly intravaginal metronidazole gel can reduce recurrence rates.[33] Treatment of male sex partners is not recommended, but condom use by male sex partners may reduce the rate of recurrence.

Pregnancy – BV has been associated with preterm labor and complications during delivery, but whether treatment of asymptomatic infection in pregnant women reduces the frequency of adverse outcomes is unclear. Symptomatic BV in pregnant women should be treated with either oral or intravaginal metronidazole or clindamycin. The safety of tinidazole in pregnancy has not been established.

VULVOVAGINAL CANDIDIASIS — Vulvovaginal candidiasis, typically caused by *Candida albicans*, is common in women being evaluated for STIs. Short courses of topical azoles are effective for treatment of uncomplicated vulvovaginal candidiasis in immunocompetent women. A single oral dose of fluconazole (*Diflucan*, and generics) is as effective as 7 days of intravaginal clotrimazole or miconazole and is preferred by many patients; severe episodes may require additional doses of fluconazole. Prophylaxis with oral fluconazole every 3 days for 3 doses and then once weekly can reduce the number of recurrences, but recurrences are common once prophylactic therapy has been stopped.[33,34]

Pregnancy – Vulvovaginal candidiasis is common during pregnancy. Intravaginal treatment with an azole is recommended.

Alternative Treatments for Vaginal Infections – Probiotics such as *Lactobacillus* spp. and dairy products such as yogurt are not effective for treatment or prevention of BV or vulvovaginal candidiasis. Douching is not effective for prevention or treatment of vaginal infection; it may lead to upper genital tract infection, is unnecessary for hygiene, and should be discouraged.

CHANCROID — Chancroid, caused by *Haemophilus ducreyi*, is currently rare in the US. A single dose of azithromycin or ceftriaxone is

Table 2. Human Papillomavirus (HPV) Vaccine[1]

Vaccine[2]	Protection Against HPV Types
Gardasil 9 (Merck)	6, 11, 16, 18, 31, 33, 45, 52, and 58

1. *Gardasil* and *Cervarix* are no longer available in the US.
2. Inactivated vaccine.
3. Two doses of the vaccine are recommended for boys and girls receiving the vaccine at 9-14 years old.
4. Previously unvaccinated adult females ≤26 years old and males ≤21 years old should receive a 3-dose series. Males 22-26 years old who have immunocompromising conditions (including HIV infection) or those who have sex with men should also receive a 3-dose series. Those above who received 2 doses ≥5 months apart before age 15 years do not need an additional dose. All those above who received only 1 dose or 2 doses <5 months apart before age 15 years should receive 1 additional dose.

usually effective, but prolonged therapy or retreatment may be required in uncircumcised men and HIV-infected patients.[4,35] Sex partners should be treated if they have had sexual contact with the infected person within 10 days of symptom onset.

GENITAL HERPES — Acyclovir (*Zovirax*, and generics), famciclovir (*Famvir*, and generics), or valacyclovir (*Valtrex*, and generics) taken orally for 7-10 days can shorten the duration of pain, systemic symptoms, and viral shedding in patients with initial genital HSV infection. Episodic treatment of symptomatic recurrent lesions with the same drugs can speed healing if treatment is started immediately upon symptom onset. Continuous suppressive therapy substantially reduces symptomatic recurrences and subclinical shedding. Valacyclovir has been more effective than famciclovir for virologic suppression of recurrent genital herpes[36] and suppressive therapy with valacyclovir has been shown to reduce the frequency of HSV transmission to sex partners.[37] HIV-infected persons may need higher doses of antivirals.

Pregnancy – First episodes of genital HSV that occur during pregnancy should be treated. Suppressive therapy with acyclovir or valacyclovir beginning at week 36 can reduce the risk of recurrence at delivery and possibly the need for cesarean section, but its efficacy in reducing the risk of neonatal HSV infection is unclear.[38,39] Acyclovir, valacyclovir, and famciclovir are classified as category B (no evidence of risk in ani-

FDA-Approved Age Range	Dose	Schedule
Females and males 9-26 years old	0.5 mL IM	2 (0, 6-12 mos)[3] or 3 (0, 2, and 6 mos)[4,5] doses

5. Minimum interval between 1st and 2nd dose is 4 weeks, between 2nd and 3rd dose is 12 weeks, and between 1st and 3rd dose is 24 weeks.

mals; no adequate studies in pregnant women) for use during pregnancy. Use of acyclovir or valacyclovir during pregnancy, even during the first trimester, has not been associated with an increased risk of congenital abnormalities to date.[40]

GENITAL WARTS AND HUMAN PAPILLOMAVIRUS INFECTION — External **genital warts** are caused by human papillomavirus (HPV) infection, usually type 6 or 11; persistent infection with other types (16, 18, or others) may cause dysplasia and neoplasia of the anogenital tract and oropharynx. No treatment has been shown to eradicate HPV or to modify the risk of cervical dysplasia or cancer, and no single treatment is uniformly effective in removing warts or preventing recurrence. Trichloroacetic acid and cryotherapy (with liquid nitrogen or a cryoprobe) remain the most widely used provider-administered treatments for external genital warts. Imiquimod 3.75% cream *(Zyclara)* and 5% cream (*Aldara*, and generics), podofilox 0.5% solution or gel (*Condylox*, and generics), and sinecatechins 15% ointment *(Veregen)* offer the advantage of self-application.[41] For all treatments except surgical removal, the initial response rate is 60-70%; 20-30% of responders will have a recurrence, but many of them will respond to a different regimen.

No treatment is recommended for **subclinical HPV** infection in the absence of dysplasia or neoplasia. The transient nature of most HPV infections in young women suggests that these infections should be treated conservatively because they usually regress spontaneously.

Pregnancy – Topical trichloroacetic acid and cryotherapy can be used during pregnancy. Podofilox and sinecatechins are not recommended for use during pregnancy. Imiquimod appears to have a low risk of fetal abnormalities, but should be avoided until more safety data become available.[4]

Prevention – *Gardasil 9* is the only HPV vaccine currently available in the US (*Gardasil* and *Cervarix* are no longer available). It is a 9-valent inactivated vaccine with protection against HPV types 6, 11, 16, 18, 31, 33, 45, 52, and 58. Vaccination against HPV does not influence the course of established infection.

The Advisory Committee on Immunization Practices (ACIP) recommends routine HPV vaccination for all girls and boys by age 11-12 years.[42] Vaccination is also recommended for females 13-26 years old and males 13-21 years old who were not fully vaccinated previously. The ACIP also recommends vaccination of MSM and immunocompromised men 22-26 years old who were not fully vaccinated previously.

In December 2016, the ACIP reduced the number of scheduled doses to two for girls and boys receiving the vaccine at ages 9-14 years old; a 3-dose series is still recommended for those who start the series at 15-26 years old and for immunocompromised persons.[43,44]

PEDICULOSIS AND SCABIES — *Sarcoptes scabiei* (scabies) and *Phthirus pubis* (pubic lice), which can be found on eyelashes, axillary, back, and leg hairs, as well as in the pubic area, can both be transmitted by intimate exposure. Topical treatment options include 1% permethrin (*Nix*, and others) or pyrethrins with piperonyl butoxide (*Rid*, and others) for pubic lice and 5% permethrin (*Elimite*, and generics) for scabies. Oral ivermectin *(Stromectol)* is an effective, more convenient alternative for treatment of both lice and scabies.[45] Crusted scabies, a serious complication usually seen in patients with AIDS or other immunodeficiencies, can be treated with 5% permethrin plus oral ivermectin (3-7 doses depending on severity).

Pregnancy – Topical permethrin and pyrethrins with piperonyl butoxide can be used in pregnant women. Oral ivermectin is not recommended for use in pregnant women; animal studies have shown adverse effects on the fetus.[46]

Partner Treatment – Sex partners and those who had close personal contact with the infected person within the last month should be treated.

1. American College of Obstetricians and Gynecologists. Committee Opinion 632: expedited partner therapy in the management of gonorrhea and chlamydial infection. Obstet Gynecol 2015; 125:1526.
2. WM Geisler et al. Azithromycin versus doxycycline for urogenital Chlamydia trachomatis infection. N Engl J Med 2015; 373:2512.
3. FY Kong et al. The efficacy of azithromycin and doxycycline for the treatment of rectal chlamydia infection: a systematic review and meta-analysis. J Antimicrob Chemother 2015; 70:1290.
4. KA Workowski et al. Sexually transmitted diseases treatment guidelines, 2015. MMWR Recomm Rep 2015; 64:1.
5. MD Eberly et al. Azithromycin in early infancy and pyloric stenosis. Pediatrics 2015; 135:483.
6. R Martin-Iguacel et al. Lymphogranuloma venereum proctocolitis: a silent endemic disease in men who have sex with men in industrialised countries. Eur J Clin Microbiol Infect Dis 2010; 29:917.
7. BP Stoner and SE Cohen. Lymphogranuloma venereum 2015: clinical presentation, diagnosis, and treatment. Clin Infect Dis 2015; 61 Suppl 8:S865.
8. LH Bachmann et al. Advances in the understanding and treatment of male urethritis. Clin Infect Dis 2015; 61 Suppl 8:S763.
9. LE Manhart et al. Standard treatment regimens for nongonococcal urethritis have similar but declining cure rates: a randomized controlled trial. Clin Infect Dis 2013; 56:934.
10. LE Manhart et al. Efficacy of antimicrobial therapy for Mycoplasma genitalium infections. Clin Infect Dis 2015; 61 Suppl 8:S802.
11. A Lau et al. The efficacy of azithromycin for the treatment of genital Mycoplasma genitalium: a systematic review and meta-analysis. Clin Infect Dis 2015; 61:1389.
12. D Getman et al. Mycoplasma genitalium prevalence, coinfection, and macrolide antibiotic resistance frequency in a multicenter clinical study cohort in the United States. J Clin Microbiol 2016; 54:2278.

13. RD Kirkcaldy et al. The efficacy and safety of gentamicin plus azithromycin and gemifloxacin plus azithromycin as treatment of uncomplicated gonorrhea. Clin Infect Dis 2014; 59:1083.
14. GA Bolan et al. The emerging threat of untreatable gonococcal infection. N Engl J Med 2012; 366:485.
15. VG Allen et al. Neisseria gonorrhoeae treatment failure and susceptibility to cefixime in Toronto, Canada. JAMA 2013; 309:163.
16. H Fifer et al. Failure of dual antimicrobial therapy in treatment of gonorrhea. N Engl J Med 2016; 374:2504.
17. T Deguchi et al. New clinical strain of Neisseria gonorrhoeae with decreased susceptibility to ceftriaxone, Japan. Emerg Infect Dis 2016; 22:142.
18. M Unemo. Current and future antimicrobial treatment of gonorrhoea - the rapidly evolving Neisseria gonorrhoeae continues to challenge. BMC Infect Dis 2015; 15:364.
19. V Levy et al. A case of persistent and possibly treatment resistant pharyngeal gonorrhea. Sex Transm Dis 2016; 43:258.
20. AR Katz et al. Cluster of Neisseria gonorrhoeae isolates with high-level azithromycin resistance and decreased ceftriaxone susceptibility, Hawaii, 2016. Clin Infect Dis 2017 May 26 (epub).
21. CDC. Guidance on the use of expedited partner therapy in the treatment of gonorrhea. Available at: www.cdc.gov/std/ept/gc-guidance.htm. Accessed June 22, 2017.
22. R Duarte et al. A review of antibiotic therapy for pelvic inflammatory disease. Int J Antimicrob Agents 2015; 46:272.
23. RC Brunham et al. Pelvic inflammatory disease. N Engl J Med 2015; 372:2039.
24. ME Clement et al. Treatment of syphilis: a systematic review. JAMA 2014; 312:1905.
25. A Ganesan et al. A single dose of benzathine penicillin G is as effective as multiple doses of benzathine penicillin G for the treatment of HIV- infected persons with early syphilis. Clin Infect Dis 2015; 60:653.
26. R Andrade et al. Single dose versus 3 doses of intramuscular benzathine penicillin for early syphilis in HIV: a randomized clinical trial. Clin Infect Dis 2017; 64:759.
27. EW Hook. Syphilis. Lancet 2017; 389:1550.
28. E Meites et al. A review of evidence-based care of symptomatic trichomoniasis and asymptomatic trichomonas vaginalis infections. Clin Infect Dis 2015; 61 Suppl 8:S837.
29. RD Kirkcaldy et al. Trichomonas vaginalis antimicrobial drug resistance in 6 US cities, STD Surveillance Network, 2009-2010. Emerg Infect Dis 2012; 18:939.
30. AC Seña et al. Persistent and recurrent Trichomonas vaginalis infections: epidemiology, treatment and management considerations. Expert Rev Anti Infect Ther 2014; 12:673.
31. CA Muzny and JR Schwebke. Pathogenesis of bacterial vaginosis: discussion of current hypotheses. J Infect Dis 2016; 214 Suppl1:S1.
32. JR Schwebke and RA Desmond. Tinidazole vs metronidazole for the treatment of bacterial vaginosis. Am J Obstet Gynecol 2011; 204:211.
33. P Nyirjesy. Management of persistent vaginitis. Obstet Gynecol 2014; 124:1135.
34. JD Sobel et al. Maintenance fluconazole therapy for recurrent vulvovaginal candidiasis. N Engl J Med 2004; 351:876.
35. DA Lewis. Epidemiology, clinical features, diagnosis and treatment of Haemophilus ducreyi - a disappearing pathogen? Expert Rev Anti Infect Ther 2014; 12:687.

36. A Wald et al. Comparative efficacy of famciclovir and valacyclovir for suppression of recurrent genital herpes and viral shedding. Sex Transm Dis 2006; 33:529.
37. L Corey et al. Once-daily valacyclovir to reduce the risk of transmission of genital herpes. N Engl J Med 2004; 350:11.
38. Antiviral drugs. Treat Guidel Med Lett 2013; 11:19.
39. American College of Obstetricians and Gynecologists Committee on Practice Bulletins. ACOG Practioce Bulletin. No. 82 June 2007. Management of herpes in pregnancy. Obstet Gynecol 2007; 109:1489.
40. B Pasternak and A Hviid. Use of acyclovir, valacyclovir, and famciclovir in the first trimester of pregnancy and the risk of birth defects. JAMA 2010; 304:859.
41. Veregen: a botanical for treatment of genital warts. Med Lett Drugs Ther 2008; 50:15.
42. Gardasil 9 – a broader HPV vaccine. Med Lett Drugs Ther 2015; 57:47.
43. E Meites et al. Use of a 2-dose schedule for human papillomavirus vaccination — updated recommendations of the Advisory Committee on Immunization Practices. MMWR Morb Mortal Wkly Rep 2016; 65:1405.
44. In brief: New adult immunization recommendations. Med Lett Drugs Ther 2017; 59:70.
45. Y Panahi et al. The efficacy of topical and oral ivermectin in the treatment of human scabies. Ann Parasitol 2015; 61:11.
46. IM el-Ashmawy et al. Teratogenic and cytogenetic effects of ivermectin and its interaction with P-glycoprotien inhibitor. Res Vet Sci 2011; 90:116.
47. JM Bohbot et al. Treatment of bacterial vaginosis: a multicenter, double-blind, double-dummy, randomised phase III study comparing secnidazole and metronidazole. Infect Dis Obstet Gynecol 2010 Sep 15 (epub).

Index

Index

B

C

G

H

N

O

Q

R

T

U

Z